PRACTICAL JOINT ASSESSMENT
LOWER QUADRANT
A Sports Medicine Manual

PRACTICAL JOINT ASSESSMENT
LOWER QUADRANT
A Sports Medicine Manual

Anne Hartley, B.P.H.E., Dip A.T.M., C.A.T.(C)
Professor Sheridan College of Applied
Arts and Technology
The Sports Injury Management Program
Oakville, Ontario
Canada

Second Edition

with 219 *illustrations*

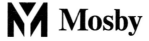 **Mosby**

St. Louis Baltimore Berlin Boston Carlsbad Chicago London Madrid
Naples New York Philadelphia Sydney Tokyo Toronto

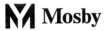

Mosby
Dedicated to Publishing Excellence

Executive Editor: Martha Sasser
Associate Developmental Editor: Kellie F. White
Project Manager: Carol Sullivan Wiseman
Production Editor: Florence Achenbach
Designer: Betty Schulz
Manufacturing Supervisor: Karen Lewis
Cover Art: Rip Kastaris

SECOND EDITION
Copyright © 1995 Mosby–Year Book, Inc.

Previous edition copyrighted 1990

Printed in the United States of America
Composition by Digital Prepress, Inc.
Printing by Von Hoffmann Press, Inc.

Mosby–Year Book, Inc.
11830 Westline Industrial Drive
St. Louis, MO 63146

Library of Congress Cataloging-in-Publication Data

Hartley, Anne
   Practical joint assessment: lower quadrant: a sports medicine manual/ Anne Hartley, -- 2nd ed.
      p.   cm.
   First ed. published in 1 v.
   Companion v. to: Practical joint assessment: lower quadrant, 2nd ed. 1994.
   Includes bibliographical references and index.
   ISBN 0-8151-4238-2
   1. Joints Examination.   2. Joints—Wounds and injuries--Diagnosis.   3. Sports injuries—Diagnosis   I. Title.
   [DNLM: 1. Joints—physiology.   2. Muscles--physiology.
3. Athletic Injuries—diagnosis.   4. Physical Examination—methods.
5. Sports Medicine.   WE 300 H332pd 1994]
RD97.H374   1994
617.4′72—dc20
DNLM/DLC   94-11608
for Library of Congress   CIP

97 98   /   9 8 7 6 5 4 3 2

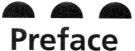

Preface

This manual was originally written for the students in Sports Injury Management Program in athletic therapy at Sheridan College in Oakville, Ontario, and for the Certification Candidates of the Canadian Athletic Therapist Association. The manual is designed to give a hands-on approach to the assessment of the joints of the body. Each chapter is divided into these sections: history, observations, functional tests, special tests, accessory tests, and palpations. On one side of the page the instructions are outlined and on the opposing side of the page are the possible interpretations of the patient's responses or results. It allows the reader to develop a systematic and thorough approach to assessing musculoskeletal disorders. Line drawings throughout the manual help to clarify hand placements or body positions for testing, as well as depicting anatomical structures and mechanisms of injury.

The upper and lower quadrant practical assessment manuals are useful clinical tools for all therapists, physicians, osteopaths, chiropractors, or other allied health professionals with a basic understanding in sports medicine. They are especially valuable for instructors and students in sports medicine or orthopaedics. The hands-on practical nature of the manuals allows the students to progress at their own pace.

Wherever possible, I have attempted to recognize the originators of the assessment techniques in my references and bibliography. However, in the course of twenty years of clinical experiences, the origins of some techniques have faded from memory. To any of the originators that I have inadvertently overlooked, please accept my sincere apologies.

ACKNOWLEDGMENTS

I would like to acknowledge and sincerely thank:

Mark Hartley, my husband, for his patience, encouragement, and time during this lengthy undertaking. Any valuable time lost will be regained.

Paul and **Dean Hartley**, my children, who allowed for maternity leave time and afternoon naps when most of my writing was accomplished. Heavens knows what more I could write by having another.

Alfred Chalmers, my father, for his advice and financial expertise in helping to develop, market, and originally publish these manuals.

Janet Chandler, my good friend and computer specialist, who never complained even when called on to rush things. Her advice was invaluable and her ideas on layout paramount.

Sheridan College of Applied Arts and Technology for providing the classroom and clinical environment in which to learn.

The Sports Injury Management students who kept me challenged and motivated daily. Most of their questions are still unanswered.

My college program colleagues who encouraged and humored me.

My medical illustrators, **Beverley Ransom** and **Susan Leopold**, who can work magic with a pen.

Anne Hartley

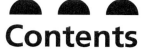

Contents

Introduction

GUIDELINES FOR USE OF THIS TEXT

The plan given in this text is a menu for assessing a joint. The order of the functional testing routine should be varied according to the history and observations recorded.

Not all of the tests may be necessary for each assessment. It will depend on your findings as you progress.

The left column is the guide for questions, instructions for hand placements, and general instructions. The right column presents the different interpretations of the findings and directs the assessor to possible damaged structures.

The interpretation section is designed to gear your thinking toward all the alternatives and allow the different possibilities to be incorporated into your assessment procedures.

Never rush your interpretation. Always rule out other possible conditions and structures.

Record all the limited joint ranges, end-feels, and painful movements, because these are the keys to determining the condition. But more importantly, these are the keys to help determine how to design an effective rehabilitation program.

GENERAL ASSESSMENT GUIDELINES

Always observe and functionally assess the joints bilaterally,

Begin with the uninjured limb first, then repeat the test on the injured limb. Compare ranges of motion, end feel, and muscular strength.

It may be necessary to retest the normal or injured site more than once, Differences in mobility can be very small (2 to 10 mm) yet very significant.

Try to arrange your testing so that the most painful test is last. This ensures that the condition will not be aggravated by your testing procedure or make the athlete apprehensive.

Your testing should be influenced by the history and observations to rule out needless testing, but you must be thorough enough to rule out all other possible injured structures, the possibility of multiple injuries, and visceral, vascular, or systemic conditions.

Always support the injured limb securely to gain the athlete's confidence and prevent further injury. If the injury is inflamed or swollen, it may be necessary to elevate the area while taking the history and between tests.

Rule out the joint above and below, especially if the history or observations suggest other joint involvement.

A scan of the entire quadrant may be necessary if the onset of the problem is insidious, if the pain is diffuse and nonspecific, or, if during testing, several joints or body parts seem to be implicated.

It may be necessary to analyze the entire quadrant's kinetic chain because any weak link can lead to dysfunction, or conversely, dysfunction can alter the normal kinetic chain.

Be aware of *radicular pain syndromes* in which the spinal nerves or nerve roots are irritated. The *radicular referred pain* is lancinating and travels down the limb in narrow bands. With radicular pain syndromes there are definite segmental neurological signs that include: dermatome numbness or paresthesia, myotome weakness, and/or reflex changes.

Be aware of somatic pain syndromes in which the source of pain comes from one or more of the musculoskeletal elements around the spine (ligament, muscle, intervertebral disc, facet joint). These syndromes have somatic referred pain that does not involve the nerve root or have neurological changes (i.e., reflexes, paresthesia). Somatic referred pain is a dull, achy pain that is perceived in an area separate from the primary source of dysfunction or pain.

Be aware that systematic disorders, visceral injuries or disease, circulatory conditions, neural disorders, and others can also affect muscle and joint function and can also refer pain.

As described above, pain is not always perceived

at the point of origin. To determine the lesion site and structure, functional structure testing must be done *before* palpation. Palpation of the painful site before functional testing not only prejudices the testing but the primary lesion may be missed.

Ask the athlete the location of the pain, nature of the pain, and any difference in the pain during the testing procedure.

Active Tests

During your active tests, the athlete should be asked to move the joint through as much range as possible. If the active range is full, an overpressure may be applied to determine the end feel of the joint. This test is important because it indicates the athlete's willingness to move the joint, as well as the range of motion of the joint and the strength of the surrounding structures.

Passive Tests

These tests are designed to test the inert structures.

During your passive tests, you move the joint until an end feel or end range is felt.

The type of end feel at the end of the range of motion is important because it assists in determining the condition, the structure at fault, and the severity of the injury. Cyriax defines six end feels.

1. **Bone-to-bone** is an abrupt hard sensation when one bone engages with another bone. This can be a normal or an abnormal end feel.
   - normal (e.g., elbow extension)
   - abnormal (e.g., when the boney end feel occurs before the end of the joint range). This can indicate an osteophyte or abnormal boney development.
2. **Spasm** is a vibrant twang as the muscles around the joint spasm to arrest movement. A knee extension with hamstring spasm is one example. This is an abnormal end feel and it is contraindicated to force the joint through more range to mobilize or manipulate. It can indicate acute or subacute capsulitis or severe ligamentous injury.
3. **Capsular feel** is a firm arrest of movement with some give to it (i.e., stretching leather). This can be normal or an abnormal end feel.
   - normal (e.g., glenohumeral lateral rotation)
   - abnormal (e.g., talocrural plantar flexion with joint effusion)

This can indicate chronic joint effusion, arthritis, or capsular scarring.

4. **Springy block** causes the joint to rebound at the end of range due to an internal articular derangement catching between the joint surfaces. This is an abnormal end feel. A knee extension with a meniscal tear or an elbow extension with a bone chip are two examples. This can indicate an intra-articular loose body.
5. **Tissue approximation** is range limited because of tissue compression. This is a normal end feel. A knee flexion with the lower leg against the posterior thigh is one example. Elbow flexion with the lower arm against the biceps muscle is another example.
6. **Empty end feel** occurs when considerable pain stops the movement before the end of range is met. There is no tissue resistance, yet the athlete arrests movement due to pain. This is an abnormal end feel. Acute bursitis, extra-articular abscess, or neoplasm can be suspected. Extreme apprehension or fear of pain by the athlete may also cause this end feel.

Not mentioned by Cyriax, but commonly found, is a normal **tissue stretch end feel**. This is due to a muscular, ligamentous, or fascial stretch (i.e., hip flexion with hamstring stretch).

Do **not** force the joint if the athlete is unwilling to move it due to pain or muscle spasm, but attempt to determine the range and what is limiting the range.

Record the quality of the motion and the presence of painful arc, crepitus, and snapping or popping that occurs during the passive movement. Also record the type and quality of the end feel.

Resisted Tests

During your resisted tests, do **not** allow joint movement. The best testing position of the joint is usually in mid-range or neutral position (resting position). Your hand placements must stabilize the joint and prevent joint movement. It may be necessary to stabilize the body part above or below the joint being tested.

Instruct the athlete to build up to a strong contraction gradually and then relax gradually as you resist, to prevent overpowering or underpowering the muscle group that you are testing.

The athlete should contract the muscles strongly. If the contraction appears weak, repeat the test. Make sure that the weakness is not from unwillingness, fear, or lack of comprehension. With this test, you are looking for strength or weakness and a pain-free or painful contraction.

The contraction may be repeated several times if the therapist suspects that there is a neural or circulatory insufficiency to the muscle that will display pain or weakness with repetitions.

Position yourself at a mechanical advantage over the limb that you are testing.

Resist more distally on the limb for better leverage with very strong athletes.

If you have determined that the injury is in a contractile tissue, specialize your testing for the muscle involved. Test the inner, middle, and outer ranges, if possible, to determine what part of the range is limited by pain or weakness.

Weakness may also be due to nerve involvement, vascular insufficiency, disuse atrophy, stretch weakness, apprehension, pain, or fatigue.

It may be necessary to position the limb so gravity assists the muscle if there is considerable weakness (Grades 1 and 2).

The strength can be graded and recorded on a scale from 0 to 5.

0 = no contraction felt
1 = muscle can be felt to tighten but cannot produce movement
2 = produces movement with gravity eliminated but cannot function against gravity
3 = can raise against gravity
4 = can raise against outside moderate resistance, as well as against gravity
5 = can overcome a great amount of maximal resistance, as well as gravity.

Record the strength and whether it is painful or pain free. Record the weakness for inner, middle, or outer range of the joint. Record the muscle or muscles causing the weakness.

Special Tests

The special tests are uniquely designed to test a specific anatomical structure for dysfunction.

Accessory Movements (Joint Play Tests)

Most joints have very small but precise joint movements that are not controlled by muscles. These movements are important for normal articular cartilage nutrition, for pain-free range of motion, and for the muscles to work through their full range. If these small joint play movements are decreased (hypomobile), increased (hypermobile), or lost, dysfunction will develop.

The therapist must test these accessory movements with the athlete relaxed and in a comfortable position. A small amount of traction is needed to open the joint space and the joint must be in its resting or loose-packed position (muscles, ligaments, capsule lax). The grip should be close to the joint surface with one hand on each side of the joint. One hand must stabilize one bone while the other hand gently moves the opposite bone in the desired direction. It must be determined if the joint play movement seems normal, hypermobile, or hypomobile compared to the other side. Often these movements are very small (about $1/8$ of an inch). The accessory movements should be assessed whenever the active and passive range is limited, yet resisted tests are full. Record the degree of joint play movement (hypomobility, normal, or hypermobility) if the movement elicits pain. This helps in assessing the joint and in designing the rehabilitation program.

For each joint described in the assessment book, the close-packed, resting or loose-packed positions, and capsular patterns are given. The reasons for their inclusion are described next.

Close-packed Joint Positions

- The *close-packed positions* for the joints occur when the joint surfaces fit together tightly (maximally congruent).
- The joint, ligament, and capsule are taut and often twisted to cause firm approximation of the articular cartilage involved.
- The closer the joint is toward its close-packed position, the greater the joint restriction.
- According to Kaltenborn, when in the close-packed position, the joint surfaces cannot be separated by traction.
- This joint position is not indicated for most joint assessments, especially for joint accessory movement or joint play movement tests.
- On occasion some joints may be locked in the close-packed position while more proximal or distal joints are tested (i.e., lock PIP joints while testing DIP joints of the hand).
- When direct trauma or overstretch forces are applied to a joint in its close-packed position,

the joint structures have no joint play, or give, and therefore have more serious injuries associated with them (fractures, maximal internal derangements).

- In close-packed position, the capsule and ligaments are already taut; therefore they are more susceptible to sprain or tear, depending on the external forces involved.
- The articular cartilages (and menisci in some cases) of each joint are tightly bound; therefore, in the case of close-packed position, boney or articular cartilage damage is more likely.

Resting or Loose-packed Joint Positions

- The *resting* or *loose-packed position* is the position where the joint and its surrounding structures are under the least stress.
- The joint capsule and surrounding ligaments are lax while the articular cartilages (and menisci in some joints) that make up the joint have some space between them.
- This is the position that the joint will assume if there is intracapsular swelling or joint effusion and it is often in the joint's midrange.
- It is important to learn this position for each joint because:
  1. It is the ideal position to test the accessory or joint play movements for that joint.
  2. It is a good position in which to place the joint to allow it to rest from stress.
  3. It can indicate to the therapist the presence of joint swelling.
  4. It is an ideal position in which to place the joint to ensure stress reduction in an acute joint injury or when immobilizing the joint.

Capsular Patterns (Cyriax)

- A *capsular pattern* is the limitation of active and passive movements in characteristic proportions for each joint.
- It is a total joint reaction that occurs only in synovial joints.
- It is characterized by an abrupt muscle spasm end feel stopping the joint motion during active and passive motion at the exact same ranges.
- The limitations in ranges can be progressively more restrictive with eventual capsular and ligamentous adhesion formation, osteophyte development, and even eventual joint fusion.
- In early capsular patterns, the restriction may appear in only one range (the one with eventu-

al greatest restriction if not rehabilitated) and later progress to more ranges.

- The capsular pattern does not indicate the injured structure. Further testing, as well as a thorough history and observations, is needed to help determine the lesion site.
- These capsular patterns are important to learn because they can confuse your joint testing interpretation due to their combination of restrictions if you are not aware of the capsular patterns. If the pattern progresses, there are serious consequences because of the multiplane restriction. They require gentle testing and rehabilitation to regain normal joint function.

Palpations in General

Palpations are a very important part of the assessment and should confirm your functional testing results. They are always carried out *bilaterally*. The injured anatomical structure should be palpated its entire length. This ensures that avulsions or partial tears can be recognized. Any temperature changes, abnormal contours, thickening, swelling, nodules, or any other palpable difference from the contralateral limb should be documented and may need further investigation.

When palpating, begin superficially and attempt to palpate each layer of tissue (i.e., from skin to fat, to fascia, to muscle, to bone) to the deepest underlying structures. It is best to visualize anatomically the structures that are being palpated as the lesion site is being examined. The entire surface of the hand should touch the injured area, although the finger pads may probe for smaller structures. Do *not* use the tips of the fingers or use *too* much force. Very careful and thorough palpations are needed to determine the lesion site, the extent of the injury, the stage of healing (inflamed-hotter than opposite side), the depth of the lesion, and potential complications.

Palpation of Myofascial Trigger Points

In the palpation section for each muscle the myofascial trigger point locations are given, as well as the areas of somatic referred pain. This information is taken from Janet Travell and David Simons' work in this area and their book (*Myofascial Pain and Dysfunction—The Trigger Point Manual*). This is important in determining the structure at fault and in realizing that the areas of referred pain may be remote from the lesion site.

According to Travell and Simons, a myofascial "active" trigger point has several characteristics:

- It is a hyper-irritable spot within a tight band of skeletal muscle.
- When compressed, it can cause referred pain, an autonomic response, a local muscle twitch or "jump sign" (intense, quick body movement).
- The referred pain can be from a low-grade dull ache to a severe incapacitating pain.
- The referred pain follows specific patterns for each muscle.
- It is caused by acute overload, overwork, fatigue, chilling, or gross trauma.
- Passive or active stretching of the involved muscle increases the pain.
- Resisted maximal contraction force of the muscle involved will be weakened.

PERSONAL MEDICAL HISTORY

The athlete's personal medical history is important to obtain before getting the history of the injury. Many athletes have previous injuries of medical conditions that are important to the new injury and its rehabilitation.

These facts help to develop a rapport with the athlete and determine their immediate concerns and expectations. During the history-taking:

- Keep the questions simple.
- Ask relevant questions in a natural progression.
- Listen attentively and clarify inconsistencies.
- Encourage cooperation and confidence.
- Remain professional at all times.

The necessary facts are:

Athlete's Name
- Introduce yourself at this time.

Age
- Many conditions develop at a certain age. Age is important because of the vulnerability of the epiphyseal plates in a growing athlete.

Address
- An address is important in case further correspondence is necessary (i.e., medical or legal).

Telephone
- A phone number is important in case an appointment needs to be changed or a follow-up is necessary.

Occupation
- Occupation can indicate time spent in certain postures (i.e., sitting, standing), and lifting or repetitive movement patterns.

Sport

- Level of competition (intramural, local, national, international, professional, recreational).
- Warm up – cool down.
- Years in sport.
- Type of training (i.e., frequency, duration).
- Position (i.e., forward, defense).

Previous Injuries

- Injury to the same quadrant or relevant information from a previous injury.
- Injury with resulting adaptations.

Previous Surgery

- Any previous surgery can cause scar tissue or postural adaptations, which may predispose the athlete to injury or problems.

Family Background

- History of similar problem that runs in the family.

Pre-existing Medical Condition(s)

- Certain conditions can affect the nature or extent of injury (i.e., hemophilia, rheumatoid arthritis, diabetes, ankylosing spondylitis).
- Certain conditions can affect healing rates (diabetes, hemophilia).

Previous Surgery

- Any previous surgery can cause scar tissue or postural adaptations, which may predispose the athlete to injury or problems.

Medication Being Taken

- Certain medications can affect the testing or mask symptoms (i.e., anti-inflammatory medication, pain killers, muscle relaxants, insulin).

CHAPTER 1

Lumbar Spine and Sacroiliac Joint Assessment

There is an integral network between the lumbar vertebrae, sacrum, ilium, and lower extremity. Any alteration in one of these affects the others so it is important to be aware of these interrelationships when assessing and rehabilitating a patient.

Symmetry of the body is important when observing and assessing but asymmetry does not always indicate pathology or dysfunction:

- Boney and muscular asymmetry is not uncommon and is usually symptom free.
- Asymmetry plus pain and mechanical dysfunction in an area or segment is important and should be investigated further with selective testing.

Specific balanced muscle groups are fundamental to balancing the pelvis and lumbar spine in the **sagittal plane**. These muscle groups include the following:

- Abdominals (rectus abdominis, transverse abdominis, and obliques), which pull the anterior pelvis upward and backward
- Hip flexors (iliopsoas and rectus femoris), which pull the anterior pelvis downward
- Erector spinae, which pull the posterior pelvis upward or create an extension force on the lumbar spine
- Deep erector spinae (including the thoracic and lumbar iliocostalis and the lumbar longissimus), which cause a posterior shear force and a compression force on the lumbar spine when contracted
- Hip extensors (gluteus maximus and the hamstrings), which pull the posterior pelvis downward
- Multifidus, which is a very significant muscle that has an excellent lever arm for extending the lumbar vertebrae

These muscles must all work together for a balanced and stable lumbopelvic unit. If any one group of muscles becomes hypertrophic or atrophied the pelvic position will become altered and all the other groups of muscles will be affected. A facilitated lumbar segment, one fatigued muscle group, one muscle injury, or one overused muscle group will affect the synergistic interrelationship of the muscles. For example, if the psoas majors are tight the lumbar spine will move into extension (excessive lordosis) and the pelvis will rock anteriorly, causing hip flexion.

Motions of the pelvis directly influence the thoracolumbar fascia—anterior pelvic movements tighten it and posterior pelvic movements loosen it. The thoracolumbar fascia attaches to the lumbar spinous processes (superficial layer) and the lumbar transverse processes (deep layer). It also serves as an attachment for the internal oblique, transversus abdominis, and latissimus dorsi muscles. Thus the thoracolumbar fascia can influence and be influenced by lumbar spine and pelvic positions and their surrounding muscles. It is therefore important to test each group in your assessment and to rehabilitate each group when there is a problem.

The ilia can be altered in the sagittal plane in an anterior or posterior position (anterior iliac rotation, posterior iliac rotation) (Mitchell, Moran, and Pruzzo):

- This can be unilateral or bilateral and often leads to sacroiliac dysfunction.
- Bilateral anterior iliac rotation usually carries the sacrum with it, leading to increased lumbar lordosis; bilateral posterior iliac rotation can lead to a lumbar flat back posture.

The structures around the pelvis, sacrum, lumbar spine, and lower extremity must also be balanced in the **frontal plane**.

If one leg is longer than the other, then one half of the pelvis is elevated and unbalanced forces go through the sacroiliac joint, the symphysis pubis, the lumbar facets, and intervertebral discs. Unequal leg length and the associated scoliosis has been linked with structural changes in the vertebral end plates, intervertebral discs, and asymmetrical changes in the facet joints (articular cartilage and subchondral) (Giles and Taylor). This can also lead to stretching of the muscles on one side and shortening of the muscles on the other side. The hip adductor and abductor muscles, the quadratus lumborum, psoas major, latissimus dorsi, and even the hip lateral rotators can be affected by this.

Specific muscle groups are also important in balancing the pelvis and lumbar spine in the **frontal plane**. These muscle groups include the following:

- Quadratus lumborum, which pulls the pelvis upward laterally and contributes to the dynamic stability of the lumbosacral junction (since it attaches to the superior and anterior bands of the iliolumbar ligament) (Bogduk and Twomey)
- Gluteus medius, which controls the pelvis from dropping on the opposite side
- Tensor fascia lata, which pulls the upper pelvis downward
- Femoral adductors (longus, brevis, magnus), pectineus, and gracilis, which pull the lower pelvis outward

These muscles must work in a synergistic manner to ensure lumbopelvic balance and stability. A change in muscle tone (hyperactive or hypoactive) of any one muscle will affect all the others and can lead to dysfunction in the lumbar spine, pelvis, or hip joint. For example, if there is one weak abductor, the pelvis will drop excessively on the opposite side, leading to compressive forces through side bending in the lumbar spine.

The ilium can be altered in the frontal plane so that one side is more superior (upslip) or inferior (downslip) from the opposite ilium (Mitchell, Moran, and Pruzzo). This can lead to sacroiliac dysfunction, symphysis pubis dysfunction, and adductor and hamstring muscle imbalance. The lumbar spine on one side will be forced into side bending coupled with rotation and the resulting compressive forces.

The pelvis, sacrum, lumbar spine, and lower extremity must be balanced in the **horizontal plane** (or transverse plane) also. The muscles that help to control the lumbar spine and pelvis in the horizontal or transverse plane include the following:

- The internal oblique, transversus abdominis, and external oblique can pull laterally
- Sartorius can pull the pelvis inward (unilaterally)
- The adductors can exert a medial rotational force on the pelvis if the femur is fixed

- Gluteals and lateral hip rotators can also affect the pelvis position when the femur is fixed
- Piriformis can influence the sacral position and, in turn, the lumbar spine (see section on sacrum)

Any muscle problems will lead to lumbar, pelvis, or hip joint dysfunction. There can be rotation of the ilium, causing inflares (one ilium ASIS is closer to the midline than the opposite ilium), outflares (one ilium ASIS is farther from the body midline than the opposite ilium), or rotation of the sacrum, causing sacroiliac dysfunction, (according to the osteopaths Mitchell, Moran, and Pruzzo).

Movements of the lumbar spine depend on several variables:

- Thickness of the intervertebral disc
- Strength, weakness, or synchronization of the muscle groups
- Shape and alignment of the facet joints
- Shape of the vertebral end plates
- Ligaments and their degree of tautness or laxity

In assessing chronic lumbar pain it is difficult to determine the lesion site. Pain can be referred down to the sacroiliac joint, buttock, posterior thigh, and even the lower leg or foot. For example, pain from trochanteric bursitis can be referred along the L5 dermatome but so can any L5 spinal segment disorder (i.e., L5 facet dysfunction, L5 nerve root irritation). A full asssessment is needed to determine which structure is at fault. Problems with the L3 spinal segment can cause groin and anterior thigh discomfort but so can a degenerative hip joint. Because of the radiation of pain from the hip joint, sacroiliac joint, and other musculoskeletal structures, a thorough assessment must be done to eliminate the possibility that other structures of the kinetic chain are responsible for the patient's symptoms.

It is difficult to determine the cause of lumbar pain, especially when it is characterized by an insidious onset.

Biomechanical dysfunction in the lumbar spine or sacroiliac joint can originate from a leg-length discrepancy, a scoliosis, a sacral torsion, poor postural habits, muscle imbalances, sports activities, excessive body weight, incorrect lifting techniques, or even functional or structural lower leg malalignments. Yet to assess and rehabilitate the athlete fully, the cause of the discomfort must be determined, and often the history-taking can be an arduous task.

Because of the complexity of chronic low back problems it is important to rule out the possibility of neoplastic, infections, structural or developmental abnormalities, or hip or kidney problems.

According to Goodman and Snyder, metastatic lesions of the lumbar spine can be secondary cancer from primary cancer of the breast, ovary, lung, kidney, and thyroid or prostate gland. Cancer of the prostate gland often presents with sciatic pain caused by metastasis of the bones of the pelvis, lumbar spine, or femur. A thorough history-taking may show that the athlete has previously had cancer.

Low back pain from cancer will not fit the typical musculoskeletal pattern. The pain is usually intense and will not respond to rest. Gross motor weakness and pain distribution that does not fit a nerve root pattern may emerge. Neoplasms may affect the sympathetic nerves also.

Kidney disorders can cause low back and flank pain. Other symptoms will indicate kidney problems such as urinary tract problems, raised temperature, pain that radiates to the groin, or blood in the urine. Athletes in contact sports can have direct trauma to the kidney area and present with flank pain.

Gynecological disorders can cause low back, sacroiliac joint, and midpelvic pain (ovarian cysts, endometriosis, ectopic pregnancy, cystocele, rectocele).

In the older athlete (60 to 70 years) an abdominal aortic aneurysm can cause severe back pain in the midlumbar region. This is a medical emergency.

Mid to low back pain can also develop from acute pancreatitis. The other signs and symptoms are gastrointestinal problems.

Sacroiliac pain is the most prominent symptom of ankylosing spondylitis. It also occurs with psoriatic arthritis, Reiter disease, and rheumatoid arthritis.

Paget disease (osteitis deformans) most commonly involves the pelvis, lumbar spine, and sacrum.

For more details on pain elicited from nonmusculoskeletal disorders, please refer to Goodman and Snyder: Differential Diagnosis in Physical Therapy.

Thorough laboratory testing and x-ray workup by the family physician may be indicated, especially if there is a history of increased pain at night.

LUMBAR SPINE AND FACET JOINTS

The body of the fifth lumbar vertebra is the largest in the body and weight from the upper body is transmitted through it to the sacrum and pelvis. The L5 vertebra is sloped forward and anteriorly, which causes the lumbar vertebra above to incline slightly backward in relation to the one below. This allows the normal lumbar lordotic curve— according to Bogduk and Twomey. The L5 vertebra assumes this position because of the angle of the sacrum (50° angle from top of sacrum to the horizontal plane), the wedge shape of the intervertebral disc (posterior disc height is 6 to 7 mm less than its anterior height), and the wedge shape of the L5 vertebra (posterior height is 3 mm less than the anterior height). Excessive lordosis (anterior lordotic curve or hyperlordotic curve) causes shearing forces forward and downward and uneven force is exerted through the disc. It has been a common belief that excessive lordosis leads to lumbar pathology, but some recent studies are challenging this belief (Hansson et al.; Pope).

The lumbar facets are normally in the vertical and sagittal plane, which allows forward bending and back bending but limits side bending and rotation. The facet joints can be flat or curved in the sagittal plane. The joints that are flat and parallel to the sagittal plane do not restrict anterior displacement but restrict rotation very well, while the joints that are curved into a "C" or "J" shape prevent both anterior displacement and rotation relatively well (Bogduk and Twomey).

The facet joints are reinforced with a posterior, superior, and inferior fibrous capsule. Anteriorly, the fibrous capsule is replaced by the ligamentum flavum, which is highly elastic and attaches to the articular margin and blends with the capsule. Posteriorly, the capsule is reinforced by deep fibers of the multifidus muscle. Synovium lines the capsule. The joints are lined with articular cartilage and rest on a thick layer of subchondral bone. There are meniscoid-like tissue and fatty tissue that fill the intraarticular spaces in the capsule. The capsule is presumed to be innervated by nociceptive and proprioceptive afferent nerve fibers. Joint position and movement is relayed to the central nervous system and a motor response can be triggered.

The role of the facet joints are to stabilize the spine, allow limited movement, and protect the intervertebral discs from shear forces caused by excessive forward bending, back bending, and rotation. The facet joint has many different names, including zygapophyseal joint, apophysial joint, and posterior joint.

According to Bogduk and Twomey, the term *facet joint* comes from the reference to the articular facets on the articular processes of the spine. They contend that this name is a poor one because there are articular facets in other joints of the body. Apophysial, sometimes spelled apophyseal, joints is an abbreviated version of the zygapophyseal joint. The term *zygapophyseal* identifies the spinal joints more clearly and is not an abbreviation.

In this manual the term *facet* is used because of the familiarity of this term in the North American medical community, although zygapophyseal is probably a better term.

The facet joint's resting position is midway between flexion and extension.

The close-packed position of the facet joints is extension.

CAPSULAR POSITION

The capsular pattern for the lumbar facet joints is limited side bending, rotation (both of which are equally limited), and extension. According to Fisk, the two articular facet joints and the disc bear weight and work together to make up a spinal joint complex. If the facet joints are injured (often by repeated rotation), then as dysfunction occurs in the joints, the intervertebral disc's function will also be affected. Conversely, if the intervertebral disc is damaged (with compression or repeated rotation), the disc pathology will eventually lead to dysfunction in the articular facet joints. Therefore the facet and disc structures must both be assessed to determine the problem and both must be rehabilitated to achieve success. Porterfield and DeRosa indicate that 84% of the weight-bearing forces go through the bone-disc-bone interface, while 16% go through the facet joint.

LUMBAR INTERVERTEBRAL DISC

Each disc has a peripheral annulus fibrosus, a central nucleus pulposus, and cartilaginous end plates. The annulus fibrosis consists of layers of highly organized collagen in concentric rings and laminated bands around the nucleus pulposus. The orientation of the fibers and the tough collagen makeup ensure that the disc is resistant to tensile stresses. The nucleus pulposus is a semifluid mucoid material that can deform under pressure to transmit forces in all directions (hydrostatic-like behavior). As the disc ages, there is a decrease in its water and proteoglycan content, and injury potential increases. Motion of the spine, as well as cyclic loading and unloading of the disc, is necessary for normal disc nutrition. The superior and inferior aspects of the disc are covered by cartilage called the vertebral end plate. The cartilaginous end plate allows diffusion of nutrients in and out of the disc. The end plate also helps to dissipate some of the pressure from the nucleus pulposus. The nucleus functions to dissipate forces under compressive loads; the annulus fibrosus functions to control tensile stresses (Panjabi et al.).

The functions of the disc are to augment movement between vertebral bodies, to absorb axial forces through the vertebrae, and to transmit compressive loads from one vertebra to the next.

Intradiscal pressures are affected as follows:
- Higher in sitting than standing (Nachemson)
- Less in the physiological lordotic posture than in a straight or kyphotic posture
- Increased 20% with passive lumbar flexion
- Increased further with active lumbar flexion (Nachemson)
- Increased the greatest amount with heavy lifting and with the Valsalva maneuver (Nachemson)

PELVIS AND RELATED JOINTS

Asymmetrical or unbalanced forces from the lower extremities are compensated for in the pelvic region. Chronic asymmetry or uneven stress may lead to ligamentous pain and muscle imbalances.

The pelvis is made up of four paired stable joints. They are:
1. The L5-S1 facet joints bilaterally—the body of S1 articulates with the body of L5 and the oblique facet joints (lumbosacral junction). Forces from the trunk are transferred through these joints to the pelvis. The facet joint capsule is a thick fibrous tissue that extends dorsally, superiorly, and inferiorly The posterior aspect of the capsule is one of the main restraints to forward bending and prevents anterior shear forces. The last two lumbar levels (L4-L5 and L5-S1) facet joints are designed to prevent anterior shear stresses (the intervertebral disc and ligaments also limit shear). The inferior articular process is oriented in the frontal plane to engage with the superior

articular process also aligned in the frontal plane to limit L4 sliding anteriorly on L5. A similar alignment of the facets limit L5 movement on the sacrum. The superior articular processes of the sacrum are shorter and stronger than the inferior articular processes of L5 vertebrae, which are longer and more vulnerable to injury.

Axial rotation to the right is limited by the compression of the left facet joint, as well as capsular stretch on the right facet joint (ligaments, the intervertebral disc, fascia, and muscle stretch also limit rotation).

2. The sacroiliac joints bilaterally—they are very stable joints that are more mobile in the young athlete and decrease in mobility as the athlete ages. The movement is very small, with the greatest amount occurring with forward bending in the standing position, according to Mitchell. They can become less stable with trauma or overuse. When equal amounts of force are experienced from the extremities to the pelvis, the mobility of the ilium on the sacrum is symmetrical. When uneven forces (i.e., leg-length differences or abnormal lower limb mechanics on one side) are experienced, the sacroiliac joint adapts with joint dysfunction. The sacroiliac joint is classified as a synovial joint. The sacral surface is made up of hyaline cartilage and the iliac surface is made up of fibrocartilage, according to Diane Lee.

The joint capsule has a synovial membrane and is reinforced by several ligaments (ventral and dorsal sacroiliac ligaments, interosseous sacroiliac ligament, iliolumbar ligament, sacrotuberous and sacrospinous ligament).

3. The hip joints bilaterally—all the weight-bearing forces are transmitted from the lower extremity to the pelvis through the hip joints. Decreased motion in either hip joint leads to increased forces through the pelvis and lumbar spine.

4. The symphysis pubis joint—usually very hypomobile and stable. Hypermobility problems, which develop in the sacroiliac joints, can cause symptoms at the symphysis pubis and the adductor muscles. Conversely, problems with the adductor muscles or symphysis pubis can cause discomfort at the sacroiliac joint.

SACRUM

There is a great deal of controversy regarding the biomechanics of the sacrum but most therapists agree that it is capable of forward, backward, side bending, and rotational movement. The osteopaths Mitchell, Moran, and Pruzzo describe in great detail these planes and axes of sacral motion. As the patient forward bends, there is a backward movement of the sacrum; as the patient backward bends, there is a forward movement of the sacrum around a horizontal axis.

The sacrum also has the ability to rotate around oblique axes of motion. These axes run from the upper right corner of the sacrum to the lower left corner and from the upper left corner to the lower right corner. The sacrum is also capable of a right rotation on the right oblique axis or a left rotation on the left oblique axis.

Other researchers have developed hypothetical models for sacral motion with different axes and biomechanics (Kapandji; Wilder; others).

The lower end of the sacrum is fixed by the piriformis muscle.

Dysfunction occurs when the sacrum loses its ability to rotate over one axis.

ASSESSMENT   INTERPRETATION

HISTORY

Mechanism of Injury
Direct Trauma (Fig. 1-1)

Was it direct trauma?

Contusion

The tips of the spinous processes can be contused (periosteal hematoma), as can the overlying tissue, but this is not very common. The erector spinae muscles on either side of the processes will usually absorb the force if the blow is from a large object.

Contusions of the low back (paraspinal area) are common in all contact sports but they must be distinguished from a vertebral fracture. Kidney discomfort or trauma must be ruled out.

Direct trauma to the ischial tuberosity can move the ilium upward or cause direct forces through the sacroiliac joint, causing dysfunction.

Fracture
- Spinous process
- Transverse process
- Arch fracture
- Pars interarticularis
- Vertebral end plate fracture

Occasionally the spinous process can be fractured from a direct blow or from landing on the buttock. These fractures tend to occur to horseback riders, alpine skiers, football players, luge competitors, and ski jumpers.

A direct impact to the side of the vertebral column can fracture the transverse process.

Any fracture through the vertebral arch is rare but potentially serious because of the chance of neurological involvement.

Compressional forces through the lumbar spine can fracture the end plate of the intervertebral disc. Under a compressional load the most vulnerable structures are the cancellous bone of the vertebra and the end plate. The damage can be a fissure fracture or depressed fracture. This can occur when falling on the backside or falling in the long sitting position.

According to Jackson and Wiltse, the pars interarticularis fatigue fracture has a high incidence in young athletes (e.g., female gymnasts and football linemen) who get into positions of excessive lumbar extension. It occurs four times more frequently in white female gymnasts than nonathletes.

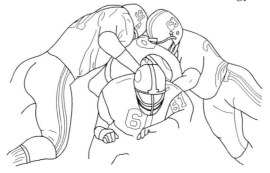

Fig. 1-1 Direct trauma.

ASSESSMENT

INTERPRETATION

According to Cyron and Hutton, the pars interarticularis fatigue fracture occurs more frequently with lumbar flexion. They feel the primary mechanism is anterior shear forces caused by repetitive flexion and extension, muscular activity, and the force of gravity on the posterior vertebral elements. The anterior position of the fifth lumbar vertebra adds to this.

There is a strong hereditary component for this defect. The average age for the appearance of symptoms is 14 years in girls and 16 years in boys, according to Grieve.

Overstretch

Was it an overstretch?

Severe injuries like fractures or dislocations of the low back are extremely rare in athletic activities.

Forced Forward Bending (Hyperflexion)

According to Kapandji, during forward bending the body of the upper vertebra tilts and slides forward (Fig. 1-2).

During forward bending, there is a straightening of the lumbar curve that occurs mainly at the upper lumbar vertebrae (Bogduk and Twomey). There is anterior sagittal rotation and anterior sagittal translation. Anterior sagittal rotation is limited by the inferior articular facet compressing against the superior articular facet. The anterior sagittal translation is limited by tension in the capsule of the facet joints.

The facet joints themselves, especially those with superior articular facets that face backward, are the most important factor limiting flexion, according to Bogduk and Twomey.

The ligament structures that are stressed in this forward bent position and thus can be injured include the following:

- supraspinous ligament, which can sprain, tear, or avulse a spinous process fragment. (There is no supraspinous ligament at L5 to S1 level, nor are there intertransverse ligaments. The latter have been replaced by the iliolumbar ligament.)
- capsular ligament of the facet joint—the posterior aspect of which is very important to prevent anterior shear during forward bending
- posterior layer of the iliolumbar ligament at L5, S1 (according to Luk et al.)

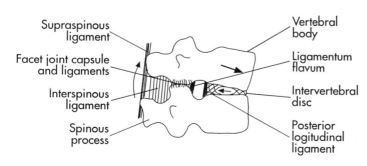

Supraspinous ligament

Facet joint capsule and ligaments

Interspinous ligament

Spinous process

Vertebral body

Ligamentum flavum

Intervertebral disc

Posterior logitudinal ligament

Fig. 1-2 Vertebral motions from forced forward bending.

ASSESSMENT   INTERPRETATION

- the interspinous ligament and ligamentum flavum are more elastic and not as readily overstretched
- posterior longitudinal ligament, (which scarcely limits flexion because it is so close to the fulcrum of movement)

Adams, Hutton, and Stott recorded the limiting factors of anterior sagittal rotation with mathematical analysis that shows the following:

- intervertebral disc resists 29%
- supraspinous and interspinous ligaments: 19%
- ligamentum flavum: 13%
- facet joint capsules: 39%

There is evidence that in the forward bent position, the nucleus pulposus of the intervertebral disc can migrate posteriorly if the annulus fibrosus is damaged or weakened in this area.

According to Adams and Hutton, the supraspinous and interspinous ligaments are damaged first, followed by the facet capsular ligaments and then the disc. However, forward bending to one side will injure the capsular ligament first.

Forced forward bending can strain the erector spinae muscles, latissimus dorsi, or lumbodorsal fascia in the low back region, especially if the athlete has tight hamstrings that contribute to the lumbar stress.

A sudden hyperflexion can avulse the tip off the spinous process. Body positions in sports that already put the spine in a flexed position (e.g., tobogganring, tuck position in skiing) predispose the T12 and L1 level to a fracture when the athlete lands. Compression fractures of the dorsolumbar junction result from this sudden jackknifing body position while falling from a height. The athlete may land on his or her feet or buttock. The vertebrae are usually crushed anteriorly and the fragments may cause severe neurological damage if they protrude into the spinal canal or cord. The vertebral cartilaginous end plates can also be fractured with these compression forces.

The lumbosacral joint allows more range of flexion and extension than the other lumbar vertebrae, according to White and Panjabi. Therefore this flexed seated body position also subjects the lumbosacral joint to sprain on landing. The end of the sacrum is pushed forward and the iliolumbar ligaments can become sprained. Falling on the buttock can cause a contusion or flexion injury to the coccyx, including the following:

- sprain of the posterior fibers of the sacrococcygeal joint capsule
- contusion to the tip of the coccyx and surrounding soft tissue
- fracture of the coccyx

Forced Back Bending (Hyperextension)

According to Kapandji, during lumbar extension the body of the upper vertebra tilts and moves posteriorly while the articu-

ASSESSMENT

INTERPRETATION

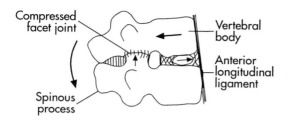

Fig. 1-3 Vertebral motions from forced back bending.

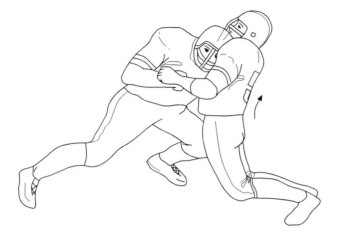

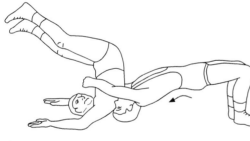

Fig. 1-4 Sports where there is forced back bending.

lar processes become more compressed and the spinous processes touch (Fig. 1-3).

Bogduk and Twomey describe a posterior sagittal rotation and slight posterior translation of the lumbar vertebrae during back bending. There is a downward movement of the inferior articular processes of the facet joints impacting against the lamina and the superior articular processes of the vertebra below.

During forced back bending the following structures can be damaged:

- compressed facet joints (capsule, synovial impingement, and articular cartilage) (this is most common)
- periosteum of the vertebrae lamina (from the inferior articular process)
- the anterior longitudinal ligament
- the vertebral arch (which can be fractured)
- a spinous process (which can be fractured when one process is forced against the other)
- the intervertebral disc (which can be damaged by tensile forces anteriorly and compression posteriorly)

Athletes running downhill throw the lumbar spine into a hyperextended position and can develop low back pain. This lumbar body extension position is assumed in sports where lumbar flexibility is required (e.g., wrestling and gymnastics) and where contact forces the assumption of this position (e.g., football, hockey, soccer) (Fig. 1-4).

ASSESSMENT   INTERPRETATION

Rotation or Side Bending (Lateral Flexion)

During rotation, the inferior articular facets of the upper vertebra impact against the opposing superior articular facet on the opposite side (i.e., right rotation left facet impaction and right facet gapping). The facet capsule on the same side is stretched (Bogduk and Twomey).

The structures that can be injured most often with a rotation are the capsular ligaments of the facet joints (one facet is compressed; the opposite facet is sheared) and the intervertebral disc (annulus fibrosis) (Fig. 1-5, *A*). The structures that are occasionally injured are the interspinous ligaments and the supraspinous ligaments.

Excessive facet compression can result in the following (Bogduk and Twomey):

- fracture of the subchondral bone
- fracture of the base of the inferior or superior articular process
- fracture of the vertebral lamina

Excessive rotation can then cause splitting of the annulus fibrosis of the intervertebral disc (especially the posterolateral aspect). According to White and Panjabi, very little rotation takes place at the upper lumbar joints because their inferior and superior articular facets prevent rotation. The most rotational motion occurs at the lumbosacral junction, which subjects the lower lumbar joints to excess stress. This may explain why disc degeneration occurs most commonly at the L4-L5 or the L5-S1 disc spaces.

Sports that involve throwing can cause problems of over rotation in the lumbar region when the athlete pivots over a fixed lower extremity (e.g., shot put, javelin, discus).

The sacroiliac joint and lumbosacral joint can be injured unilaterally by a twisting mechanism.

Combinations of forward bending and side bending cause excessive force on the facet joints and their ligamentous structures (Fig. 1-5, *B*). The iliolumbar ligament (superior band) is particularly susceptible to sprain in this position. Side bending (lateral flexion) with an increased lordotic curve leads to increased shearing forces through the facet joints.

NOTE: Side bending or lateral flexion movements are always coupled with axial rotation.

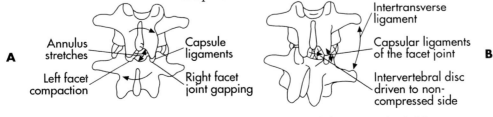

A, Annulus stretches, Left facet compaction, Capsule ligaments, Right facet joint gapping

B, Intertransverse ligament, Capsular ligaments of the facet joint, Intervertebral disc driven to non-compressed side

Fig. 1-5, A, Upper vertebral axial rotation (right). **B,** Vertebral side bending (left).

ASSESSMENT

INTERPRETATION

Overcontraction
Was it a forceful overcontraction?
Was it an eccentric contraction?

A forceful contraction against too great a resistance can cause a muscle strain of the involved muscles. This occurs most frequently to the erector spinae muscles or the lateral flexors. Muscle strains or tears occur in sports involving explosive upper-body movements over a fixed pelvis, e.g., weight lifting, javelin, discus, shot put, handball, squash, boxing, and wrestling.

An eccentric contraction against too great a resistance also leads to strains and tears, e.g., lowering a weight, causing erector spinae to strain.

Overuse
Was it an overuse mechanism?

Rotation

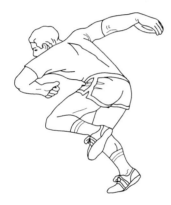

Fig. 1-6 Repeated lumbar rotation (discus throw).

This is most common among throwers (Fig. 1-6) but also occurs in racquet sports, cross country skiing, rowing, and paddling.

Repeated trunk rotation over a fixed pelvis can result in gluteus medius or piriformis syndromes.

The small lumbar spine rotator muscles can also become inflamed or result in microtearing of their attachments on the spinous processes. Repeated rotation can cause stress of the facet joints with compression of articular cartilage of the superior articular process of the lower vertebrae by the inferior articular process of the upper vertebrae. Cartilage breakdown may occur with eventual degenerative changes in the facet joint on this side and with time on the opposite side. Osteophytes can then develop at the edges of the articular cartilage that is compressed. With the failure of the facet joint to block rotation the intervertebral disc becomes very susceptible to rotational torsion and damage.

Recent literature shows that the intervertebral disc has microfailure with as little as 3° of rotation and macrofailure at 12° (Farfan et al.). The annulus fibrosis develops circumferential splits and eventually radial fissures that can allow nucleus pulposus migration and its related problems. The annulus fibrosis is most vulnerable to injury with rotation in the flexed position.

Back Bending (Extension)

Because of compression loads on the facet joints and the lamina of the vertebra below during back bending, the facet joint can degenerate or the inferior articular process may break down the periosteum of the lamina below.

Repeated lumbar spine flexion and extension with the cyclic loading of the neural arch leads to stress fractures of the pars interarticularis, resulting in spondylolysis, and, if the stress fracture is complete, to spondylolisthesis.

ASSESSMENT   ## INTERPRETATION

The sacroiliac joints can also become sprained or inflamed due to repeated back bending.

Compression

According to White and Panjabi, repeated compression forces on the lumbar spine force the spine into lordosis and can lead to breakdown of the intervertebral discs, the vertebral end plates, or even the facet joints.

Intervertebral damage occurs most commonly with a compression and forward bending position.

Sports that involve repeated lifting include pairs figure skating, weight lifting (Fig. 1-7), dance, and shot put. These are most susceptible to compression damage.

Forward Bending

Exertion for a prolonged period of time in the forward bent position can cause back pain. This is especially true if the athlete has tight hamstrings and the stress is shifted up to the lumbar spine to get the necessary flexion range. Sports in which this occurs are weight lifting, bicycling, hockey, paddling, alpine skiing, and speed skating.

Pain

Location of Pain
Where is the pain located?

Local Pain
Lumbar pain (Fig. 1-8)

Most individuals will be affected by pain in the lower back sometime in their life.

Low back pain of a local somatic origin can be caused by the following:
- facet joint (synovial membrane, capsule) (Mooney and Robertson)
- posterior vertebral ligaments (Kellgren)
- intervertebral disc (posterior aspect of annulus fibrosis) (Wiley et al.)

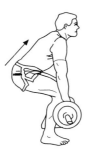

Fig. 1-7 Repeated lumbar compression.

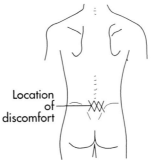

Location of discomfort

Fig. 1-8 Local lumbar pain.

ASSESSMENT   # INTERPRETATION

- anterior and posterior longitudinal ligaments (Kellgren)
- paravertebral muscles, tendon, and fascia (Travell)
- dura mater or dural sleeve (the dural sleeve is both chemosensitive and mechanosensitive, therefore traction or irritation (disc inflammatory contents) can evoke a response (Smyth and Wright)
- nerve root (previously damaged [Loeser] or under traction [Smyth and Wright])
- bone (periosteum and subchondral) (Kellgren)

According to McKenzie, a lumbar backache that starts centrally and moves unilaterally is most likely caused by an intervertebral disc lesion. In the early stages of minor disc lesions the characterisitic feature is a local backache. Most pain that stays localized in the lumbar spine is caused by lesions of a local muscle, ligament, or facet.

The onset of symptoms from lumbar spondylolysis is usually localized in the low back and, to a lesser extent, to the posterior buttocks and thighs.

A backache brought on by stretching of the ligaments in spondylolisthesis is usually aggravated by prolonged standing or repeated lumbar forward and back bending movements of the spine.

Local back pain is usually from lesions in the skeletal muscle, bone, capsule, and superficial periosteum.

According to Grieve, pain from lesions of the lumbar synovial joints and their immediate periarticular structures may be local, referred, or both.

Pain from the intervertebral disc that does not involve the neighboring tissue (especially nerve root) may also be localized. Conversely, root pain due to intervertebral herniation will cause pain in the involved limb distally with little or no pain locally.

Referred Pain

Pain can be referred to the low back from other structures or conditions, which include the following:

- visceral (kidney disorders, gynecological disorders, prostatitis, pancreatitis, small intestine disorders)
- vascular (abdominal aortic aneurysm, occlusion of iliac arteries)
- neural (infections of the neural tissue, arachnoiditis)
- cancer (prostate, spinal metastases)
- systemic disorders (rheumatoid arthritis, ankylosing spondylitis, osteoporosis, vertebral osteomyelitis)

Pain referred from intraabdominal or pelvic problems will usually have a full and pain free lumbar spine assessment, unless the problem has caused a facilitated segment in the lumbar spine. With visceral problems there are other signs and symptoms related to the organ and pain is not relieved with rest.

ASSESSMENT   INTERPRETATION

Somatic Referred Pain (Fig. 1-9)

Somatic referred pain is pain of a musculoskeletal origin that is perceived in an area remote from the lesion site (i.e., back pain can be referred to the lower limb). This pain is of a diffuse, dull nature and can be projected segmentally or along dermatomes, myotomes, or sclerotomes. For example, pain in the L4 dermatome area can be referred from an L3-L4 facet joint, the supraspinous or interspinous ligaments, the longitudinal ligaments, or any muscle structure supplied by the L4 nerve root. The referred pain patterns can vary greatly from individual to individual. Somatic referred pain can come from lumbar facet joints, capsules, ligaments, muscles, dura mater, dura sleeve, fascia, or bone.

This somatic referred pain may be caused by confusion in the central nervous system. Afferent pain messages from the lumbar spine travel to the neurons in the central nervous system at the same time as afferent messages from the lower extremity (buttock, thigh, lower leg, or foot). The central nervous system confuses the messages and interprets pain in both the lumbar spine and lower extremity.

Pain can be referred to the low back or leg from other joints such as the hip joint or the sacroiliac joint.

Radicular Pain

Radicular pain is caused by irritation of spinal nerves or nerve roots and results in neurological signs (sensory or motor changes) at that level. This pain is of shooting or lancinating

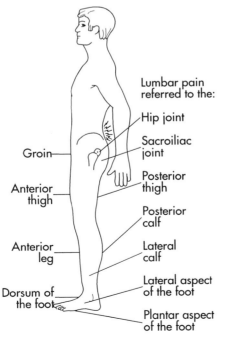

Lumbar pain referred to the:

Hip joint

Sacroiliac joint

Groin

Posterior thigh

Anterior thigh

Posterior calf

Anterior leg

Lateral calf

Lateral aspect of the foot

Dorsum of the foot

Plantar aspect of the foot

Fig. 1-9 Referred pain from lumbar pathology.

ASSESSMENT

INTERPRETATION

quality and travels down the involved limb. For example, shooting radicular pain in the S1 dermatome may also have a decreased ankle jerk and weak gastrocnemius and hamstring muscle groups. The pain is usually more severe in its distal distribution than at the irritation site. It is important to note that the dermatomes, myotomes, and scleratomes have a great deal of variation in their distribution in the general population.

Myofascial Pain

Myofascial pain is described by Simons and Travell in their discussion of myofascial trigger points. They indicate that there are point tender trigger points in muscle tissue that refer pain in specific patterns. For these point locations and pain patterns, refer to their book (see bibliography).

Referred, Radicular, or Myofascial Referred Pain
BUTTOCK, POSTERIOR THIGH, CALF, AND FOOT (FIG.1-10)

An ache in the buttock that changes sides is suggestive of sacroiliac arthritis.

Pain referred into the buttock unilaterally can be caused by myofascial trigger points in the iliocostalis lumborum, longissimus thoracis, multifidi, quadratus lumborum, and gluteus maximus muscles (according to Simons and Travell).

Buttock pain and pain felt at the posterior thigh, back of the knee, and calf (sciatica) is often seen in the presence of a posterolateral disc protrusion and associated nerve root irritation.

The L4-L5 and L5-S1 facet joints and sacroiliac joints can refer pain to the lateral lumbar and buttock region mainly.

Alternating sciatica from one leg to the other suggests the early signs of ankylosing spondylitis, intermittent claudication, bilateral osteoarthritis of the hip, spinal claudication, a large disc herniation, or malignant disease.

The sacroiliac joints are derived from the first and second sacral segments and therefore an injury to these joints can cause pain in the posterior thigh and calf. Ankylosing spondylitis can cause this posterior thigh pain but it begins with sacroiliac joint degeneration. Intermittent claudication gives rise to posterior thigh and calf pain on walking. Bilateral pain in the posterior thighs and calves is usually caused by spondylolisthesis, spinal claudication, or a neoplasm.

Pain referred down the posterior thigh can come from a myofascial trigger point in the midbelly of the gluteus medius (according to Travell and Simons). Pain referred down the posterior thigh and calf can come from a myofascial trigger point in the midbelly of the gluteus minimus. Pain referred down the posterior thigh, calf, and into the sole of the foot can come from a myofascial trigger point in the midbelly of the piriformis muscle, and pain referred into the posterior knee and calf can also

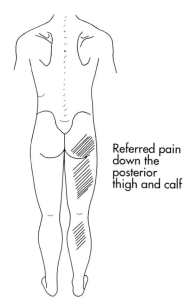

Referred pain down the posterior thigh and calf

Fig. 1-10 Posterior buttock, thigh, and calf referred pain.

ASSESSMENT

INTERPRETATION

come from myofascial trigger points in the soleus, gastrocnemius, or popliteus muscles.

GROIN

Pain in the groin and along the inner thigh with lumbar spine symptoms can be caused by pressure on the third sacral nerve root.

Groin pain usually indicates hip pathology.

ANTERIOR THIGH, LOWER LEG, AND DORSUM OF THE FOOT

Pain in the front of the thigh with lumbar symptomology characterizes a second or third lumbar root compression. If the pain spreads to the anterior aspect of the lower leg, the third lumbar root is probably involved.

Pain referred into the anterior thigh can also come from myofascial trigger points in the iliopsoas, adductor magnus, vastus intermedius, and quadriceps femoris muscles (according to Travell and Simons).

An irritation of the second or third lumbar nerve roots can cause pain in the hip joint, psoas, adductors, quadriceps, femur, or acetabulum.

A local irritation of the anterior cutaneous nerve can cause pain and/or numbness here also—the nerve is irritated as it passes under the inguinal ligament.

Pain that is referred into the anterior thigh, knee, and medial aspect of the lower leg can come from myofascial trigger points in the adductor longus and brevis muscles (according to Travell and Simons).

Pain that radiates to the dorsum of the foot, especially to the second and third toes, can be a fifth lumbar nerve root irritation.

LATERAL THIGH, LATERAL LEG, AND LATERAL FOOT

Pain in the lateral thigh with lumbar spine symptoms occurs with an irritation of the fourth or fifth nerve root—this pain can radiate to the inner and dorsal aspect of the foot.

Pain in the lateral thigh can also come from myofascial trigger points in the vastus lateralis and tensor fascia lata (according to Travell and Simons).

Pain and/or paresthesia in the skin supplying the lateral thigh is caused by an injury to the lateral cutaneous nerve—this is a local nerve irritation (meralgia paresthetica) caused by trauma as it crosses the inguinal ligament.

Lateral leg pain from pressure on the peroneal nerve is usually just from trauma or prolonged compression, such as sitting with the legs crossed.

Pain down the lateral aspect of the lower leg and foot with localized pain behind the lateral malleolus can come from a myofascial trigger point in the peroneal muscles (according to Travell and Simons). Pain reaching the lateral border of the foot

ASSESSMENT

INTERPRETATION

and the fourth and fifth toes is often caused by a first sacral nerve root compression.

PERINEAL

Pain in the perineal (rectal, penile, scrotal, testicular, vaginal, bladder) tissue is very rare but a low lumbar disc lesion compressing the fourth sacral root can cause this.

Onset

Can the athlete describe the onset of pain?

Sudden

A sudden pain following a twist or lift that becomes worse in a couple of hours or by the next day and is described as a snap, tear or click, is indicative of the following:
- muscle strain or tear
- ligament sprain or tear
- facet joint subluxation or meniscal entrapment between the articular facets (Bogduk describes an entrapment where the meniscoid material that is normally present in the facet joint does not reenter the joint and results in a strain on the joint capsule; Bogduk and Twomey)
- acute intervertebral disc protrusion

A sudden pain in the sacroiliac joint that is preceded by a sudden twisting motion can indicate a sacroiliac joint sprain.

Gradual

A gradual onset of constant lumbar discomfort or radiating pain usually indicates the following:
- chronic intervertebral disc degeneration with nerve root irritation
- degenerative facet joint
- neoplasm
- spondylolysis (Fig. 1-11, A)

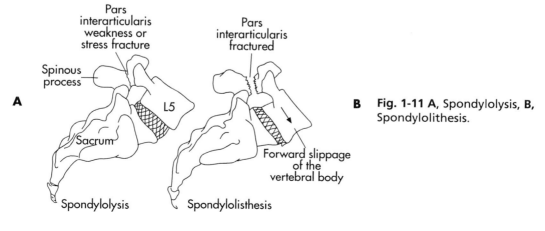

Fig. 1-11 A, Spondylolysis, **B**, Spondylolithesis.

ASSESSMENT

INTERPRETATION

- spondylolisthesis (Fig. 1-11, *B*)
- systemic or local disease

Repeated episodes of local pain usually indicates the following:

- intervertebral disc protrusion with posterior longitudinal ligament irritation
- an unstable facet joint

Radicular pain that begins as a backache, radiates unilaterally down one leg with no back symptoms, and progresses to numbness in that limb is associated with a progressing disc herniation with nerve root irritation.

Type

Can the athlete describe the pain?

Sharp

Sharp, well-localized pain suggests a superficial lesion. Generally, the closer the tissue is to the body surface the more localized the pain. Sharp pain is usually elicited from the following structures:

- skin
- superficial fascia (e.g., lumbodorsal fascia)
- tendon (e.g., the iliopsoas)
- superficial muscle (e.g., the superficial erector spinae)
- superficial ligament (e.g., the supraspinatus ligament and the interspinous ligament)
- bursa (e.g., the greater trochanteric)
- periosteum (e.g., the spinous process)
- muscle-periosteal junction (e.g., the quadratus lumborum)
- joint capsule (e.g., the facet joint)

Sharp and Shooting

This is often associated with the following:

- nerve lesion presumably affecting the A delta fibers (e.g., the sciatic nerve)
- nerve root irritation (radicular pain) with neurological changes, i.e., dermatomal paresthesia, numbness, or myotomal weakness

Dull

Dull and aching pain spread over a diffuse area is typical of a deeper somatic pathologic condition; deep somatic pain can be associated with autonomic system responses (sweating, piloerection, pallor). Dull pain is usually elicited by the following:

- deep muscle (e.g., deep erector spinae and gluteus medius)
- bone (e.g., vertebral body)

Aching

Aching pain may be felt from the following:

- fascia (e.g., lumbodorsal fascia)

ASSESSMENT	INTERPRETATION

- deep muscle (e.g., piriformis)
- deep ligament (e.g., posterior longitudinal ligament)
- chronic bursitis (e.g., iliopsoas bursitis)

Burning

This sensation is experienced from the following:
- skin (e.g., lesion or irritation)
- peripheral nerve (e.g., neuritis)

Pins and Needles, Tingling

These sensations may originate from the following structures:
- peripheral nerve (e.g., lateral cutaneous nerve of the thigh)
- dorsal nerve root (e.g., L5 nerve root pain down the lateral calf)

Tingling in both feet or all four extremities suggests involvement of the spinal cord or may be a sign of serious spinal pathologic conditions or a systemic disease.

Numbness (Anesthesia)

Numbness may be caused by the following:
- dorsal nerve root compression (e.g., S1 nerve root numbness under the lateral malleolus)
- peripheral nerve compression (e.g., obturator cutaneous nerve supply to the medial thigh)

Time of Pain
When is the pain worse?

Morning
Is it worse in the morning?

Morning pain suggests that rest does not help relieve the symptoms or that the sleeping position or the mattress is not supporting the lesion.

Morning pain and stiffness can suggest a muscular injury, an ongoing infection, or inflammatory condition (e.g., arthritis, ankylosing spondylitis, degenerative disease). Lumbar stiffness that lasts until late morning suggests ankylosing spondylitis.

Joint and disc problems are usually relieved by sleeping, especially when the sleeping position places the lumbar spine in a good resting position.

Evening or All Night
Is pain worse in the evening, or all night?

Pain at night or pain that lasts all night is a sign of a more serious pathologic condition such as a bone neoplasm, local or systemic disease, or very acute intervertebral disc lesion. The sacroiliac joint can cause night pains when the athlete lies on his or her back and when he or she turns over.

Hip joint problems or greater trochanteric bursitis can cause discomfort when lying on the affected side.

ASSESSMENT

INTERPRETATION

As the Day goes on

Does pain get worse as the day goes on?

Pain that worsens as the day goes on means that the condition is aggravated by activity. This is true of disc lesions in particular, although facet problems, arthritis, and muscular problems can also be aggravated by daily activity.

Sacroiliac dysfunction and pain is aggravated by weight-bearing postures.

Sitting (Fig. 1-12)

What effect does sitting have on the pain?

Does the pain change when rising from sitting?

Pressure on the intervertebral disc is increased in the seated position, especially when the spine is in kyphosis versus lordosis (Nachemson). If the athlete has had to remain seated for a long period of time (e.g., during a plane or car ride), the symptoms often worsen.

The slouched seated position also causes fatigue and over-stretching of the posterior ligaments of the lumbar spine and facet joint ligaments and capsule.

An athlete with spondylolisthesis may find that sitting relieves the pain but that walking or prolonged standing will increase discomfort.

When there is ligamentous instability or a muscle strain, changing positions triggers pain.

Facet joint derangements usually cause pain on movement; this pain is relieved by recumbency.

Sacroiliac joint problems are aggravated by sitting and by rising from a seated position.

Aggravating Activities

• facet
• sacroiliac joint
• spondylosis, spondylolisthesis
• intervertebral disc

Prolonged sitting, lifting, stooping, or twisting aggravate intervertebral disc lesions and pre-existing facet problems. Pain in the sacroiliac joint that is aggravated by activities involving a combination of hip and spine extension or rotation suggests a sacroiliac joint sprain, iliac rotational displacement, or sacroiliac joint hypomobility or hypermobility. Sacroiliac dysfunction

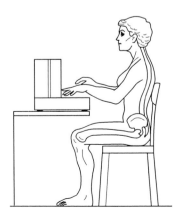

Fig. 1-12 Prolonged sitting can aggravate lower back conditions.

ASSESSMENT

INTERPRETATION

causes pain on twisting, climbing stairs, sitting and rising from a chair, and on prolonged standing with weight bearing on the affected side.

Positions of excessive lordosis aggravate spondylosis and spondylolisthesis.

Coughing or sneezing causes sharp pain whenever there is a space-occupying lesion in the spinal canal. An increase in intrathecal pressure causes pressure on the dura, which results in increased pain. An intervertebral disc herniation is the most common cause of this pain.

Alleviating Activities

Lying with the hips and knees flexed seems to alleviate most back problems (Fig. 1-13). Sitting with a lumbar roll supporting the lumbar spine in lordosis can also alleviate back pain.

Most lumbar musculoskeletal pain is alleviated by rest.

Pain Progression

In tendon and ligament injuries, the pain decreases 3 to 5 weeks after wound closure, but can last up to 6 months.

Muscular injuries have pain that decreases quickly (within a week to 10 days).

Degenerative disc problems can cause ongoing pain that can last for months or even years.

Pain caused by facet problems tends to decrease after a month to 6 weeks if the aggravating positions are avoided.

Pain that gets worse quickly can be caused by a systemic infection or an acute disc herniation.

Severity

The severity of pain is not a good indication of the degree of injury. For example, a facet joint sprain can be extremely painful, whereas a complete disc herniation may cause numbness and only slight pain.

Function

Degree of Disability

Can the athlete continue in his or her sport?

How is the athlete's daily routine affected?

Back injuries can be very debilitating or just a minor nuisance. The degree of disability is indicative of the degree of injury. Muscle spasm of the erector spinae can affect all body movements, even walking. Usually the more daily or sporting

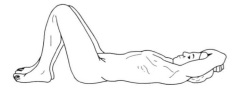

Fig. 1-13 Lying with the hips and knees flexed alleviates most back problems.

ASSESSMENT

INTERPRETATION

Are there problems with bladder or bowel function or control? Is there any anesthesia or paresthesia in the groin or genitals? Is there any gynecological problem or discomfort? Is there night pain, unexplained weight loss, or excessive fatigue?

activities that the athlete is able to perform, the less severe is the back problem. A disc protrusion affecting the sacral nerves resulting in bowel or bladder problems or numbness should be referred to a physician immediately because it may be a cauda equina compression, which is considered a medical emergency.

Since prostate cancer can cause lumbar pain, any urinary irregularities should be referred for further examination. Kidney problems can also cause back or flank discomfort and should be recognized as a potential source of pain.

Any gynecological problems, as in ovarian discomfort and intermenstrual bleeding or irregularities can indicate reproductive pathology and should be referred for further investigation with a physician. Unexplained weight loss, fatigue, and night pain are symptoms of serious back pathology (e.g. neoplasm, tuberculosis) and medical referral is imperative.

Sensations

Can the athlete describe the sensations felt at the time of injury and now?

Clicking

If the back clicked at the time of injury (usually rotational), a facet problem should be suspected.

Tearing

A tearing sensation strongly suggests a muscle injury.

Numbness

Numbness or paresthesia is a sign of a nerve root irritation or injury and the exact location of the lack of sensation must be investigated to determine the spinal segment involved.

Numbness can also be the result of a peripheral nerve injury and this will follow the local cutaneous nerve supply area.

Meralgia paresthetica (entrapment of the lateral femoral cutaneous nerve) can cause numbness in the lateral thigh.

Catching

Catching on movement is often a sign of a muscle spasm or of a facet joint problem.

Sudden backache with catching can indicate a locking of a facet joint. It usually occurs with a sudden reaching or twisting motion in the hypermobile athlete. It may be trapping of a synovial meniscoid villus of the facet joint. Muscle spasm holds the joint in flexion.

Tingling, Warmth, or Coldness

Tingling, warmth, or coldness can be caused by a neural (nerve root) or circulatory problem.

ASSESSMENT

INTERPRETATION

Particulars

Has the family physician, orthopedic surgeon, neurologist, athletic therapist, athletic trainer, physiotherapist, physical therapist, osteopath, or chiropractor been consulted in this problem?

What were their findings?

Are x-ray results available?

Were physiotherapy, prescriptions, or manipulations administered previously?

What helped or did not help the problem?

Any previous diagnosis or medical treatments (physiotherapy, chiropractic) should be recorded, including the names and addresses of the physicians concerned so that their assistance can be called on if needed.

Their findings and what worked or did not work will help to decide the best form of treatment and rehabilitation.

Any x-ray findings, prescriptions, specific exercises, or manipulations should also be recorded.

OBSERVATIONS

The athlete should be wearing only underclothing so that posture and spine can be assessed. The entire spine functions as a unit and any injury or defect can affect other structures, so a complete postural scan is necessary. Any lower limb dysfunction can alter the spine and vice versa.

A plumb line may be used to bisect the body to check for asymmetry and body alignment in the anterior, posterior, and lateral views.

The athlete's lumbar spine movements should be observed from the moment the athlete arrives in the clinic until completion of the palpations at the end of your assessment.

During postural observations, the therapist is looking for asymmetry and alignment problems. It is important to realize that asymmetry or poor alignment does not always cause symptoms or need correction. If symptoms are caused by malalignment or asymmetry, further functional assessment of the cause is indicated and correction can then be initiated.

Standing

Anterior View
Head Position
Rotated or side bent.

A head position that is rotated or side bent may mean that the athlete is compensating for a spinal deformity or an imbalance below (e.g., scoliosis, muscle imbalance, leg length).

Facial Expression

Chronic pain of an ongoing nature can cause an athlete to appear fatigued and drawn. Acute pain may cause discomfort in several positions and this can readily be seen on the athlete's face.

ASSESSMENT   INTERPRETATION

Shoulder Level

Overdevelopment of one side of the body in the athlete who, for example, plays tennis, throws a javelin or pitches a baseball can lead to a drop shoulder on the overdeveloped side, which can cause a functional scoliosis (Fig. 1-14).

Structural scoliosis may also cause the shoulders to be at different heights.

Unilateral muscle spasm in the low back can cause a functional scoliosis and the shoulders may not be level.

A leg-length difference can cause scoliosis and uneven shoulder heights.

Rib Cage Position

With structural scoliosis, the vertebrae are rotated and one side of the rib cage may be more prominent and turned closer to the midline than the other side.

Umbilicus Position

Note if the umbilicus is in the midline of the body. An off-center umbilicus can be because of the following:
- asymmetrical abdominal muscle development
- pelvic obliquity
- scoliosis
- unilateral muscle spasm
- nerve injury

Abdominal Development

The abdominals should be well developed with good muscle tone to protect and balance the pelvis. If the athlete has a pro-

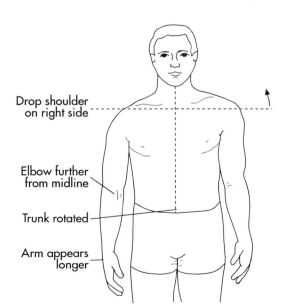

Drop shoulder on right side

Elbow further from midline

Trunk rotated

Arm appears longer

Fig. 1-14 Anterior view. Drop shoulder.

ASSESSMENT   INTERPRETATION

truding abdomen and the associated muscle weakness, the back is susceptible to excessive lordosis and its related problems.

Elbow Distance from the Trunk (Carrying Angle)

If the distance of the elbows from the trunk is different on the two sides, muscle spasm, scoliosis, or uneven unilateral development may be the cause.

Arm Length

If one arm looks longer than the other, the athlete may have a drop shoulder with associated scoliosis.

Anterior Superior Iliac Crests and Spines

The anterior iliac crests and spines should be level.

If one crest and anterior superior iliac spine is higher than the other, there could be a leg-length difference (Fig. 1-15), angulation of the femoral neck, or asymmetrical ilia.

If the anterior superior iliac spine is higher or lower than the opposite side, it can indicate iliac rotation or a leg-length difference.

Hip, Knee, and Low Back

If the hip, knee, and low back are all slightly flexed, it can be a sign of an iliosacral dysfunction with posterior iliac rotation.

Hip Anteversion or Retroversion

If the femur (sometimes even the entire leg) is rotated inward, anteversion or a posterior iliac rotation exists—anteversion causes the pelvis to tilt anteriorly. If it is bilateral, it can add to or lead to excessive lumbar lordosis. If the femur (sometimes the entire leg) is rotated outward, retroversion or an anterior iliac

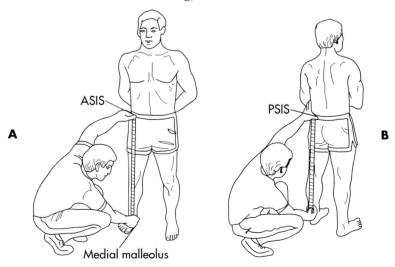

Fig. 1-15 Leg-length measurements.

ASSESSMENT	INTERPRETATION
	rotation exists. Retroversion unilaterally can cause a leg-length difference along with its lumbar problems.
Quadriceps Development	Quadriceps atrophy can result from a neurological problem at L2, L3, or L4 or at the femoral nerve. There are numerous other causes for quadriceps atrophy (such as previous knee or hip pathologic conditions).
Genu Valgum or Varum	Genu valgum is often associated with a pelvis that is rotated anteriorly. This anterior rotation leads to an increased lumbosacral angle and excessive lumbar lordosis. If one knee is in varum and the other is in valgum, a leg-length difference can result, which can lead to lumbar problems.
Tibial Torsion	Internal tibial torsion can lead to a rotation of the femur internally with a resulting anterior tilt of the pelvis and increased lumbar lordosis.
Longitudinal Arch If a leg-length difference is suspected, the leg length should be measured from ASIS to the medial malleolus (see Fig. 1-15).	If one arch is depressed or pronated and the other is supinated, a functional leg-length difference can result. Anatomical leg-length differences can be caused by previous fracture, structural differences, malalignment, and others.
Lateral View *Forward Head*	Changes occur in the muscles and soft tissue in response to the forward head position; these changes have implications down the entire spine. There is shortening of the suboccipital muscles and an increased midcervical lordosis. The thoracic spine increases its kyphosis proportionally and the lumbar spine usually then assumes a position of greater lordosis.
Excessive Thoracic Kyphosis	Excessive thoracic kyphosis can be due to ankylosing spondylitis, Scheuermann disease, osteoporosis, hereditary asymmetry in pedicle length or vertebral arch height, or adolescent epiphysitis. There is an increased incidence of spondylolysis in adolescents who have increased thoracolumbar kyphosis or Scheuermann disease.
SCHEUERMANN DISEASE (ADOLESCENT OSTEOCHONDROSIS)	Males, usually between the ages of 14 and 18, develop this as a result of anterior disc protrusion—the end plate of the vertebra is eroded, causing wedging of the thoracic vertebrae (T10 to L1 region). Usually there is only slight back pain but posture will be altered, causing thoracic kyphosis.

ASSESSMENT

INTERPRETATION

Excessive Lumbar Lordosis

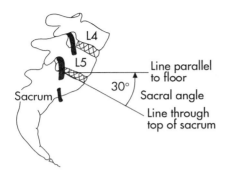

Fig. 1-16 Normal sacral angle.

Excessive lumbar lordosis is readily seen from the side with the anterior pelvic tilt. All the muscles that control the pelvis and lumbar spine must be balanced so that the angle of the top of the sacrum to a horizontal line (sacral angle) does not exceed 30° (Fig. 1-16). Although some recent research indicates that there is no correlation between the shape of the lumbar lordosis and back pain, (Hansson et al.), there is still the concern of the anterior shear forces when the curve is excessive. Grieve and Farfan do **not** believe postural excessive lumbar lordosis is a prerequisite to lumbar spine pathology. However, prolonged approximation of the posterior elements or repeated hyperextension on an excessive lordotic spine will lead to pathology (see Fig. 1-18).

The amount of lordotic curve is determined by the following:

- wedge shape of L5
- wedge shape of the L5-S1 intervertebral disc
- slope of the sacrum
- surrounding musculature
- stabilizing lumbar ligaments

The muscle groups that must be balanced for a normal curve are the abdominals, erector spinae, glutei, hamstrings, and hip flexors. A normal lumbar curve is necessary because it can absorb shock and compressive forces by giving slightly. A straight flat lumbar spine has all the forces of compression or repeated loading only through the intervertebral discs.

POSTURAL MUSCLE IMBALANCES (FIG. 1-17)

Bad postural habits or overuse of certain muscle groups can lead to the sacrum tilting forward and to the development of excessive lumbar lordosis.

The muscle imbalances are usually weak abdominals, tight hip flexors (iliopsoas, rectus femoris), tight erector spinae, weak hamstrings, and weak gluteals (see Fig. 1-17).

Postural habits like a hyperlordotic stance (accentuated if wearing high-heeled shoes) or leaning to shift weight over one leg only (in which the spine is curved excessively) are examples of poor postural habits.

Weak abdominals and tightened lumbar fascia are common causes of abnormal stress.

SPORT-RELATED MUSCLE IMBALANCES

Certain sports tend to cause imbalances through overdevelopment of one or more groups of muscles. For example, hockey causes strong, tight hip flexors, which lead to excessive lumbar lordosis. The back flop move in high jump tends to overstrengthen the erector spinae and shorten the lumbar fascia. Other sports that demand extreme positions of lumbar lordosis and cause problems include figure-skating, the butterfly stroke in swimming, gymnastics, diving, and weight lifting.

ASSESSMENT

INTERPRETATION

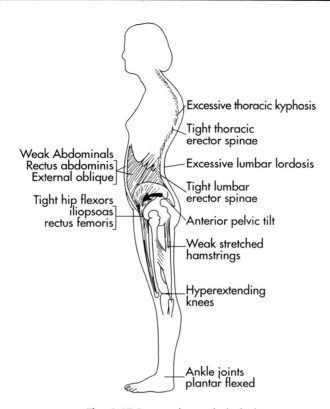

Weak Abdominals
Rectus abdominis
External oblique

Tight hip flexors
iliopsoas
rectus femoris

Excessive thoracic kyphosis

Tight thoracic
erector spinae

Excessive lumbar lordosis

Tight lumbar
erector spinae

Anterior pelvic tilt

Weak stretched
hamstrings

Hyperextending
knees

Ankle joints
plantar flexed

Fig. 1-17 Postural muscle imbalance.

Other muscle imbalances in the frontal plane caused by unilateral overuse include a tight quadratus lumborum, tensor fascia lata, and adductors or piriformis on one side, along with a weak gluteus medius on the opposite side.

Structural Causes

Excessive lordosis can also be caused by underlying structural abnormalities.

SPONDYLOLYSIS (FIG. 1-11, A)

The most common structural defect in the lumbar spine is spondylolysis. This is a defect in the pars interarticularis of the vertebrae. It can be congenital (failure of arch fusion) or the result of repeated microtrauma producing a stress fracture through the pars articularis. In adolescents, the onset of symptoms coincides closely with the adolescent growth spurt and is sometimes associated with a history of trauma (age 10 to 15 years, 14 years in girls, and 16 years in boys). Anatomic studies suggest that shear forces are greater on the pars interarticularis when the lumbar spine is extended. In adolescents, the pars interarticularis is thin, the neural arch is weak, and the intervertebral disc is less resistant to shearing forces. There is also a strong hereditary predisposition to this defect.

ASSESSMENT

INTERPRETATION

It can occur in the lumbar spine where shearing forces occur with L5 over the sacrum (occasionally with L4 over L5) during repeated hyperextension. Repeated flexion-extension motions may also cause these stress fractures by placing repeated leverage over the neural arches. This results in back pain and dysfunction problems, especially in gymnasts, offensive linemen in football, baseball pitchers, tennis players, skaters, divers, basketball players, pole vaulters, butterfly stroke swimmers, high jumpers, volleyball spikers, and weight lifters (according to Dangles).

Defects in the pars interarticularis are more common in young female gymnasts than in the general populations (according to Jackson and Wiltze). The repeated flexion-extension motions during walkovers, flips, and poses may cause this problem. These stresses may be further accentuated by the effect of side bending movements on the extended spine, which occurs with back walk-over movements.

When the lesion is at the lumbosacral level, the onset of symptoms is quicker and the lesion is more likely associated with spina bifida occulta.

SPONDYLOLISTHESIS (SEE FIG.1-11, *B*)

This is a forward slippage of the superior vertebra over the inferior one. Forward slippage can be caused by a facet deficiency, a loss of pars continuity, or attenuation of the pars interarticularis. A bilateral spondylolysis can result in spondylolisthesis if there is repeated trauma to the pars interarticularis. It occurs in the senior athlete who has disc and facet joint deterioration and frequently it occurs in young athletes between the ages of 9 and 14. It occurs more often in females; whereas spondylolysis is more likely in male athletes.

There are grades of slippage with corresponding grades of severity and complications. There is a hereditary susceptibility to this problem but repeated cyclic loading of the neural arch in certain sports is another likely cause.

The most severe degrees of forward slippage occur when there are congenital abnormalities of the sacrum or L5 arch.

SPINA BIFIDA OCCULTA

Spina bifida occulta is a birth defect but the faulty structure leads to back symptoms when the spine is subjected to repeated stress. In spina bifida occulta, there is a lack of fusion of the neural arch of one or more vertebra(e) posteriorly and there is a weakness at this level, which makes it more susceptible to problems. There can be dysplasia or absence of the spinous process of the L5 or S1 vertebra. Usually, the meninges and nervous tissue are in tact and there are no neurological abnormalities. Often there is an overlying lipoma or tuft of hair.

ASSESSMENT

INTERPRETATION

VARIATIONS IN SACRAL FUSION

The sacrum is made up of five bones that fuse during adolescence—various structural anomalies can develop if this fusion process does not proceed normally. Sacralization of the fifth lumbar vertebra (fusion of sacrum to L5) unilaterally or bilaterally can occur. If only one side fuses, a low back muscle imbalance and structural imbalance can develop. If this joint is fixed, there is more strain through the fourth lumbar joint and the sacroiliac joints. Lumbarization of the sacrum can also occur in which the top bone of the sacrum fails to fuse. It usually results in few problems but can lead to complications if lumbosacral trauma has occurred.

EXCESSIVE LUMBAR LORDOSIS PROBLEMS

Other researchers feel that this excessive lordotic position can lead to several lumbar problems (Fig. 1-18), including the following:

- lumbar strain
- disc degeneration and herniation
- lumbar sprains
- a potential for developing spondylolysis or spondylolisthesis
- facet joint degeneration
- nerve root impingement problems.

Knees
Hyperextending knees (genu recurvatum)
Flexed knees

Hyperextending knees (genu recurvatum) are often seen with an anterior pelvic tilt and the resulting excessive lumbar lordosis (Figs. 1-18 and 1-19).

A flattened lumbar curve can have a posterior pelvic tilt. The athlete often will then have tight hamstrings, which make forward bending stressful to the lower back.

Flexed knees can be caused by an acute spinal derangement such as a disc herniation or a facet joint lesion. They can also be caused by a multisegmental capsular restriction, which occurs

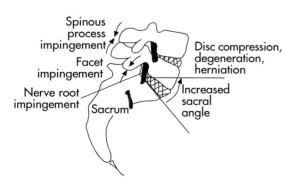

Fig. 1-18 Problems from an increased sacral angle.

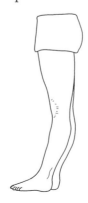

Fig. 1-19 Genu recurvatum.

ASSESSMENT   INTERPRETATION

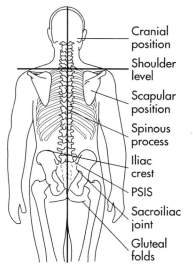

Cranial position

Shoulder level

Scapular position

Spinous process

Iliac crest

PSIS

Sacroiliac joint

Gluteal folds

Fig. 1-20 Posterior view (boney).

with significant degenerative changes (e.g., ankylosing spondylosis).

Posterior View (Fig. 1-20)
Shoulder Levels

A drop shoulder on an athlete who overuses one arm in a sport (e.g., tennis) will often be accompanied by functional scoliosis and its related back problems.

Scapular Positions (Spine and Angle)

Symmetry of the scapulae, the level of the spines, and the inferior angle help to determine bilateral muscle and boney development.

Spinous Process Alignment of Whole Spine

These processes can be felt or marked with a body marker to determine if there is any scoliosis (C or S curves of the spine) or steps.

If the spine is rotated, extra stress is placed on the facet joints, nerve roots, and intervertebral discs.

Scoliosis can be functional or structural.

Functional scoliosis can be caused by the following:
- unilateral muscle tightness, overdevelopment, or spasm
- unilateral muscle imbalances (overdevelopment of one side, e.g., in throwers)
- a leg-length difference (e.g. unilateral pronation)
- a disc protrusion or facet dysfunction impinging the nerve roots on one side

In some athletes the long leg side causes the ilium to rotate backward and to cause L5 to rotate to that side (due to attachments of iliolumbar ligament), resulting in scoliosis.

Structural scoliosis can be caused by the following:
- hereditary growth abnormality

ASSESSMENT	INTERPRETATION

- a structural leg-length difference (e.g., unilateral anteversion)
- structural pelvis obliquity
- hemivertebra in which half a vertebra develops—this usually has spontaneous correction above and below the angulation.

When the athlete has scoliosis, the facet joints are asymmetrically loaded. They will then resist shear forces unequally, and sustained or repeated loading can lead to joint rotation toward the side with the most oblique facet. This rotational tendency may overload the involved facet joint, leading to sprain or degeneration, and place additional stress on the annulus fibrosis of the intervertebral disc.

A prominent spinous process at L5 can indicate spondylolisthesis. A step deformity at L4-L5 or L5-S1 can also indicate spondylolisthesis.

Paraspinal Muscle Development

Look for paraspinal hypertrophy or atrophy.

Unilateral hypertrophy can indicate problems with the sacroiliac joint on that side. Bilateral hypertrophy will cause a furrow appearance between the muscles that can indicate the following:
- paraspinal muscle spasm
- underlying spondylolisthesis
- overdevelopment of the spinal extensors in an athlete—this can lead to a muscle imbalance and add to excessive lumbar lordosis

Waist Angles

The waist angle should be level bilaterally. If it is not, a leg-length discrepancy, a lateral pelvic tilt, or an iliac rotation may exist.

Iliac Crest

The crests should be level—one crest being higher can be caused by a leg-length difference, by a lateral pelvic tilt or an iliac rotation.

Posterior Superior Iliac Spines (PSIS) (Fig. 1-21)

The PSISs should be level.

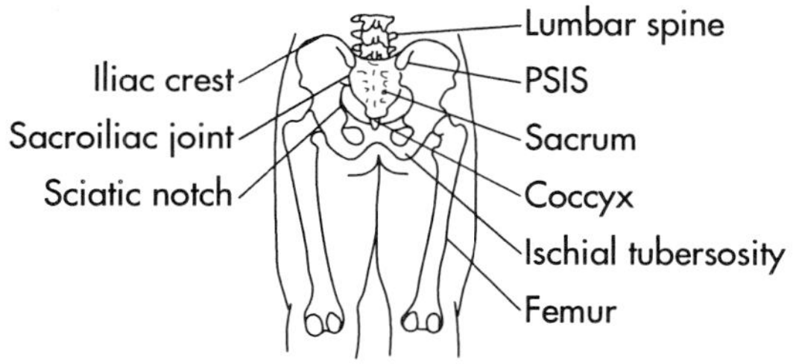

Fig. 1-21 Posterior view (pelvis).

ASSESSMENT

INTERPRETATION

LEG LENGTH DIFFERENCE

If one posterior superior iliac spine, the iliac crest, and the anterior superior iliac spine are lower on the same side there may be an anatomical leg-length difference or a rare downslip of the ilium. A quadratus lumborum muscle spasm on the opposite side can also cause this asymmetry.

If one posterior superior iliac spine is higher and the anterior superior iliac spine on that side is lower, there is a functional leg-length difference or anterior iliac rotation.

Leg-length differences are often associated with sacroiliac, facet joint, and disc pathologic conditions. The pelvis and sacral base tilt toward the short leg side while the lumbar spine rotates in the same direction but side bends in the opposite direction (Fryette's First Law); therefore the L5-S1 facet joint on the short leg side is distracted while the opposite facet is in compression. The malalignment of the sacroiliac joint and facet joints leads to dysfunction that can worsen with time and overuse. Scoliosis can also result due to the rotation and side bending.

Sports that involve repeated running or jumping can cause the spine to twist on weight bearing because of the different leg lengths. The forces on heel strike are off center on the short leg side and the force is not transmitted uniformly through the leg, ilium, sacroiliac joint, and lumbar vertebrae.

ILIUM ROTATION

The athlete with acute sacroiliac dysfunction with posterior iliac rotation (backward rotation of the ilium on the sacrum) may tend to stand with the hip and knee in compensatory extension on the injured side. The posterior superior iliac spine and iliac crest will be lower on the involved side but the anterior superior iliac spine on the involved side will be higher.

The athlete with an anterior iliac rotation (forward rotation of the ilium on the sacrum) will stand with the painful side in compensatory flexion. The PSIS and iliac crest will be higher on the involved side but the ASIS will be lower.

These rotational problems can lead to dysfunction in the spine, pelvic girdle, and the entire lower quadrant.

Boney abnormalities

If the iliac crest is low on one side but the posterior spines or greater trochanter are level, the following may exist:
- a boney abnormality of the pelvis
- a positional fault of the sacroiliac joint
- an anomaly of the femoral neck
- a slipped capital femoral epiphysis

Gluteal Folds (Fig. 1-22)

Gluteal folds should be level and the gluteal muscle tone should be equal. Sagging of one buttock can be caused by an L5

ASSESSMENT   INTERPRETATION

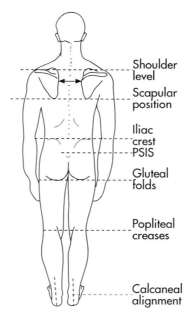

Shoulder level

Scapular position

Iliac crest

PSIS

Gluteal folds

Popliteal creases

Calcaneal alignment

Fig. 1-22 Posterior view (soft tissue).

or S1 nerve root impingement or lesion. Hip joint conditions can also lead to gluteal atrophy. A lower gluteal mass can indicate a leg length difference. The gluteal cleft is tilted to the short leg side.

Hamstring Development

Atrophy of the hamstrings and gastrocnemii on one side can be a sign of chronic S1 or S2 radiculopathy.

Atrophy of the buttock and hamstring can also develop from a hip arthritis. Other knee and hip conditions can lead to atrophy.

Popliteal Creases

These creases should be level—uneven creases can be caused by a functional or structural lower leg difference.

Gastrocnemii Development

Atrophy of either gastrocnemius can also be a sign of an S1 or S2 nerve root irritation or lesion. Ankle, gastrocnemii, and achilles tendon injuries can also lead to atrophy.

Calcaneal Alignment

A unilateral calcaneal valgus will cause a slight functional leg-length difference because of the loss of the longitudinal arch (pronation). If one calcaneus is in valgus and the other is in varus the leg-length difference may be significant.

ASSESSMENT

INTERPRETATION

Excessive pronation can lead to excessive internal rotation up the limb with resulting anterior pelvic tilt and increased lumbar lordosis.

Skin Markings

Skin markings on the back often indicate underlying pathologic conditions. Lipoma (fatty lumps), faun's bears (tufts of hair), or birth marks may be a sign of underlying spina bifida. Skin tags and café-au-lait spots can indicate that a tumor or collagen disease exists.

A hair patch can also indicate an underlying boney defect—congenital boney bar separating the lateral halves of the spinal cord.

The skin, paraspinally, may have an "orange skin" (dimpled) appearance that has a tougher, thickened texture. This usually indicates pathology at that segmental level.

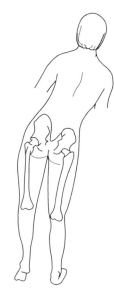

Fig. 1-23 Trendelenburg gait. The gluteus medius weakness causes the body to lean toward the weak side.

Gait

Observe the athlete's gait throughout the entire assessment. If the athlete is a runner, running mechanics should also be observed. The gait involves complex neuromuscular coordination of the lumbar spine, hips, and pelvis in all three planes. Any dysfunction in the lower quadrant will become observable during gait.

The athlete who has a weak push-off on one side may have gastrocnemius weakness from an S1 nerve root problem. The athlete with a Trendelenburg gait may have a gluteus medius weakness from an L5 nerve root problem (Fig. 1-23). The athlete with an acute disc or facet problem will have a shortened stance on the involved side and the knee may stay in slight flexion with loss of full extension of the hip and back on push off. Lumbar erector spinae spasm may shorten the stride length because the lumbar spine may stay in a kyphosis (flat back) position. Gait is slightly altered by lumbar spine problems, but if there is hip or pelvis dysfunction, walking is altered significantly and usually contributes to the pain. During gait, the ilium appears to move posteriorly during the swing phase and this converts to an anterior rotation during the stance phase. (For more detail see section on Gait-Pelvic movements in the Hip and Pelvis Assessment chapter.)

Sitting, Standing, and Lying Postures

During the history taking, observations, and functional testing, mentally note or record what movements cause the athlete pain and what postures relieve the pain.

Sitting is uncomfortable for most people with low back problems, especially if an intervertebral disc lesion exists. Sitting discomfort is worsened if there is no lumbar support given to the lumbar spine. Pain with an acute facet joint derangement is aggravated by being up and about and is relieved by sitting or reclining.

ASSESSMENT   INTERPRETATION

An athlete with an acute disc herniation with nerve root irritation will not be able to long sit (legs stretched out) without a great deal of discomfort because of the stretch on the dural sheath. Prolonged standing will aggravate most backs.

The most extreme movement of the sacroiliac joints occurs when a person rises from the sitting position—this will cause pain if a sacroiliac pathologic condition exists.

Lumbar spasm and pain can make it difficult to move from the supine to the prone position and back again.

SUMMARY OF TESTS

FUNCTIONAL TEST

Rule Out
    Hip Joint
    Thoracic Spine
    Systemic Disorders
Tests in Standing
    Active forward bending
    Active return from forward bending
    Active backward bending
    Repeated active forward bending and back bending
    Active side bending
    Active side bending and back bending
Tests in Sitting
    Active trunk rotation
    Active forward bending in sitting
Tests in Prone Lying
    Resisted hip extension with knee flexion
    Active spinal extension
    Resisted hip extension with knee flexion
    Active double leg raise
Tests in Side Lying
    Active side bending or lateral flexion
    Resisted hip abduction
    Passive lumbar flexion and extension

SPECIAL TESTS

Neurological Tests
    Passive straight leg raise
    Bowstring sign
    Femoral nerve stretch (passive)
    Neuromeningeal mobility test
Myotome testing
    Heel and toe walking
    Resisted plantar flexion

ASSESSMENT   INTERPRETATION

    Resisted knee extension
    Resisted hip flexion
    Resisted foot dorsiflexion and inversion
    Resisted hallux extension
    Resisted foot eversion
    Resisted knee flexion
    Resisted hallux flexion
    Resisted foot intrinsics
    Urogenital region tests
Dermatome Testing
Cutaneous Nerve Supply Testing
Reflexes
    Knee reflexes
    Ankle reflexes
    Babinski reflex
    Ankle clonus
Lower Limb Girth Measurements
Intrathecal Pressure Tests
    Valsalva Maneuver
    Cough test
Muscle Imbalance Tests
    Long sitting toe touching
    Abdominal strength
Sacroiliac Joint Tests
    Kinetic test
    Pelvic rocking test
    Gapping test
    Hip flexion and adduction test
    Gaenslen's sign
    Sacroiliac joint test
    Patrick's or Faber test
    Sit up test for iliosacral dysfunction
    Ankylosing spondylitis test
    Leg length measurement tests
    Circulatory tests

Rule Out

Hip Joint

Perform these tests if the history-taking, observations, and functional tests suggest the possibility of a hip joint dysfunction.

Hip Joint Test (Hip Flexion and Medial Rotation With Overpressure)

In supine lying, the athlete actively flexes the hip and the therapist applies an overpressure until pelvic motion

During the hip "clearing" test, joint range of motion and end feel should be noted. If there is asymmetry, abnormal mobility, or pain on either side, hip dysfunction exists. With hip joint

ASSESSMENT

INTERPRETATION

begins. Your stabilizing hand is on the pelvis to prevent pelvic movements, yet feel when the pelvic motion wants to begin.

The athlete then internally rotates the hip, and the therapist applies an overpressure until pelvic rotation begins. Look for asymmetry bilaterally and whether or not there is abnormal motion or pain. If the hip "clearing" test is positive you must carry out a full hip joint assessment.

Laguerre Test

Position the athlete as in the Faber test. With the athlete's hip externally rotated and abducted and the knee flexed, gently externally rotate the hip until an end feel is reached.

Thoracic Spine

Rule out thoracic spine dysfunction throughout history-taking and observations. In observations look for excessive thoracic kyphosis, gibbus deformity (sharp localized posterior angulation of the thoracic curve) or dowager's hump (osteoporosis causing excessive kyphosis). Look for scoliosis (C- or S-shaped curve in the thoracic and/or lumbar spine).

If an upper thoracic dysfunction is suspected, have the athlete forward bend, back bend, side bend, and rotate the lower cervical spine while you observe the thoracic function and determine if local pain or dysfunction is present.

If a midthoracic spine dysfunction is suspected, test the athlete with the following motions. With the athlete seated in a low back chair and the lumbar spine supported, have the athlete clasp hands with fingers interlaced behind the head. The fingers should run from the occiput to the cervical thoracic junction in a position to prevent motion of the cervical spine. The flexed elbows are together in front of the athlete's

problems, excessive force will be transmitted through the pelvis and lumbar spine during numerous weight-bearing activities. Every time the hip joint is moved to full rotation or flexion during weight bearing in sport, the forces will be transmitted into the pelvis and spine, with less shock dissipation occurring through the hip joint.

Any hip joint pain or asymmetry confirms a hip joint condition.

Restrictions of the thoracic spine can cause problems or compensatory motions in the lumbar spine.

Scoliosis can cause rotatory curves throughout the spinal vertebrae that will limit some motions and make the spine and its components more susceptible to injury.

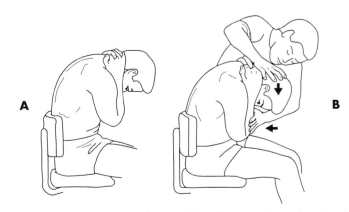

Fig. 1-24 A, Thoracic spine forward bending. **B,** Thoracic spine forward bending overpressure.

ASSESSMENT   INTERPRETATION

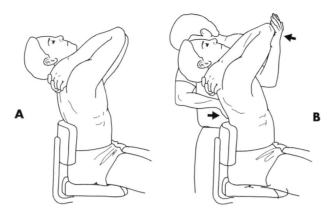

Fig. 1-25, A, Thoracic spine back bending. **B**, Thoracic spine back bending overpressure.

Fig. 1-26 A, Thoracic spine side bending. **B**, Thoracic spine side bending overpressure.

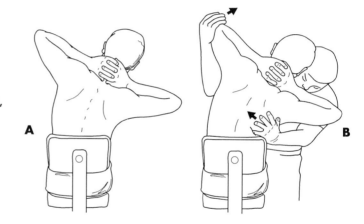

chest (Fig. 1-24, *A*). Have the athlete forward bend, moving the elbows toward the groin. There should be no lumbar flexion. The athlete then back bends as far as possible over the back of the chair without extending the lumbar spine (Fig. 1-25, *A*). For thoracic side bending the athlete moves the flexed elbows out laterally in the frontal plane and side bends as far as possible without lifting the pelvis or side bending the lumbar spine (Fig. 1-26, *A*). For thoracic rotation, (Fig. 1-27) the athlete's arms are crossed in front of the body with the elbows flexed. The athlete flexes partially then rotates as far as possible. If the

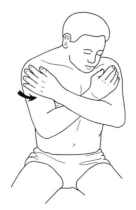

Fig. 1-27 Thoracic spine rotation.

ASSESSMENT   ## INTERPRETATION

range is restricted in any of these motions, without pain, overpressures can be done (see Figs. 1-24, *B*, 1-25, *B*, and 1-26, *B*).

Systemic Disorders

Is there a systemic problem?

Test the joints involved, but if a systemic condition is suspected, send the athlete for a complete medical checkup with his or her family physician. This checkup should include blood work, x-rays, and urine testing.

Systemic conditions that affect the lumbar spine must be ruled out with a thorough medical history and observations. Systemic conditions can exist with any of the following responses or findings:
- painful back at night with joint stiffness in the morning
- poor general health, especially during periods when the injury flares up
- problem continually getting worse without an apparent cause
- problem having an insidious onset
- painful limb joints with lumbar discomfort
- problem not responding to rest or activity

The systemic disorders next discussed can affect the lumbar spine.

Ankylosing Spondylitis

This is an inflammatory autoimmune disorder of the connective tissue of the body that begins with pain around the sacroiliac joints. It is a form of polyarthritis that progresses with involvement of the sacroiliac joints and then into the spinal joints with eventual ossification. Proximal joints like the hip and shoulder may be affected but the distal joints are rarely involved. It eventually affects several different areas, including the cardiovascular and pulmonary systems. The range of lumbar extension decreases, as well as the amount of chest expansion (due to costovertebral joint involvement) during inhalation. Chest expansion measurements from full exhalation to inhalation drop to less than 2.5 cm. The vertebral ligaments and capsule ossify, and sclerosis of the iliac and sacral bones develops later. This occurs most commonly in healthy and often athletic males from 18 to 20 years and is a progressive condition with restricted spinal mobility by the third to fifth decade of the athlete's life. Other joints can be affected occasionally (shoulders, hips). The main initial symptom is low back and sacroiliac pain with severe morning stiffness. The stiffness is relieved by exercise and aggravated by rest. Side flexion bilaterally is often markedly restricted. The stiffness progresses up to the thoracic spine and chest. The sacroiliac joint changes usually appear radiographically first.

Leukemia

The initial phases of leukemia can cause back pain.

ASSESSMENT

INTERPRETATION

Rheumatoid Arthritis

Although rheumatoid arthritis initially appears in the hands and wrists, it can cause back pain.. However, this condition is usually seen in other joints first.

Neoplastic Disorders

Neoplasms, primary or secondary, are uncommon in the lumbar area. When rare tumors of the spine are involved, the lesions occur in the spinous processes, transverse processes, neural arches, or articular facets. Secondary malignant tumors of the spine can occur from kidney and prostate primary sites in men and breast, ovary, lung, or thyroid in women.

Cancer of the prostate is the second most common site of cancer in men. Sciatic pain can be caused by metastasis of the cancer to the lumbar spine or pelvis. The pain from this disorder is unrelenting and does not alter with postural changes. There are usually other signs that include night pain, weakness, weight loss, and fatigue. Always inquire regarding previous illnesses or cancer.

Infectious Disorders

Osteomyelitis of the vertebrae is rare.

Bacterial or tuberculosis infections have pain that is constant whether at rest or with activity. The pain increases quickly and usually there is a fever and changes in the blood sedimentation rate.

Osteoporosis

This is a metabolic bone disorder that commonly affects the spine, especially in postmenopausal women (five times more common in women than men). It is most visible in the thoracic spine where marked kyphosis develops. There is a reduction of the mineral content of bone with a resulting decrease in bone mass. There is persistent aching pain in the low thoracic area and there can be low back pain also.

Paget Disease

This metabolic bone disorder, sometimes called osteitis deformans, can affect any of the vertebrae but the most common site is the lumbosacral joint. Unexplained acceleration of deposition and reabsorption of the bone occurs. The sacrum is the most commonly affected bone. The athlete is usually over 55 years old and there are no distinctive clinical features except aching pain in the lesion site. Referred pain down the leg can occur if the sacrum is involved. The pain does not ease with rest.

Gout

Sacroiliac joint and spinal gout can occur with pain, intense muscle guarding, and gross limitations of movements. It usually

ASSESSMENT

INTERPRETATION

occurs (90%) in the metatarsophalangeal joint of the great toe. It is an inherited metabolic disorder in which uric acid is not dissolved and excreted but is converted into crystals that deposit in joints and other tissues.

Tests in Standing

Active Forward Bending (40° to 60°) (Fig. 1-28)

The athlete tucks his or her chin on the chest and forward bends as far as possible.

The movement should be done slowly, attempting to progressively flex through the cervical, thoracic, and lumbar vertebrae.

Observe and feel the movement at each vertebral segment and between the spinous processes.

There should be a degree of separation between the processes without any flat sections (from muscle spasm or hypomobility).

You can palpate the transverse process of the L5 vertebra bilaterally as the athlete forward bends. The symmetry of motion is noted. There should **not** be any rotation or side bending with the forward bending.

An overpressure into forward bend-

This movement is initiated by a contraction of the psoas and abdominal muscles; then gravity and an eccentric contraction of the sacrospinalis muscles take over (according to Kapandji). Multifidus is believed to assist this movement with an eccentric contraction (according to Twomey and Taylor).

During forward bending, the vertebrae rotate anteriorly (anterior sagittal rotation) and translate forward (anterior sagittal translation) (Bogduk and Twomey). As the lumbar spine leans forward further, the inferior articular facet of the upper vertebra can not move and therefore the upper surfaces of the vertebral bodies lean downward. This increases the anterior shear that the facet joint is designed to prevent. The anterior rotation is limited by the facet joint capsule, as well as the supraspinous ligament, infraspinous ligament, and ligamentum flava (Fig. 1-29).

According to Yamamato et al., flexion motion in the lumbar spine occurs from L1 to L5, and L5 to S1 has the greatest range of motion. The L4-L5 and L5-S1 segments combine for 45° of motion.

The capsular ligaments of the facet joints have a very important role in preventing anterior shear forces caused by the body weight. They provide 39% of the joint's resistance according to Adams, Hutton, and Stott. The ligamentum flavum, interspinous, and supraspinous are all stretched. The intervertebral disc resists forward bending by 29%, the supraspinous and infraspinous resist by 19%, and the ligamentum flavum resists by 13%.

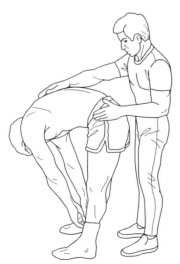

Fig. 1-28 Active lumbar spine forward bending.

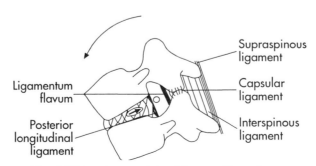

Fig. 1-29 Lumbar vertebral forward bending.

ASSESSMENT

ing can be applied at the end of range if the movement was painfree yet limited.

On occasion, it is important to hold the full range of forward bending for a period of time. This may become a necessary part of your lumbar assessment when the history indicates that symptoms are produced only after activities involving prolonged forward bending have occurred, e.g., field hockey, ice hockey, rowing.

During all active, passive, and resisted tests, the athlete should be asked if there is any pain or change in sensations during the test. During the passive tests you should ask the athlete if and where the stretch or pain is felt.

In a middle-aged or elderly athlete who has multisegmental bilateral lumbar facet joint restrictions or degenerative joint disease, several tests will be restricted and/or painful. There will be aching in the low back and sometimes in the hips. These athletes are stiff in the morning and pain is increased with prolonged walking or standing. The restrictions will follow a general capsular pattern with marked limitations in back bending and side bending bilaterally and mild limitations in rotations and forward bending.

INTERPRETATION

Twomey and Taylor believe the joint capsule and ligaments limit lumbar flexion, but they believe the greatest restraining influence is the pressure between the apposed articular facet joints.

If the annulus fibrosis is weakened posteriorly, the nucleus pulposus may move posteriorly, stretching its posterior fibers.

The hip joint is important to the athlete's ability to complete forward bending. Athletes with a serious or acute problem of the lumbar spine will flex mainly at the hips while the lumbar spine is held in lordosis by spasm of the sacrospinalis muscles.

There should be a good lumbopelvic rhythm, with spinal flexion and pelvic rotation following a smooth pattern forward. During the initial forward bending the pelvis is locked by the hip extensors; the lumbar vertebrae move as described until the lumbar lordotic curve is flattened. The sacrum is believed to follow the lumbar movement. After the lumbar movement, the pelvis rotates anteriorly over the hip joints. The lumbosacral joint offers the most sagittal plane movement when compared with the ranges of the other lumbar joints (according to White and Panjabi). This is difficult to see but the fact that most movement occurs at the lower lumbar region is important to remember. With age the amount of this movement decreases.

A painful arc (pain through part of the range) may be a sign of a herniated disc fragment, which catches during this forward bending or when the nerve root catches on the protruded disc.

If structural scoliosis is present, the thoracic area will twist during forward bending and one side of the thoracic cage will appear higher than the opposite side (Adam's Test) when viewed from behind the athlete.

Not only is the range of motion during forward bending important but how each lumbar vertebra moves on one another is also important. Lumbar segments that do not seem to move (hypomobile) or move excessively (hypermobile) should be recorded.

If, while palpating the L5 vertebra transverse process during forward bending, there is asymmetrical motion with side bending or rotation, a lower quadrant dysfunction is present. Further functional testing can be done to determine the cause.

Prominent spinous process steps and gaps between spinous processes should be looked for when performing this test.

With full forward bending the normal lumbar lordosis should be straightened but not reversed. Incomplete straightening may be caused by the following:
- muscle spasm or tightness of the low back
- local or generalized facet capsular restriction
- degenerative disease causing sacrospinalis muscle spasm
- rigidity of the entire spine present with advancing ankylosing spondylitis

ASSESSMENT

INTERPRETATION

Pain at the limit of range of motion may be caused by the following:

- dura mater stretch (i.e., when there is a disc herniation or protrusion)
- sciatic nerve root irritation or nerve compression
- lumbodorsal muscle strain or thoracolumbar fascia strain (erector spinae, transversospinalis, intertransversarii, sacrospinalis, latissimus dorsi)
- a hip problem
- apposition of the caudal edges of the vertebral bodies anteriorly due to osteophyte formation

Central backache at the end of range of motion may indicate a joint problem or a sprain of the following ligament(s):

- posterior capsular ligaments of the facet joint
- supraspinous ligament
- ligamentum flavum
- interspinous ligament (rare)
- posterior longitudinal ligament (rare)
- superior band of the iliolumbar ligament

Unilateral pain during forward bending may cause the athlete to deviate toward or away from the painful side. Side deviation toward the painful side may indicate a medial intervertebral disc protrusion into the nerve root, and side deviation away from the painful side may indicate a lateral protrusion. These deviations toward and away from the painful side are controversial.

Deviations to the involved side on forward bending and away from the involved side on back bending may be caused by a facet joint asymmetry or unilateral facet joint capsule tightness.

Deviations to one side can also occur if there is unilateral hip joint pathology or a gluteal muscle injury.

Pain felt down one limb posteriorly during forward bending usually indicates a disc herniation with nerve root irritation.

The gentle overpressure at the end of the active forward bending determines the end feel or if it changes the symptoms. A bone-to-bone end feel can suggest an osseous restriction. A muscle spasm may limit the range of motion. A capsular or springy end feel can indicate underlying joint dysfunction. A dural restriction may cause shooting or burning pain with the overpressure.

The range of forward bending can depend on the flexibility of the hamstrings because of their origin on the ischial tuberosity. Some athletes with tight hamstrings will not have full range of motion in forward bending. To gain more range forward, the lumbar and thoracic spine are subjected to extra stress—this is important to note in the athlete who does a lot of bending in his or her sport or occupation. If hamstring tightness is limiting the range of motion, the athlete can flex his or her legs slightly, then

ASSESSMENT

INTERPRETATION

forward bend. Sharp, local pain with digital pressure on the spinous process can indicate dysfunction at that spinal segment.

A deep, aching or throbbing pain with pressure can indicate a disease state at that spinal level.

Active Forward Bending Test (Mitchell, Moran, and Pruzzo) (Fig. 1-30)

The athlete repeats the movement while you palpate just inferior to the posterior superior iliac spines bilaterally with your thumbs during the forward bending. The pelvis must be level for this test. If there is a leg-length discrepancy the shorter leg should be elevated with a lift under the foot until the iliac crests are level before doing the test. With the athlete in the full forward bent position, determine if the boney depressions inferior to the PSIS where your thumbs are resting are level. Determine if one depression rides up higher during the final range of forward bending. You may close your eyes during the movement to enhance the palpatory findings. This test may have to be repeated several times.

When forward bending is done with thumb palpation inferior to the posterior superior iliac spine, you are determining if the iliosacral movement is symmetrical or if one side rides higher at the end of range of motion. This tests ilium movement around a relatively fixed sacrum, therefore the term *iliosacral movement* is used. If the right side is blocked or hypomobile the right *posterior superior iliac spine* migrates further upward and forward than the left posterior superior iliac spine. The right ilium in this example is locked on the sacrum and rides upward at the end of forward bending.

The lesions that can cause this locking can be the following:
- right anterior iliac rotation
- left posterior iliac rotation
- pubic or iliac subluxation (superior or inferior)

During normal forward bending, the sacrum should move forward smoothly on the ilium with the lumbar vertebrae because of the ligamentous attachment of the sacrum and L5.

There is controversy concerning this test because many therapists often get false positives.

With iliosacral dysfunction or a lack of mobility, problems arise when the athlete bends forward repeatedly or during the end of the swing phase of walking or running.

Active Return from Forward Bending (Fig. 1-31)

The athlete should keep his or her chin on the chest and slowly return to the upright position. You monitor

The lumbopelvic rhythm should be smooth during lumbar reversal and pelvic rotation. The lumbar vertebrae should evenly return to the upright while the pelvis rotates around the hip

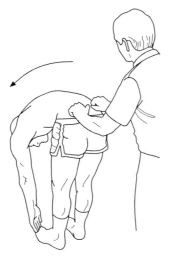

Fig. 1-30 Standing forward bending test.

ASSESSMENT   INTERPRETATION

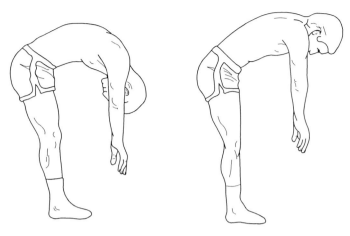

Fig. 1-31 Active return from forward bending.

smoothness and ease of the movement while observing the lumbopelvic rhythm.

joints. The hip joints must be painfree for a smooth pelvic rotation to take place. According to Cailliet, if the athlete attempts to stand upright by flexing the knees and tucking the pelvis under the spine, it is often because of disc degeneration, lumbar spine instability, severe muscle spasm, or a posterior facet problem. The lumbar region is forced to remain lordotic as the athlete stands up. The pelvic swing may be done to avoid putting pressure on the sensitive posterior facet joints. If severe enough, the athlete may have to use the hands on the knees to push the body upright.

If the body deviates to the right or left in the same pattern as in forward bending, often the body is moving around the spasm caused by disc herniation or disc fragment in the joint.

Interruption of a smooth pelvic rotation can also imply the following:
- tight or spasm of hamstrings
- irritated sciatic nerve (disc herniation, piriformis syndrome)
- hip joint pathologic conditions
- sacroiliac dysfunction
- gluteal strain or spasm

A painful arc (pain during part of the range and then the pain is eased as the movement continues) may be present in the return from forward bending that was not present in forward bending. This can indicate a problem with the posterior elements of the lumbar spine or lumbar joint instability.

Active Backward Bending (Extension 20° to 35°) (Fig. 1-32)

The athlete bends the head, neck, shoulders, and spine backward while you place a hand on the crest of the

The movement is initiated by contraction of the long back extensor muscles, then controlled eccentrically by the abdominal group, according to Twomey and Taylor.

ASSESSMENT

INTERPRETATION

pelvis to stabilize it. During this, the pelvis should not tilt nor should the hips extend. Areas of the spine that appear to bend easier (hypermobility) and areas that seem restricted (hypomobility) should be recorded. Overpressure or sustained overpressures may be necessary if active back bending is pain free yet symptoms occur with forced extension or after prolonged extension positions.

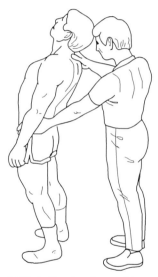

Fig. 1-32 Active backward bending.

During back bending the vertebral bodies undergo posterior sagittal rotation and slight posterior translation (Bogduk and Twomey). The inferior articular processes move downward and impact against the lamina of the vertebra below so that there is a bone-on-bone end feel. According to Yamamoto et al., in lumbar extension there is a similar range of motion at L1-L2, L2-L3, and L3-L4, and more motion at L4-L5 and L5-S1.

The intervertebral disc is acted on by compressive forces posteriorly and tensile forces anteriorly. If the annulus fibrosis is weakened anteriorly, the nucleus pulposus may be pushed anteriorly, which stretches the anterior fibers of the annulus and the anterior longitudinal ligament.

Minor pain at the end of range of motion may indicate the following:
- a posterior facet joint problem
- a sacroiliac joint problem

More forces act on the facet joints during back bending if the intervertebral disc height is decreased by injury.

With multisegmental capsular restrictions the range will be limited due to premature close packing of the facet joints, as occurs in ankylosing spondylitis or following osteophyte formation. This may be accompanied by a painful or painless end feel, depending on the presence of any inflammation.

If back bending causes pain in the buttock or lower limb, it could be because of the following:
- articular derangement in a lumbar facet joint
- intervertebral disc herniation
- articular derangement of the hip joint
- sacroiliac joint sprain

Back bending that causes pain in the front of the thigh can occur because of a third lumbar disc lesion, iliopsoas strain, or osteoarthritis of the hip.

If hip pain limits back bending, repeat the lumbar back bending with one of the athlete's legs resting on a stool or repeat it while the athlete is sitting.

The thoracolumbar fascia may play a part during lumbosacral back bending.

Repeated Active Forward Bending and Back Bending (McKenzie)

The active forward bending and active back bending test can be repeated about 10 times according to McKenzie's work (MacQueen—see workshop reference).

If the repeated test is used, you must record if the lumbar pain centralizes into the back area or radiates or refers distally.

Does the pain increase or decrease?

Lumbar pain caused by postural problems usually does not increase during these repeated movements.

Lumbar pain caused by mechanical dysfunction in the lumbar spine usually does not increase during the repeated movements but may increase slightly during the movement at the end of range. With mechanical dysfunction, there is no peripheralization (referred pain into the buttock or leg) of the pain. (Peripheralization of pain in McKenzie's work indicates that the injury is aggravated, whereas centralization of pain indicates the condition is relieved.)

ASSESSMENT

Is the pain felt during the movement or only at the end of range?

These repeated movements should **not** be done in the lumbar patient with acute pain or spasm.

These repeat tests are done to help the therapist design a rehabilitation program that will relieve pain.

Active Side Bending (Lateral Flexion, 15° to 20°) (Fig. 1-33)

The athlete is asked to side bend the head, shoulders, and spine to one side while sliding the arm down the lateral aspect of the leg. Measure the amount of bending by comparing the distance from the fingertip to the fibular head. If there is no limitation of range of motion or pain, apply a gentle overpressure to see if pain or other symptoms are reproduced.

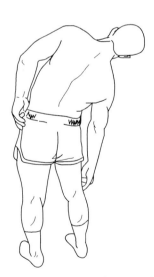

Fig. 1-33 Posterior view of active side bending.

INTERPRETATION

Lumbar pain caused by derangement of the intervertebral disc will usually have increased pain with the repeated movements and the pain will often radiate or peripheralize into the buttock or leg. With a posterior herniation the pain usually increases and peripheralizes with forward bending and decreases and centralizes with back bending—although the reverse may be true and forward bending may relieve pain while back bending aggravates (peripheralizes) it. Lumbar pain from nerve root adhesions usually causes no change in back bending but causes an increase of distal pain with repeated forward bending, especially at the end of range.

Quick catches during the repeated movements or when changing direction can occur with segmental instability.

Pure side bending does not occur; there are complex coupling movements of rotation and side bending that are beyond the scope of this manual. According to Kapandji, the body of the upper vertebra tilts and the nucleus of the disc is displaced to the opposite side during side bending. Twomey and Taylor describe a cephalad movement of the inferior facet joint of the superior vertebra on the superior facet joint of the vertebra below during active side bending.

Yamamato et al. found equal ranges in lateral bending bilaterally with the greatest motion at L2-L3 and the least motion at L1-L2.

Range of motion is limited by the following:
- lumbosacral fascia
- capsular facet ligaments
- iliolumbar and iliofemoral ligament
- intertransverse ligament
- latissimus dorsi, quadratus lumborum, deep spinal muscles, lateral fibers of the external and internal oblique muscles

Serious diseases of the lumbar spine can result in limitation of side bending on both sides (e.g., tuberculosis, ankylosing spondylosis, neoplasm, osteomyelitis).

With increasing age the amount of side bending decreases, and there will be painless limitation from osteophyte formation in the elderly.

Pain on the side toward which the athlete bends indicates that compression of the lesion is causing pain. This is true of a chronic lumbar disc lesion, a facet joint impingement, or a sacroiliac injury. Usually with an acute disc lesion there will be lateral deviation away from the involved side when the athlete stands.

Pain on the opposite side away from the direction that the athlete bends can indicate a lumbar joint (interspinous ligament, joint capsule) or muscle injury (quadratus lumborum,

ASSESSMENT   INTERPRETATION

sacrospinalis, intertransverse muscles). An iliac crest contusion will be acutely painful when the muscle fibers pull on the crest during side bending. A localized capsular restriction will limit side bending slightly toward the involved side, but a multisegmental capsular restriction can cause restrictions on both sides.

A painful arc during side bending usually suggests a disc lesion that catches the dura mater—this is usually at the fourth lumbar level. An athlete with a herniated disc causing a nerve root irritation may have radiating pain with side bending toward or away from the herniation. The herniation can be medial or lateral to the nerve root and this determines which direction of side bending causes the pain.

Pain from overpressure is most likely from a capsular restriction, especially in chronic disorders such as ankylosing spondylosis.

The greater the lumbar lordosis the greater the coupled shearing forces through the disc and facet joints during side bending.

Active Side Bending and Back Bending

The athlete side bends and back bends to each side. Any pain or changes in sensation are noted. You can overpressure the back bending and side bending position if there is no pain on the active test. Guide the athlete into the back bending and then side bending position to the right with your hands on the athlete's shoulders. Pressure is exerted down the left shoulder through the thoracic spine and lumbar spine and into the right leg.

This test increases the shearing forces through the facet, disc, and sacroiliac joint.

If the athlete indicates pain in the region of the sacroiliac joint during the movement, sacroiliac joint pathologic conditions are probable.

If the athlete indicates pain in the region of the facet joint at the end-of-range, facet pathologic conditions should be suspected. With acute facet joint derangement, the lumbar back bending and side bending combination on the involved side compresses the joint and causes pain. If the facet joint is involved, forward bending and contralateral side bending will be slightly restricted and dural signs will be negative.

This test also stresses the iliolumbar ligament that can cause pain and dysfunction in the lumbar spine.

Tests in Sitting

Observe posture, noting any changes or any signs of discomfort in this position. Sitting is painful for most people who have back problems, especially if the lumbar curve is not supported.

If scoliosis is observed when the athlete is standing and disappears when the athlete is sitting, the asymmetry is caused by the lower limbs and is therefore functional. However, if the scoliosis remains when the athlete is in the seated position, it is likely to be structural.

Active Trunk Rotation (3° to 18°) (Fig. 1-34)

The athlete sits with arms crossed in front of the chest and with his or her hands placed on the opposite shoulder.

The athlete rotates the upper body while you stabilize the pelvis.

The lumbar spine is not built for rotation because of the position of the articular facets of the vertebrae. Therefore the primary limiter to rotation are the facet joints (Ahmed et al.) and secondarily the intervertebral disc. Most trunk rotation occurs at the cervical and thoracic levels.

ASSESSMENT   INTERPRETATION

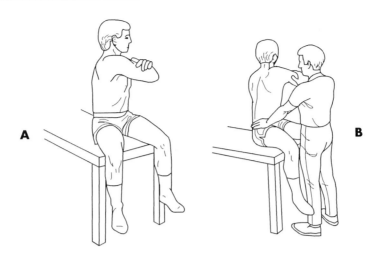

Fig. 1-34 A, Active trunk rotation. **B**, Trunk rotation with overpressure.

The athlete rotates to the right and then to the left—a gentle overpressure can be applied if the range of motion is full and pain free.

According to Kapandji, when trunk rotation occurs the vertebrae tilt forward slightly, opening the posterior facets and stretching the posterior lateral annulus of the disc.

According to Yamamoto et al., the maximal range of axial rotation is under 3° with the least amount of motion at L5-S1.

This rotation movement may be slightly limited by the following inert tissue:
- supraspinous ligament
- interspinous ligament

This movement is also somewhat limited by the following muscles:
- the opposite deep rotators
- the opposite internal oblique
- the external oblique on the same side
- the lumbofascia that is stretching on the opposite side

Limitation of range of motion and/or pain on the side that is opposite the direction of rotation suggests a muscle strain, usually of the obliques or lumbofascial tissue.

Limitation and/or pain on the same side as the rotation suggest a facet lesion or a disc protrusion.

The overpressure may help pinpoint the location of pain or restriction (Fig. 1-34, *B*). For example, an acute sacroiliac dysfunction will be painful with this rotation test and the pain will be localized in the involved sacroiliac joint region.

Active Forward Bending in Sitting

Long sitting

This test should be done if there is a restriction in forward bending in the standing position.

If forward bending in the long-sitting position causes buttock or limb pain, a disc herniation in which the disc material protrudes into the dural section of the nerve root can be suspected.

ASSESSMENT

The athlete is long sitting and forward bends, starting gradually at the head, shoulders, and then the trunk, attempting to touch his or her head to the knees.

Short Sitting (Fig. 1-35)

If a sacroiliac lesion is suspected, this forward bending test is repeated in short sitting with feet elevated on a stool (Mitchell, Moran, and Pruzzo) (Fig. 1-35, *A*).

The athlete must forward bend the upper body as far as possible while you palpate just inferior to the posterior superior iliac spine joints (the iliac crests must be level for this test; if they are not, put a lift under the ischial tuberosity until the pelvis is level) (Fig. 1-35, *B*).

Determine if the posterior superior iliac spine moves symmetrically and equally on each side.

If there is dysfunction, one side may ride up higher than the opposite side. This rise usually occurs at the end of range of motion.

You may need to close your eyes to increase your palpatory sensitivity.

You may need to repeat this test several times.

INTERPRETATION

The test in this position fixes the pelvis and allows more lumbar spine movement.

Any of the findings from the active forward bending in standing should occur again to verify your findings (e.g., muscle spasm, painful arc, hypomobility).

Active seated forward bending tests the sacroiliac motion.

The ilium is fixed because of the weight through the ischial tuberosities in sitting. Therefore during forward bending the sacrum is moving on the ilium.

If there is normal sacral movement on the ilium, the level of the posterior superior iliac spine will remain the same.

If there is a *sacroiliac lesion*, the standing posterior superior iliac spine will move normally on forward bending in the standing position but one will move higher on the seated forward bending test. The higher one is hypomobile because the sacrum and ilium move as one at the end of range of motion rather than independently.

If there is an *iliosacral lesion*, the standing forward bending test will bring one posterior superior iliac spine higher, while in the sitting forward bending test both spines will remain level. These findings are based on Mitchell, Moran, and Pruzzo's research.

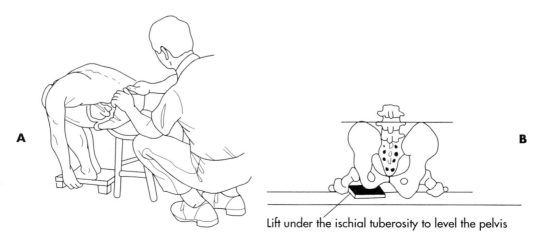

Lift under the ischial tuberosity to level the pelvis

Fig. 1-35 A, Active forward bending in sitting. **B,** Lift under the ischial tuberosity to level the pelvis.

ASSESSMENT   INTERPRETATION

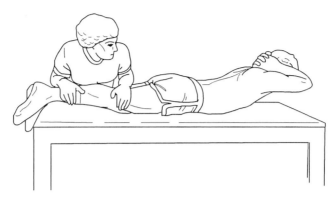

Fig. 1-36 Active spinal extension.

Tests in Prone Lying

Resisted Hip Extension with Knee Flexion

Resist the athlete's hip extension with one hand stabilizing the pelvis and the other hand resisting the thigh.

During this test, any signs of weakness of the gluteus maximus, which is associated with lumbar or referred low back pain, can come from an L5 nerve root problem or an inferior gluteal nerve injury. It will also be weak if the gluteus maximus muscle is injured.

Active Spinal Extension (Kendall and McCreary) (Fig. 1-36)

Firmly stabilize above the posterior knee and midcalf. If necessary, lean over the athlete with your body weight to stabilize his or her lower extremities.

The athlete is asked to put his or her hands behind the head and raise the chest off the plinth.

If the athlete is unable to do this, he or she may place hands down at the side or clasp them behind the back and then lift the upper body upward.

The athlete should be able to complete spinal extension with hands behind the head if the back extensors, latissimus dorsi, quadratus lumborum, and trapezius muscles are functioning normally. The ability to complete spinal extension with hands clasped behind the head is considered normal and is indicative of 100% of muscular function capacity. The ability to complete spinal extension with hands behind the back is good, or 80% of muscular function capacity. The ability to lift the thorax so that the xiphoid process of the sternum is raised slightly from the plinth is considered fair and is 50% to 60% of muscular function capacity.

When the low back is strong and the upper back is weak, attempts to raise the thorax will not be successful.

Spinal extension may relieve or increase back or leg pain with an intervertebral disc herniation.

If a lumbar facet joint irritation is present there will be pain during movement and at the end of range of motion, localized mainly in the vicinity of the joint.

Active Double Leg Raise (Fig. 1-37)

This test should not be done if an acute lumbar problem exists. Stabilize the athlete's pelvis.

The athlete is asked to lift both legs off the plinth approximately 10°—lift-

When the legs are raised, the back extensors must stabilize the hip joint, and any weakness of or injury to the back extensors will elicit pain.

Any hip extensor strain or weakness may cause pain in the glutei or hamstrings.

ASSESSMENT

INTERPRETATION

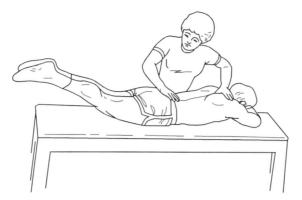

Fig. 1-37 Active double leg raise.

ing the legs at an angle that is greater than 10° involves lumbar hyperextension, which is not desired.

Pain, weakness, or limitation of range of motion indicates a problem with the muscles or their nerve supply.

The prime movers are:

- Erector spinae muscles (sacrospinalis)—dorsal rami of lower cervical, thoracic, and lumbar spinal nerves
- Transversospinalis—dorsal and ventral rami of the spinal nerves

Tests in Side Lying

Active Side Bending or Lateral Flexion (Kendall and McCreary)

The athlete lies on the side with arms crossed over the chest. Using your body weight, apply vigorous pressure over the pelvis and thigh.

The athlete attempts to lift the upper body off the plinth.

Trunk raising in this position is a combination of side bending and hip abduction.

The grading by Kendall and McCreary is the ability to raise the trunk laterally to a point of maximum lateral flexion in normal muscle function (100%). The ability to raise the lower shoulder 4 inches from the table is good muscle function (80%). To raise the lower shoulder 1 to 2 inches is fair muscle function (50%).

Pain weakness, or limitation of range of motion can come from the muscles or their nerve supply.

The prime movers are:

- Internal and external obliques—ventral rami of lower sixth thoracic and first lumbar spinal nerves
- Quadratus lumborum—ventral primary divisions (T12-L4) spinal nerves

The accessory movers are the latissimus dorsi and the hip abductors.

If you hold the trunk firmly but the thorax is rotated forward as the trunk is side bending, the external oblique is stronger.

If the thorax rotates backward during the side bending, the internal oblique is stronger.

If the back hyperextends as the athlete rises, the quadratus lumborum and latissimus dorsi show a stronger pull.

According to McNab, the athlete with a sacroiliac joint sprain

ASSESSMENT

INTERPRETATION

or any sacroiliac disease may find this movement painful because the contracting glutei tend to pull the pelvis away from the sacrum.

Resisted Hip Abduction

Resist hip abduction on the athlete's upper leg with one hand resisting the tibia and the other hand stabilizing the pelvis.

The athlete's lower hip and knee should be flexed.

Pain, weakness, or limitation of range of motion can come from the muscles or their nerve supply.

The prime mover is the Gluteus medius—superior gluteal nerve (L4, L5, S1).

The accessory movers are the gluteus minimus, gluteus maximus, tensor fascia lata, and the sartorius muscles.

Weakness can come from the superior gluteal nerve or from a L4, L5, or S1 nerve root problem.

Passive Lumbar Flexion and Extension (Fig. 1-38)

The athlete is side lying close to the side of the plinth, with knees flexed and over the edge of the plinth.

The hip of the lower leg is flexed at an angle of 45° to stabilize the trunk.

Face the athlete and with the index finger palpate the gap between adjacent spinous processes, starting at the lowest levels.

With the other hand, flex the athlete's upper hip and knee to an angle of 90°.

Move the athlete into varying degrees of hip flexion (in a rocking fashion) while palpating the spinous processes and the gapping between them.

At 90° of flexion, movement is felt at the lumbosacral joint.

More flexion of the hip allows palpation of interspinous motion at progressively higher levels of the lumbar spine.

Palpate for normal spinous process movement, mobility of each vertebra, and the degree of gapping between the processes. This movement is very subtle and careful palpatory skills are necessary.

Pain felt during the movement and on palpation of the supraspinous or interspinous ligament may indicate a sprain of the ligament.

Each level should have a smooth, painless symmetry of movement.

The inability of a lumbar level to have gapping indicates a hypomobility dysfunction.

If one level of the lumbar vertebrae or the ligaments surrounding the joint are tender it usually indicates dysfunction at that level.

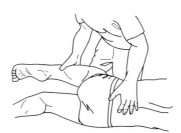

Fig. 1-38 Passive lumbar flexion and extension.

ASSESSMENT

INTERPRETATION

SPECIAL TESTS

Neurological Tests

If you suspect from the history-taking, observations, or previous functional tests that the athlete is suffering from a neurological problem (i.e., a nerve root problem, the following tests should be done).

Passive Straight-Leg Raise (Laseque's Test)
Part 1

The athlete is asked to slide back on the plinth to a long-sitting position before assuming the supine position. If the athlete cannot sit comfortably and must lean backward, it indicates that there could be a nerve root and disc herniation problem. This result is compared to the straight-leg test results to help identify the malingering patient.

The athlete should be relaxed with the knees fully extended. With one hand on the athlete's knee to keep it extended and the other hand under the heel, passively raise the leg slowly (the limb should not be internally or externally rotated) (Fig. 1-39, *A*). The limb is lifted as one unit with the knee extended until pain is produced in the lower extremity and/or the back. The athlete's pelvis must not rotate or lift off the plinth. It is important to record the exact range that the leg is raised before pain or other symptoms are experienced. With the leg within that range of discomfort, perform these tests:
- passive dorsiflexion of the ankle (Fig. 1-39, *B)*
- passive plantar flexion and inversion
- forward bending of the athlete's neck (Fig. 1-39, *C*)
- passive hip medial rotation and adduction

Record any changes in sensation or pain that these movements may cause. All this should be repeated bilaterally.

The straight-leg raise (SLR) is a key tension test for all spinal or leg symptoms that appear to involve the neural system. It can stress neural tissue from the brain to the toes.

The SLR test for lumbar symptoms stresses the following:
- mobility of the dura mater and the dural sleeve of the spinal nerves for the fourth lumbar level caudally
- mobility of the fourth and fifth lumbar nerve roots
- mobility of the first and second sacral nerve roots
- tension in the hamstrings due to injury or spasm
- dysfunction of the hip joint and its capsule
- dysfunction of the lumbosacral or sacroiliac joint

Ankle dorsiflexion will add tension to the neural structures especially along the tibial tract. Further tension can be added by everting the foot.

The SLR with dorsiflexion and inversion stresses more of the sural nerve component.

Plantar flexion and inversion with the SLR stresses the neural network along the common peroneal nerve.

Forward bending of the cervical spine tends to stress the neural structures throughout its entirety but especially bringing in the meningeal or dural segments around the brain, the cervical spine, and the thoracic spine.

Passive hip adduction and medial rotation will stress more of the sciatic nerve segment of the nervous system.

ASSESSMENT   INTERPRETATION

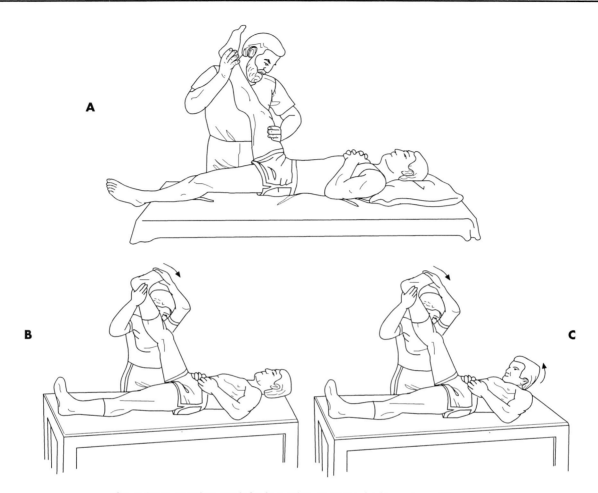

Fig. 1-39 A, Passive straight leg raise. **B**, Straight leg raise with passive ankle dorsiflexion. **C**, Passive straight leg raise with passive ankle dorsiflexion and cervical forward bending.

NORMAL RESULTS

The normal pain-free SLR varies from an angle of 60° to 120° with muscle tension behind the knee, thigh, or calf limiting the range of motion. If the athlete has a pronounced lumbar lordosis the range of motion will be less, whereas an athlete with a flat back will have more range.

There should be no increase in symptoms or pain with cervical forward bending, dorsiflexion of the ankle, or palpation of the peroneal nerve.

HAMSTRING SPASM LIMITATION

The cause of limitation can be spasm of the hamstrings, which is an involuntary protective mechanism that prevents, for example, a painful stretch of the dura mater or the nerve root. Hamstring spasm may also be caused by a facet joint or lumbar

ASSESSMENT	INTERPRETATION

ligament injury. A protective spasm in the lumbar or buttock region may also be present.

To do this test there must be good extensibility of the hamstrings and good mobility of the lumbosacral and sacroiliac joints.

To ensure that a hamstring spasm, tightness, or lesion is not limiting the range of motion, a hold/relax technique to relieve the hamstring spasm can be done before the SLR test is carried out. If there is a hamstring lesion, the pain will be very localized and a mechanism of injury will be present.

To overcome the protective spasm, lower the athlete's leg slightly and dorsiflex the foot or forward bend the neck to test the nerve sensibility versus the muscle extensibility.

Extremely tight hamstrings can occur because of spondylolysis or spondylolisthesis.

MENINGEAL IRRITATION LIMITATION

The SLR is limited in a meningeal irritation and neck forward bending is impossible.

A dural problem anywhere along its length will cause pain when the cervical spine is forward bent during the SLR.

NERVE ROOT, DURAL, NERVE, OR JOINT LIMITATIONS

A limitation due to the nerve root is usually caused by a disc protrusion.

If there is a nerve root irritation the SLR is usually limited at an angle of 30° of hip flexion. There is a high correlation between pain and a positive SLR test with a lower lumbar disc protrusion. According to Shiquing this correlation is as high as 98.2%. The prolapsed disc can bulge into the dural sac of the caudal equina or prolapse into some part of the dural investment of the nerve root. The larger the herniation the more the SLR is limited. There will also be pain during common peroneal nerve palpations.

There is little dural movement at an angle of 30° but tension gradually develops from angles of 30° to 70°. At an angle of 70°, the sciatic nerve and its nerve roots are fully stretched. Pain that is experienced at angles greater than 70° is probably joint pain of the hip, lumbosacral, or sacroiliac joints. The supporting structures of the pelvis and the lumbopelvic ligaments are stressed at this range.

If SLRs bilaterally cause pain at angles greater than 70°, the lesion is probably in the sacroiliac joints.

The dural sheath is a structure that is very sensitive to pain. The dura can be moved upward by forward bending the neck or caudally by flexing the hip and dorsiflexing the ankle. Any dural lesion will cause pain with these actions.

Neck flexion or hip medial rotation with the straight-leg test also increases tension in the lumbosacral nerve roots.

ASSESSMENT

INTERPRETATION

PAIN

A passive SLR may produce pain in the leg, back, or both.

Back pain during the SLR test along with other disc-protrusion symptoms is usually from central protrusions due to tension on the dura. Back and leg pain during the SLR test is usually from an intermediately located protrusion. Leg pain during the SLR test is usually from a lateral disc protrusion due to tension on the nerve roots. On this basis the distribution of pain during the SLR test accurately predicts the location of the intervertebral disc lesion—the literature shows a very high correlation. Pain patterns during the test do **not** predict the level of the protrusion.

A painful arc on a SLR at angles between 45° to 60° with a painfree range of motion above and below this may indicate a small localized disc protrusion that catches the nerve root and then slips over it.

The SLR can be full even with a disc lesion if the lesion is at the second or third lumbar nerve root.

A limited SLR without a disc lesion can be caused by the following:
- any interspinous ligament damage
- hip, sacroiliac, or lumbosacral joint problems
- low back or posterior leg fascial restriction
- malignant disease or osteomyelitis of the ilium or femur
- ankylosing spondylitis
- fractured sacrum
- contusion or strain of the hamstring muscle group
- adhesions epidurally or within the dura will alter the normal nerve mobility
- tumor at or above the fourth lumbar level

Part 2

Perform the SLR test on the athlete's nonpainful side. This is called the *well-leg raising test*.

Your findings can indicate several things.

Pain in the opposite side or on the well-leg-side test (cross straight-leg raising) indicates a large posteromedial prolapsed disc or a centrally located protrusion. If a disc lesion exists, pain is often felt in the opposite thigh or buttock because of the tension transmitted through the dura mater, especially if the protrusion lies between the dura mater and the nerve root at the fourth level.

A central posterior prolapsed disc into the dura will usually cause pain during the following:
- ipsilateral leg raising
- contralateral leg raising
- cervical forward bending

A medial disc herniation with nerve root irritation will usually cause pain with bilateral leg raising, but neck forward bending is painless. A lateral disc herniation with nerve root irritation will usually cause pain with leg raising ipsilaterally but not contralaterally, and neck forward bending may or may not be painful.

ASSESSMENT

Bowstring Sign (Fig. 1-40)

This test is done if the passive straight leg test was positive. The athlete's straight leg is raised until pain is produced. The leg is then flexed until the pain abates. Rest the athlete's leg on your shoulder with your thumbs placed in the popliteal fossa over the common peroneal nerve (just medial to the biceps femoris tendon). Apply gentle pressure to the nerve.

Femoral Nerve Stretch (Passive) (Fig. 1-41)

This test is recommended for an athlete with upper lumbar symptoms, anterior thigh, or hip pain.

With the athlete prone lying, hold the front of the knee with one hand and stabilize the pelvis with the other hand.

INTERPRETATION

Pressure on the common peroneal nerve that causes pain in the back or down the leg confirms that a nerve root tension problem exists.

If the athlete feels pain in the front of the leg during the test, the femoral nerve may be damaged.

If the low back hurts, the third lumbar nerve root may be irritated. Usually pain is experienced at full range. The third lumbar nerve root can be irritated by a disc protrusion. The amount of range of motion before pain is experienced may help to assess

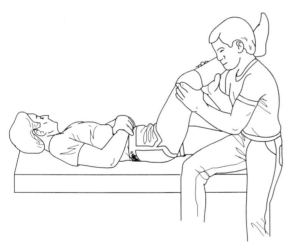

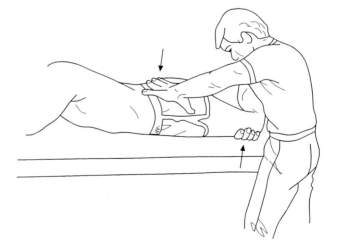

Fig. 1-40 Bowstring sign.

Fig. 1-41 Femoral nerve stretch.

ASSESSMENT

INTERPRETATION

Passively flex the knee to an angle of 90° and extend the hip until an end feel or pain limits the range of motion. The pelvis must be firmly stabilized to prevent pelvic and lumbar spine extension. Record the range and symptoms produced. Compare bilaterally.

the degree of protrusion of disc material from the L3 to the L4 interspace.

If the hip flexors are tight a stretch in the nerve may not be possible and getting the knee flexed to an angle of 90° may be difficult.

Neuromeningeal Mobility Test (Slump Test [Maitland])

The slump test can **not** be done on every spinal condition. An acute intervertebral disc herniation is at risk in the forward bent position and may not be tolerated. If the neural condition is inflamed or worsening, pain may restrict this test. Dizziness from vertebrobasilar insufficiency or spinal cord or cerebrovascular accidents are contraindications for the slump test.

This is a progressive test. If any of the positions cause strong pain, do not go to the next step. Always ask if there is any pain. Ask where it is and how severe it is.

The athlete is high sitting on the end of the plinth with the knees flexed 90° and the posterior thighs supported by the table. Ask the athlete to clasp his or her hands together behind the back. Then instruct the athlete to slump the lumbar and thoracic area of the back forward. Attempt to bow the spine rather than flex at the hips (Fig. 1-42, *A*).

Apply pressure with axilla and forearm of your right arm over the athlete's shoulder area to achieve the maximum slump in the spine. Ask about symptoms.

While you maintain the slumped back at its maximum curve, ask the athlete to flex his or her head to the chest (chin to chest) (Fig. 1-42, *B*). Record any symptoms. If significant pain rather than stretch discomfort is elicited, do **not** progress with the slump test. Apply pressure with your hand to his or her head to achieve full cervical flexion. Record any change in symptoms.

While you maintain this position, ask

During this test the spine is placed in maximum lumbar, thoracic, and cervical flexion combined with hip flexion, knee extension, and ankle dorsiflexion. The neuromeningeal structures (any pain-sensitive tissue in the spinal canal or intervertebral foramen) are placed on full stretch and any inflammation or mechanical dysfunction can elicit pain. Neural symptoms produced with thoracic and lumbar flexion can suggest an irritation of the neuromeningeal structure in this part of the spine. The following can be irritated:

- sciatic nerve
- dura or dural sheath
- spinal cord
- nerve roots or nerve root sleeve

Flexion of the cervical spine stretches these structures cephalically while knee extension and foot dorsiflexion increases the tension caudally. If the athlete cannot fully extend the knee because of the reproduction of the pain, a neural structure above is implicated.

Research has shown that some hamstring injuries can also give the neural pain sensation with knee extension (Kornberg and Lew). The majority of patients should experience some pain in the T8 or T9 area with neck flexion, or behind the knee in the hamstring area with knee extension and ankle dorsiflexion, but full range and relief of pain should be achieved when tension is released with neck extension. The restrictions should be symmetrical. The release of one component (i.e., neck flexion) reduces the tension in the pain-sensitive structure and allows further range in another component (i.e., knee extension). Some subjects will feel an instant ease of symptoms, whereas others may need to extend the neck further to relieve their symptoms. When the neck is extended, if the neural signs decrease and the knee can extend or the ankle dorsiflex further, it indicates a neuromeningeal structure problem. The test is considered positive if one side reproduces more symptoms than the opposite side. Detailed analysis of the test are beyond the scope of this book and one is referred to Grieve's book (Massey) or Butler DS.

ASSESSMENT	**INTERPRETATION**

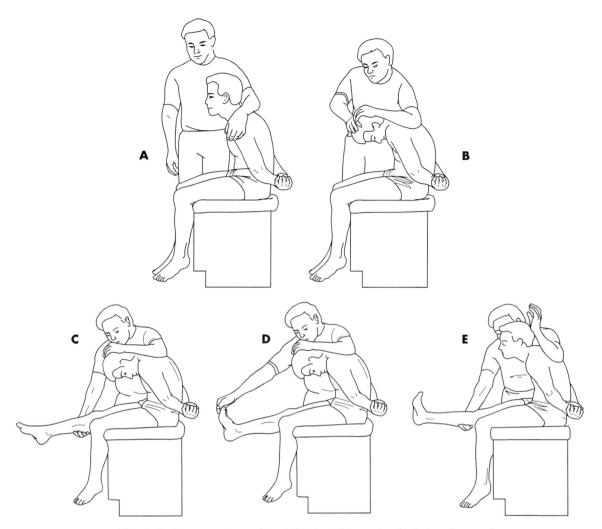

Fig. 1-42 Neuromeningeal mobility test (slump test). **A,** Lumbar and thoracic forward bending. **B,** Cervical forward bending. **C,** Knee extension. **D,** Ankle dorsiflexion. **E,** Cervical back bending.

the athlete to extend the knee actively as far as possible (Fig. 1-42, *C*). Record the response. Then ask the athlete to dorsiflex the ankle as far as possible (Fig. 1-42, *D*).

Hold the dorsum of the athlete's foot with your left hand to push the athlete's knee into maximal extension and foot into maximal dorsiflexion. Record the results.

Release the cervical flexion and assess the response carefully. Ask the

ASSESSMENT

INTERPRETATION

athlete to tilt the head back (extend the neck) and try to extend the knee further (Fig. 1-42, *E*).

The test is repeated bilaterally. The range of motion, symptoms, and pain responses are compared.

Myotome Testing

These tests are done if nerve root involvement is suspected. Provide resistance with an isometric test of key muscles that receive innervation from a specific segmental innervation. Because each muscle group receives innervation from more than one spinal segment, disc protrusions may cause only subtle muscle weakness. The strength of the contraction must be sufficient for you to overcome the athlete's contraction so that even a minor motor weakness can be detected. All these tests must be done bilaterally and should be graded very carefully.

Myotomes are musculature supplied by each spinal nerve. Most muscles are innervated by more than one spinal segment—the noted spinal level is the predominant segmental origin for most individuals.

Heel and Toe Walking

Walking on the heels and then the toes for 10 steps is a good gross motor test for myotome weakness.

Weakness of the L4 myotome will make it difficult for the athlete to walk on the heels, since the foot drops. Difficulties in toe walking or excessive dropping of the heel in midstance indicates an S1 myotome problem.

Resisted Plantar Flexion (While Standing) (Fig. 1-43)

The athlete goes up and down on his or her toes, one foot at a time, placing one finger on the plinth for balance. The athlete should be able to do a minimum of 10 to 20 repetitions on each foot.

This test is done to test the S1, S2 neurological level. Since most limb muscles are innervated by more than one spinal segment, only slight motor loss may result from a disc problem.

Disc herniation usually affects only one spinal segment. The strong gastrocnemii must be tested by repeated resistance of the entire body weight before weakness may be apparent. One leg fatiguing faster can be indicative of an S1 nerve root irritation from a herniated disc. Most athletes can perform 20 repetitions easily if no pathological condition exists.

The inability to go up on the toes at all or cramping of the calf can indicate a chronic disc herniation or a more serious neural condition.

An injury to the gastrocnemius, Achilles tendon, or ankle joint will also cause weakness.

Resisted Knee Extension (While Standing)

The athlete performs repetitive one-legged halfsquats and returns to a

This is a test mainly of the L3 neurological level.

This myotome test is necessary with the body weight because

ASSESSMENT

INTERPRETATION

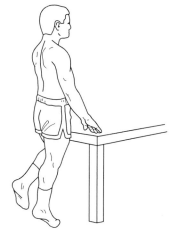

Fig. 1-43 Resisted plantar flexion.

standing position. A minimum of 10 to 20 half/squats on each leg should be done easily.

of the multisegmental innervation of the quadriceps (L2, L3, L4) and the muscle's strong nature.

Any difference in strength bilaterally can indicate an L3 nerve root irritation from a herniated disc.

The ability to perform a minimum of 10 resisted knee extensions is normal.

It is necessary to rule out knee pathological conditions, which may affect this test. Several athletes have injured knees and this test may not be suitable for them. It may be necessary to resist knee extension manually in these athletes.

The prime movers and their nerve supply are:
- Rectus femoris—femoral N (L2, L3, L4)
- Vastus lateralis—femoral N (L2, L3, L4)
- Vastus medialis—femoral N (L2, L3,L4)
- Vastus intermedius—femoral N (L2, L3, L4)

Resisted Hip Flexion

Have the athlete supine lying and resist hip flexion with one hand above the knee and one hand at the ankle.

This mainly tests for weakness of the second lumbar neurological level but weakness from a disc lesion here is rare.

A neuroma or secondary neoplasm is a possibility.

The prime movers and their nerve supply are:
- Psoas major—ventral rami of lumbar nerves (L1, L2, L3)
- Psoas minor—branch from first lumbar nerve (L1)
- Iliacus—femoral N (L2, L3)

It is necessary to rule out hip dysfunction, which may affect this test.

Resisted Knee Extension (Lying)

Have the athlete supine lie with their knees flexed to 90°, put one hand on the athlete's opposite knee with the athlete's closest leg flexed over your arm. Resist knee extension at the ankle on

This tests for neurological problems at L3. The prime mover and the nerve supply is the Quadriceps—femoral N (L2, L3).

ASSESSMENT   INTERPRETATION

the knee draped over your arm. The athlete meets your resistance with a strong contraction. This test is better than the standing test if the athlete has knee pathology. The test can be done with the knee at 30° flexion or less if patellofemoral pathology exists. There is less patellofemoral joint compression at 0° to 30° of knee flexion.

This test is done bilaterally.

Enquire regarding previous knee injuries that may affect the results.

Resisted Foot Dorsiflexion and Inversion (Fig. 1-44)

Resist dorsiflexion and inversion of the athlete's foot bilaterally.

This tests for weakness at the fourth lumbar neurological level (usually caused by a disc herniation). A lateral disc herniation at the fourth level will impinge the fourth nerve root.

The prime mover and its nerve supply is the Tibialis Anterior—deep peroneal N (L4, L5).

Resisted Hallux Extension (Fig. 1-45)

The athlete dorsiflexes the ankle and extends the great toe. Resist extension of the athlete's great toe at the distal phalanx by placing the index fingers against the toe nail. Repeat on the other side.

This tests for weakness at the fifth lumbar neurological level (usually caused by a disc herniation).

Disc lesions are fairly common at the fifth lumbar level but disc herniation at the fourth or fifth level can compress the fifth nerve root.

A protrusion that is off center at the fourth level can catch and compress the fifth root.

A full root syndrome at this level can cause weakness of the extensor hallucis longus, the peroneals, and the gluteus medius.

The prime movers and their nerve supply are:
- Extensor hallucis longus—deep peroneal N (L5, S1)
- Extensor hallucis brevis—deep peroneal N (S1, S2)

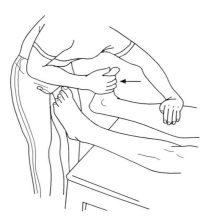

Fig. 1-44 Resisted dorsiflexion and inversion.

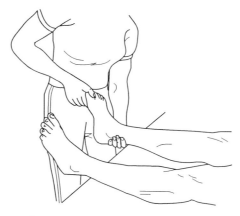

Fig. 1-45 Resisted hallux extension.

ASSESSMENT

INTERPRETATION

Resisted Foot Eversion (Fig. 1-46)

Resist on the lateral border of the athlete's foot while the athlete attempts to turn the foot outward. Repeat bilaterally and compare strength.

Resisted foot eversion can be weak from a fifth lumbar or first sacral level.

If there was also weakness with hallux extension, the L5 root is involved. If resisted plantar flexion in standing and foot eversion are both weak, the S1 nerve root is irritated.

A disc herniation of the fifth lumbar disc can compress the first and second sacral roots. This causes weakness in plantar flexion in standing, foot eversion, and resisted knee flexion.

The prime movers and their nerve supply are:
- Peroneus longus—superficial peroneal N (L5, S1, S2)
- Peroneus brevis—superficial peroneal N (L5, S1, S2)

Resisted Knee Flexion (Fig. 1-47)

Resist knee flexion by the athlete.

Resistance is applied at the athlete's ankle with your other hand resting on the thigh to prevent pelvic movement.

The athlete pulls the heel backward while you pull it forward. Make sure that there is no joint movement (isometric test). Repeat and compare bilaterally.

This tests the L5, S1, and S2 neurological levels but is mainly used to test S1.

This motor or myotomal test for knee flexion tests the hamstring strength for any segmental deficits at L5, S1, and S2.

The strength is compared bilaterally—a disc herniation at L5 or S1 can cause the nerve root problem.

The prime movers and their nerve supply are:
- Biceps femoris—sciatic N (L5, S1, S2)
- Semimembranosus—sciatic N (L5, S1, S2)
- Semitendinosus—sciatic N (L5, S1, S2)

Resisted Hallux Flexion (Fig. 1-48)

Resist great toe flexion in midposition. Place the tips of your thumbs on the pads of the great toes and ask the athlete to flex the toes against your resistance.

Repeat on the other side.

This is primarily a test for the S2 neurological level.

A disc herniation at L5 to S1 can cause S1 and S2 weakness.

The prime movers are:

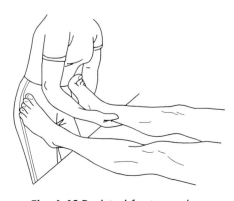

Fig. 1-46 Resisted foot eversion.

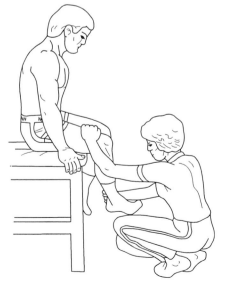

Fig. 1-47 Resisted knee flexion.

ASSESSMENT

INTERPRETATION

- Flexor hallucis brevis—medial plantar N (S2, S3)
- Flexor hallucis longus—tibial N (S2, S3)

Resisted Foot Intrinsics (Fig. 1-49)

Resist flexion of all the toes. Place the tips of your fingers against the pads of the athlete's toes and ask the athlete to flex the toes against your resistance.

Repeat on the other side.

This primary tests the S3 neurological level.

All the intrinsics of the foot are served by the S2 and S3 neurological levels.

Urogenital Region

This can be tested by questions pertaining to pain in the perineum or genitals and weakness of the muscles of the bladder or rectum.

Most problems in this area result from the fourth sacral root. All the muscles of the urogenital region are supplied by the perineal branch of the pudendal nerve (S2, S3, and S4). Any problems here indicate a medical emergency and the athlete should be referred to a nearby medical facility.

Dermatome Testing (Fig. 1-50)

The skin is checked for cutaneous analgesia.

Dermatomes can overlap and vary greatly in individuals.

Instruct the athlete to look away while you touch the surface of the skin with a pin, asking the athlete if the sensation is sharp or dull. Touch the athlete with the pin in comparable areas in both extremities. Five to ten pinpricks in each dermatome.

See the diagram for dermatome areas.

The dermatome is an area of skin (and hair) supplied by the afferent or sensory fiber of a single spinal segment.

The dermatomes of each spinal nerve overlap and vary in each individual—only gross changes can be detected by a pin.

If the results show areas of lack of full sensation, the area can be retested with sharp, hot and cold objects (e.g., test tubes). Texts vary on these dermatomes (Gray's text is referred to below).

The dermatomes are the following:

L1

- lower abdomen and groin
- lumbar region from the second to the fourth vertebrae
- upper and outer aspect of the buttock

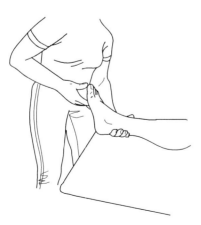

Fig. 1-48 Resisted hallux flexion.

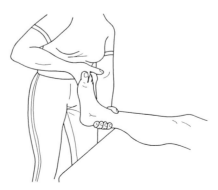

Fig. 1-49 Resisted foot intrinsics.

ASSESSMENT

INTERPRETATION

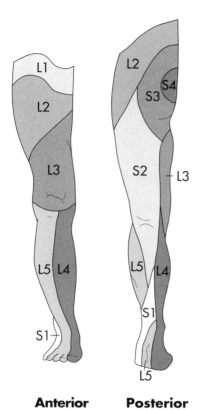

Anterior **Posterior**

Fig. 1-50 Dermatomes.

L2
- lower lumbar region
- upper buttock
- anterior aspect of the thigh (not medially)

L3
- medial aspect of the thigh to the knee
- anterior aspect of the lower one third of the thigh to just below the patella

L4
- medial aspect of the lower leg and foot
- inner border of the foot
- great toe

L5
- lateral border of the leg
- anterior surface of the lower leg
- second, third, and fourth toes
- central portion of the sole of the foot

S1
- posterior aspect of the lower one quarter of the leg
- posterior aspect of the foot, including the heel
- lateral border of the foot and sole
- fifth toe

S2
- posterior central strip of the leg from below the gluteal fold to three quarters of the way down the lower leg

S3
- central gluteal area

S4
- a saddle shaped area, including the anus, perineum, scrotum and penis, and labium and vagina

Dermatome or Cutaneous Nerve Supply

Sometimes it is difficult to determine if the analgesia is of a dermatomal or cutaneous origin (e.g., the great toe and second toe, all the toes).

Sometimes it is difficult to determine the cause of the analgesia. For example, paresthesia in the great toe and second toe can be caused by the following:
- fifth lumbar root problem
- anterior tibial compartment problem
- second digital nerve problem

Paresthesia in all the toes can indicate the following:
- lateral tibial compartment problem
- fifth lumbar or first sacral compression

Nerves originate at the spinal cord and exit through the intervertebral foramen. The angle of exit of the nerve from the spinal cord and the size of the foramen is a factor with disc protrusions—these two variables may affect the dermatomal and myotomal areas affected.

A disc lesion affects only one nerve root (in general), and a protrusion just to one side of the midline tends to compress the root at the same level. A protrusion at L5-S1 interval space quite

ASSESSMENT   ## INTERPRETATION

often produces a fifth lumbar motor weakness and first sacral sensory deficiency. A large protrusion can affect two roots but seldom three—three roots affected could mean the presence of a neoplasm.

The motor and sensory components of the nerve root emerge separately. If the protrusion compresses from below, the palsy occurs in motor function; large protrusions compress the entire root and cause both motor and sensory impairment.

Bilateral weakness of muscle or bilateral loss of sensation is rarely caused by a disc lesion because when the protrusion herniates, it protrudes to one side or the other of the posterior longitudinal ligament, which causes unilateral changes. Bilateral changes can occur with a central disc protrusion, claudication, or central spinal cord problem.

Cutaneous Nerve Supply Testing (Fig. 1-51)

The skin is checked for cutaneous analgesia as above but check for numbness in the cutaneous areas served by the peripheral nerves. See the diagram of cutaneous nerve supply areas.

If the lateral border (from the greater trochanter to about the middle of the thigh) feels numb but the athlete has no

If the lateral border (from the greater trochanter to about the middle of the thigh) feels numb but the athlete has no back symptoms, this can be *meralgia paresthetica*. This is an irritation of the lateral cutaneous nerve (posterior branch).

If the lateral and half of the anterior surface of the upper thigh feels numb but there are no back symptoms, this can be an irritation of the lateral cutaneous nerve (anterior branch). This cutaneous nerve can be irritated as it passes under the inguinal

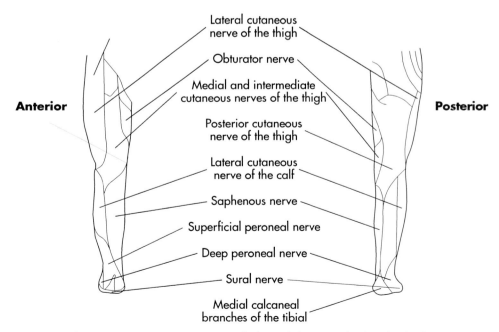

Anterior

Posterior

Lateral cutaneous nerve of the thigh
Obturator nerve
Medial and intermediate cutaneous nerves of the thigh
Posterior cutaneous nerve of the thigh
Lateral cutaneous nerve of the calf
Saphenous nerve
Superficial peroneal nerve
Deep peroneal nerve
Sural nerve
Medial calcaneal branches of the tibial

Fig. 1-51 Cutaneous nerve supply (meralgia paresthetica shaded).

ASSESSMENT

back symptoms, this can be meralgia paresthetica. This is an irritation of the lateral cutaneous nerve (posterior branch).

Reflexes

To test the reflexes the following factors are required:
- the athlete must be relaxed
- the tendon must be placed on stretch
- the muscle must receive an adequate stimulus
- reinforcement is sometimes necessary

Knee Reflexes

With the athlete high sitting, tap the patellar tendon with a reflex hammer and observe the patellar reflex bilaterally.

This should be repeated 8 to 10 times to test the reflex fatigability or to uncover the fading reflex response, which indicates developing root signs.

If there is no response the athlete is asked to carry out an upper body isometric contraction by interlocking fingers and pulling the hands away from one another (with the elbows flexed), or clenching the jaw.

A bilateral comparison should be done.

Ankle Reflexes

With the athlete high sitting, gently push the foot into slight dorsiflexion.

Leave one hand under the ball of the foot while the Achilles tendon is tapped to cause an involuntary plantar flexion of the ankle. A bilateral comparison should be done.

Tap repeatedly as above.

INTERPRETATION

ligament and is not to be confused with numbness from a disc lesion.

The lack of sensation from a cutaneous nerve supply is different from the dermatomes and therefore the therapist must memorize the different patterns or refer to mapping diagrams.

The deep tendon reflex tests are done to determine if there is any segmented neurological deficit causing a diminished reflex on one side. These tests are important because a change in the quality of the reflexes can indicate nerve root compression versus an irritation. Reflex testing is based on the fact that a normal skeletal muscle that is suddenly stretched will result in a reflex contraction of that muscle.

A reflex will be decreased in a lower motor neuron injury and may be exaggerated with an upper motor neuron disease or injury.

The knee reflex is mediated through the nerves from L2, L3, and L4 nerve roots (primarily by L4).

Because of its multisegmented input the response is not absent but will be diminished if the nerve root is compressed.

A disc herniation at L3-L4 is the usual cause for diminished knee reflexes.

This is a deep tendon reflex for the S1 neurological level.

If the reflex is diminished or absent on one side compared to the other, this indicates a neurological deficit.

Usually a disc herniation at the L5-S1 level is the cause.

ASSESSMENT   INTERPRETATION

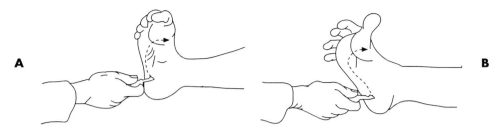

Fig. 1-52 Babinski reflex. **A,** Negative. **B,** Positive.

Babinski Reflex (Fig. 1-52)

Run a sharp instrument (end of reflex hammer) across the plantar surface of the athlete's foot from the calcaneus along the lateral border of the forefoot.

This test is done if upper or lower motor neuron involvement or spinal cord involvement is suspected. Cord signs are pins and needles in the extremities bilaterally, or all four extremities and altered movement patterns.

The Babinski sign is part of a primitive flexion reflex.

A positive response to this test is a sign of upper motor neuron disorder that indicates some dysfunction of the motor area of the brain or the corticospinal tracts, which suppresses the flexion response.

The positive Babinski causes the great toe to extend while the other toes plantar flex and splay.

The negative response causes the toes to bunch up uniformly or to flex and adduct.

Ankle Clonus

With the athlete supine lying, flex the athlete's knee slightly, then rapidly dorsiflex the ankle. This is a test for spinal cord function.

A positive clonus response is a "cogwheel" type rigidity.

Lower Limb Girth Measurements

Perform this test if muscle atrophy from a nerve root problem is suspected.

The maximum girth of the calf and thigh are measured on both legs at the joint line at 3", 6", and 9" above the joint line and 2", 4", and 6" below the joint line. Rule out atrophy in these measurements from previous or existing hip, knee, or ankle injuries.

Atrophy of the quadriceps can be due to a neurological problem at the L3 level—this is rare. Atrophy of the hamstrings can be caused by a disc herniation at the L5 or S1 level. Atrophy of the gastrocnemii can be caused by an L5 or S1 disc herniation. It is important to realize that athletes often have lower limb (especially knee) injuries that can also affect these measurements.

Intrathecal Pressure Tests

These tests are performed if a neurological problem with pressure on the dural sheath is suspected.

ASSESSMENT

INTERPRETATION

Valsalva Maneuver

The athlete is asked to hold his or her breath and then to bear down, creating increased intra-abdominal pressure.

If pain increases and/or radiates it can indicate that there is increased intrathecal pressure, which is pressure within the dura around the spinal cord. This increased pressure is usually due to a herniated disc, tumor, or osteophyte occupying space in the spinal cord area.

Cough Test

The athlete is asked to cough and then to comment on any pain or sensation changes.

If pain increases it indicates that the dura is compressed (i.e., there is increased intrathecal pressure).

This test is often positive in the presence of disc lesions.

The sudden increase of intrathecal pressure stresses the nerve endings in the dura, which is already irritated due to the disc protrusion.

This is not as conclusive of a disc protrusion as once thought because EMG studies have shown that the erector spinae also increase their activity during coughing. If the erector spinae are in spasm, a cough can add to the discomfort. However, if the pain radiates down a nerve root or along pain pathways, a disc protrusion is the more likely cause.

Muscle Imbalance Tests

These tests are performed if a muscle imbalance is suspected.

Long Sitting Toe touching (Kendall and McCreary) (Fig. 1-53)

Ask the athlete to lie supine and then to reach for the toes while keeping the knees straight and the head tucked in.

Look from the side at the athlete's back, pelvis, and knees.

Upper and Lower Back

Look at the contours in the upper and lower back.

The curve of the back should occur evenly from the lumbar to the cervical vertebrae.

If there is extra curving of the upper back and a flat lower

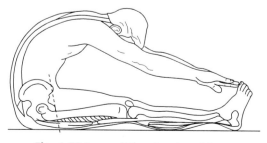

Fig. 1-53 Long sitting toe touching.

ASSESSMENT

INTERPRETATION

back, a muscle spasm or shortened muscles in the lower back should be suspected. These could add to or cause the lower back problem.

The upper back curves the extra amount to make up for the lumbar restriction.

Pelvis
Look at the position of the pelvis.

If the pelvis is rotated forward and the hamstrings are overstretched, this can add to low back pathology.

Knees
Look at the position of the knees.

If the knees are flexed, suspect tight hamstrings that could add to low back discomfort. The knees can also flex to take the stretch off the sciatic nerve (if disc or nerve root irritation is involved). Extremely tight hamstrings can occur in cases of spondylolysis and spondylolisthesis.

Ankles
Look at the position of the ankles.

If the ankles plantar flex during this test, the gastrocnemii may lack flexibility.

These muscle imbalances in groups of muscles like the hamstrings, the gastrocnemii, or the erector spinae can cause mechanical low back problems, which usually accentuate lumbar lordosis. Muscle imbalances between each limb can also cause torsional mechanical problems for the lumbar spine. Recording the bilateral and group imbalances will help determine mechanical causes of injury and help in the design of a rehabilitation program.

Hip Flexor Tightness (Thomas Test) (Fig. 1-54)
The athlete is supine lying with his or her knees over the end of the plinth.

Flex the athlete's hip and knee, bringing the knee to the chest, and leave the other leg over the edge of the plinth.

If the nonflexed hip comes up off the plinth, the hip flexor (iliopsoas) on that side is tight. If the knee extends and/or the hip flexes, the rectus femoris is tight.

If the hip flexes but the knee remains flexed, there is an iliopsoas tightness.

If the hip abducts, the tensor fascia lata is tight.

Any hip flexor tightness can add to lumbar lordosis while the athlete is standing. Excessive lumbar lordosis can cause or accentuate several low back conditions.

Abdominal Strength (Curl Sit up) (Fig. 1-55)
The athlete is hook lying with knees flexed comfortably and with fingers on the temples.

Instruct the athlete to put the chin on the chest by curling up gradually and attempting to get the head and shoulders off the plinth about 30°.

If the athlete cannot raise the head and hold the curl position, weak abdominals exist. Abdominal strength is necessary to help prevent an excessive anterior pelvic tilt that can lead to lumbar lordosis and lumbar pain.

The athlete should be able to hold this position for 5 or more seconds. The rotational component tests the abdominal oblique muscles. Any difficulty twisting to one side more than to the

ASSESSMENT

INTERPRETATION

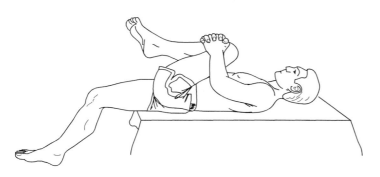

Fig. **1-54** Thomas test for hip flexor tightness.

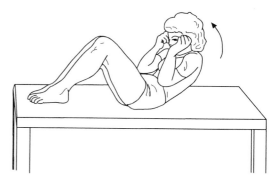

Fig. **1-55** Abdominal strength (curl sit up).

This position should be maintained for 5 seconds (scapula just off the plinth).

If the athlete can do this partial curl sit up, have him or her attempt it with a twist, so that the right shoulder goes toward the left knee and vice versa.

The athlete still just curls up 30° in each case.

Sacroiliac Joint Tests

Perform these tests if the history-taking, observations, or previous functional tests suggest sacroiliac or iliosacral dysfunction.

Kinetic Test

This tests for iliac and sacral rotation during one-legged standing. The athlete stands with weight evenly distributed through both legs. Palpate and locate the inferior posterior iliac spine bilaterally with your thumbs and the spinous process of S2, which is parallel to the PSIS. The athlete then stands on one leg and flexes the opposite knee toward the chest. Observe weight transfer and balance. Palpate inferior to the PSIS on the nonweight bearing side with one thumb and the other thumb on the S2 spinous processes. The PSIS should move down or caudally (posterior ilium rotation)— the sacral process is relatively a fixed

other can be caused by an imbalance in the oblique abdominal muscle strength.

Testing the abdominals is very important for the athlete with low back pain because reflex inhibition can be caused with ongoing muscle spasm in the erector spinae.

The abdominals must be retrained or they will quickly atrophy, which will worsen the problem.

If there is sacroiliac joint hypomobility or fixation, the PSIS will move cephalically (upward) rather than caudally (downward) on the nonweight bearing side.

ASSESSMENT   INTERPRETATION

reference point. As the foot returns to the ground the PSIS should move back upward or cephalically.

Repeat on the opposite side.

Pelvic Rocking Test

Place your palms on both anterior superior iliac spines and initiate a gentle rocking motion.

One hand holds the iliac crest while the other hand pushes down gently posteriorly, feeling for the amount of movement.

Then the crest is held still and the other side is gently pushed. During this, feel for a symmetry of motion.

If the sacroiliac joint is injured this test may cause pain and the motion on the injured side may be reduced or increased in comparison to the other side.

If there is right posterior iliac rotation the right anterior superior iliac spine may appear to be higher and the left anterior superior iliac spine may appear to be more prominent and lower.

This test stretches the sacroiliac ligaments and tests for hypomobility and hypermobility in the sacroiliac joint.

Gapping Test (Fig. 1-56)

Cross your hands over the pelvis with the palms against the anterior superior iliac spines and take up the slack.

Pressure is then applied downward and outward on the ilia.

The test is positive if it causes unilateral sacroiliac pain or posterior leg pain.

The test helps determine if hypomobility or hypermobility exists in the sacroiliac ligaments.

Hip Flexion and Adduction Test (Fig. 1-57)

With the athlete's knee flexed, flex and adduct the leg—this stresses the sacroiliac joints.

Place your finger medial to the PSIS to monitor the ligamentous tension.

In this hip position, the sacroiliac joint on that side is stressed and dysfunction will elicit pain. Hip joint problems may also cause discomfort during this test. Stretching the S1 nerve root can also occur with this test and elicit pain if acute nerve root irritation exists.

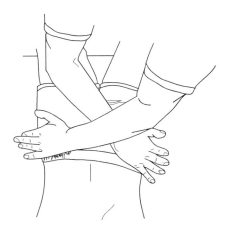

Fig. 1-56 Sacroiliac joint gapping test.

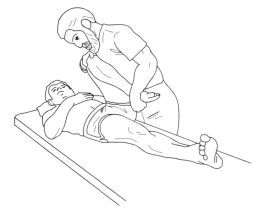

Fig. 1-57 Hip flexion and adduction test.

ASSESSMENT

INTERPRETATION

Gaenslen's Sign

Instruct the athlete to draw both legs onto the chest while lying supine.

Shift the athlete to the edge of the plinth with the buttock on one side off the plinth and allow the leg on the same side to extend over the edge while the opposite leg is held to the chest by the athlete.

When the leg is dropped over the side of the plinth, the sacroiliac joint rotates forward on the same side and posteriorly on the contralateral side. This causes pain if there is sacroiliac joint dysfunction.

Sacroiliac Joint Test (Side lying Gaenslen's Test)

The athlete is lying with the non-painful side down. On the nonpainful side the hip and knee are flexed and the athlete hugs the knee to lock the pelvis and lumbar spine.

The uppermost hip is now extended to its limit while the knee is kept extended.

Pain indicates a positive test.

As the upper hip is extended, there is a rotary stress applied to the ilium on that side against the sacrum.

This movement causes pain in the sacroiliac region if a sacroiliac joint sprain or dysfunction exists.

Pain in the hip joint during this test can indicate hip joint dysfunction.

Patrick's or Faber Test

(F) lexion, (Ab) duction, (E) xternal (R) otation (FABER)

The athlete is lying supine with one leg straight. Take the other hip into abduction and external rotation.

The knee and hip are flexed so that the heel is placed on the knee of the straight leg.

Observe the hip range of motion and knee position.

Apply pressure to the flexed knee while the opposite hand stabilizes the pelvis over the opposite anterior superior iliac spine for stabilization.

Repeat and compare bilaterally.

Pain from the hip or sacroiliac joint indicates a positive test.

A negative test occurs when the flexed knee drops down parallel to the opposite leg or to the plinth.

A positive test occurs when the flexed knee is unable to fall into full abduction.

A positive test can indicate the following:
• hip joint pathological condition
• sacroiliac joint dysfunction
• iliopsoas muscle injury
• adductor muscle injury

Inguinal pain suggests a hip pathological condition.

If the athlete experiences pain in the sacroiliac joint with the overpressure, there is dysfunction to this joint.

With the hip in this position the flexibility of the adductor muscles is tested, as is the integrity of the iliofemoral and pubofemoral ligaments.

Sit up Test for Iliosacral Dysfunction (Fig. 1-58)

The athlete is supine with the body straight and legs symmetric. The athlete flexes the knees, lifts the pelvis off the plinth about 4 inches, then drops the pelvis down to the table.

Passively extend the knees and lower the legs one at a time to the plinth.

The legs are then rolled medially and released.

The sit up test can also be used to determine if anterior or posterior iliac rotation exists.

As the athlete forward bends, the spine segments lock together and the sacrum allows for the end mobility. Once the lumbar forward bending reaches the sacrum, the sacroiliac joint should move 2° to 6° in a mobile joint.

If the right sacroiliac joint is blocked or hypomobile in a position of posterior iliac rotation, the following will occur:
• sacrum and ilium will move together as a unit

ASSESSMENT

INTERPRETATION

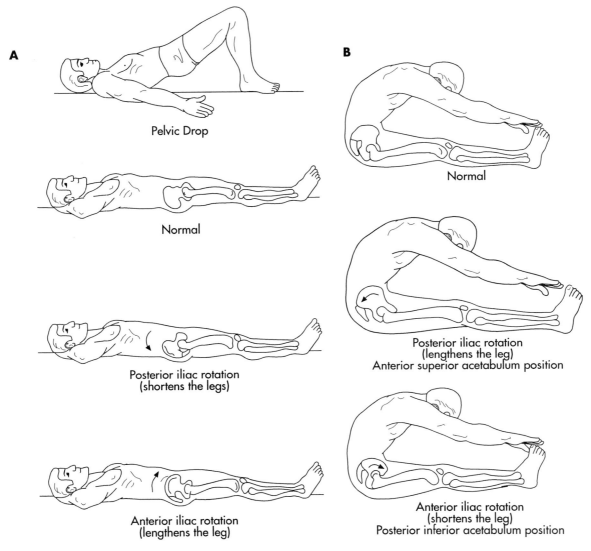

A

Pelvic Drop

Normal

Posterior iliac rotation
(shortens the legs)

Anterior iliac rotation
(lengthens the leg)

B

Normal

Posterior iliac rotation
(lengthens the leg)
Anterior superior acetabulum position

Anterior iliac rotation
(shortens the leg)
Posterior inferior acetabulum position

Fig. 1-58 Sit-up test for iliosacral dysfunction.

Palpate and observe the level of the distal medial malleoli.

The athlete is instructed to sit up, and the level of the malleoli are checked again.

- the acetabulum is thrust forward on the right side, making the leg appear to lengthen when the athlete sits up
- the right malleolus goes from a shortened length in the supine position to a longer length in the sitting position

If the right sacroiliac joint is in an anterior iliac rotation, the leg may appear longer or the same length in supine lying but the leg will get shorter when the athlete sits up.

ASSESSMENT

INTERPRETATION

NOTE: According to Hesch; Mitchell; and others, the iliosacral dysfunction will have these other clinical signs:

Anterior Iliac Rotation

- ASIS is inferior, anterior, and medial to opposite ASIS
- PSIS is superior and anterior on that side
- medial sulcus (formed by ilium overlapping the sacrum) is shallow
- anterior iliac crest is inferior on the same side as the dysfunction
- posterior iliac crest is superior
- pubic tubercle on that side may be lower
- ischial tuberosity is superior

Posterior Iliac Rotation

- ASIS is superior, posterior, and lateral to opposite ASIS
- PSIS is inferior and posterior
- medial sulcus is deeper
- anterior iliac crest is superior
- posterior iliac crest is inferior
- pubic tubercle may be higher
- ischial tuberosity is inferior

Ankylosing Spondylitis Test (Fig. 1-59)

This test should be done if ankylosing spondylitis is suspected. The chest girth is measured at expiration and then at maximum inspiration.

With ankylosing spondylitis the chest expansion ability decreases.

There should be a difference of at least an inch between the inspiration and expiration girth measurements.

Leg-Length Measurement Tests (Fig. 1-60)

This test is performed if a leg-length difference is suspected.

Stand at the end of the plinth and ask

Look for a difference in leg length and record the difference.

Determine if the difference occurs in the femur or the tibia.

Look for problems of pelvic asymmetry or muscle imbalances

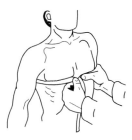

Fig. 1-59 Ankylosing spondylitis test (chest girth measurement).

ASSESSMENT

the athlete to flex the knees and to lift the pelvis off the plinth about 4 inches, then drop it.

Extend the athlete's legs and measure the distance from the anterior superior iliac spine to the medial malleolus bilaterally.

To determine whether the discrepancy lies in the tibia or femur, have the athlete lie supine with the knees flexed to 90° with feet flat on the plinth.

Compare the height of the tibias and determine if one is longer (Fig. 1-60, *A*). If, in this position, one knee appears more anterior, the femur is longer (Fig. 1-60, *B*).

If a discrepancy exists, the length of the tibias can be compared by measuring from the medial joint line to the malleolus, or the lengths of the femurs can be compared by measuring from the greater trochanter to the lateral femoral condyle.

Measurements can be taken initially in standing (see Fig. 1-15).

Circulatory Tests (Fig. 1-61)

If a circulatory problem is suspected, check the following pulses:
- Femoral artery
- Popliteal artery
- Posterior tibial artery
- Dorsalis pedis artery

PALPATIONS

Palpate areas for point tenderness, temperature differences, swelling, adhesions, calcium deposits, muscle spasms, and muscle tears. Palpate for muscle tenderness, lesions, and trigger points.

INTERPRETATION

that affect the body position during measurement. A posterior iliac rotation, for example, can cause the upward and forward position of the acetabulum, which can make that leg appear shorter.

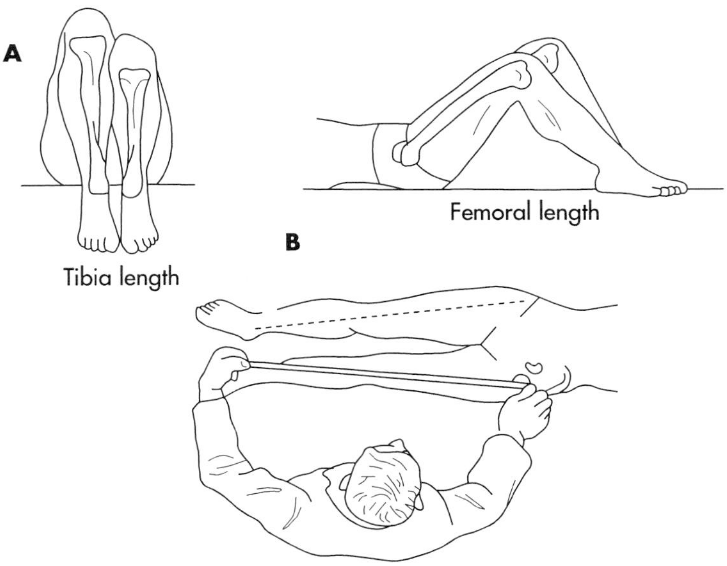

Fig. 1-60 Leg-length measurement tests. **A**, Tibial height. **B**, Femoral length.

Diminished pulses can suggest circulatory deficiencies or neural deficiencies that can be caused by sympathetic nervous system involvement.

According to David Simons and Janet Travell, myofascial trigger points in muscle are activated directly by overuse, overload, trauma, or chilling, and are activated indirectly by visceral disease, other trigger points, arthritic joints, or emotional distress. Myofascial pain is referred from trigger points that have specific patterns and locations for each muscle. Trigger points are hyperactive spots, usually in a skeletal muscle or the muscle's fascia, that are acutely tender on palpation and that evoke a muscle twitch when palpated. These points can also evoke autonomic responses (i.e., sweating, pilomotor activity, local vasoconstriction).

ASSESSMENT

INTERPRETATION

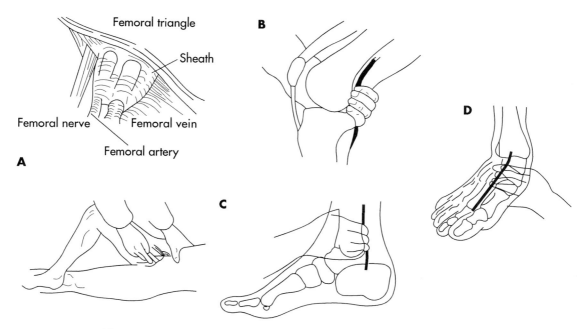

Fig. 1-61 Circulatory tests. **A**, Femoral artery. **B**, Popliteal artery. **C**, Posterior tibial artery. **D**, Dorsalis pedis artery.

Posterior Structures (Prone)

Boney
Spinous Processes (Fig. 1-62)
SPRINGING TEST (ANTERIOR-POSTERIOR PRESSURE)

The spinous processes are palpated for any irregularities. Start at the first lumbar segment and work toward the sacrum. Pressure is applied downward gently with the thumb over each spinous process. The amount of rigidity or movement of each vertebral segment should be noted.

You are looking for the amount of motion at each spinal segment. Rigidity usually indicates hypomobility and springing usually indicates hypermobility.

You may find hypermobility above or below a hypomobile segment or hypermobility in each segment in some individuals.

When estimating the lumbar level, often the fifth lumbar spinous process is small and recessed and difficult to locate.

Any lumbar joint dysfunction can cause some discomfort or pain with pressure at the involved level.

LATERAL PRESSURE

Each spinous process can be pushed laterally with the side of the thumb to see the rotational mobility of the segment.

The L4-L5 interspace is level with the top of the iliac crests. Rotational restriction or pain can indicate dysfunction at the involved level.

Large gaps between the spinous processes or the absence of spinous processes can suggest spina bifida.

A palpable step or ledge can suggest spondylolisthesis.

ASSESSMENT

INTERPRETATION

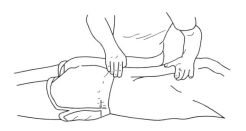

Fig. 1-62 Palpation of spinous processes and paraspinal muscles.

Transverse Processes of Lumbar Vertebrae

Palpate on either side of the spinous processes from T12 to L5. The rotational status of the lumbar segment can be determined.

Rotation of one vertebral segment on another can occur because of muscle spasm or scoliosis.

Lumbosacral Junction

Palpate the spinous process of L5. Palpate for point tenderness from the location of the iliolumbar ligaments to the transverse processes.

Palpation of the spinous process and the transverse process helps to determine if this lumbar vertebra is rotated.

Posterior Pelvis and Sacral Triangle

The sacral triangle is formed by the two posterior superior iliac spines and the top of the gluteal cleft. Palpate the entire sacrum, locating the sacral hiatus, the inferior lateral angle, median crest, the spinous tubercles, and the cornua of the sacrum (see Fig. 1-63).

Palpate the length of the sacrum 1 cm from the midline. Place the thumbs over the sacral cornua bilaterally, noting the location and symmetry. Palpate the sacroiliac ligaments running from the iliac crest to the sacral tubercles.

Palpate the erector spinae muscle, multifidus, and fascia in the area (longissimus thoracis). Palpate the posterior superior iliac spines and determine their location and symmetry.

The sacrum has the freedom to move in the sagittal plane about a transverse axis (Fig. 1-63). This axis is approximately at the second sacral vertebra. According to Hesch, there is also an oblique and vertical axis.

If the sacrum is rotated one cornua may feel more prominent while the other feels deeper. The sacrum can be rotated because it has adapted to abnormal stresses through the lumbar vertebrae or to asymmetrical forces through the limbs (e.g., leg length problem). The rotation of the sacrum in turn can cause problems in the pelvis and the low back. Point tenderness in the sacroiliac ligaments or muscles overlying them suggests dysfunction in this area. The posterior superior iliac spines are points of attachment for the sacrotuberous ligaments and dorsal sacroiliac ligaments. These ligaments are important to the stability of the sacrum and sacroiliac joint. Pain in this area often indicates a sacroiliac joint dysfunction.

If one posterior inferior iliac spine is more prominent than the other, posterior rotation of the ilium or an iliac outflare may be present.

On deep palpation of the sacrum's midsection you may feel spongy sensation or increased tissue tension if right or left sacral torsion exists. The depth of the sacral cornua or the prominence of the cornua can also indicate torsion; e.g., in the case of a left rotation on a left oblique axis, the sulcus on the left will feel shallow and tense while the right sacral sulcus will feel deep. With normal tissue tone, pain in this area can indicate problems

ASSESSMENT

INTERPRETATION

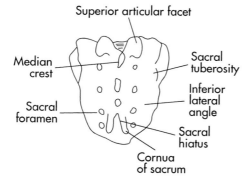

Fig. 1-63 Dorsal aspect of sacrum.

with the longissimus thoracis, the attachment of the iliolumbar ligament, the posterior sacroiliac ligaments, or dysfunction of the sacrum or the L5-S1 joint.

Ischial Tuberosities

With the athlete prone lying, raise the athlete's lower legs and flex the athlete's knees. The athlete's legs are then lowered to the plinth. This helps to balance the pelvis before palpation is initiated. Palpate the levels of the ischial tuberosities bilaterally to determine if they are level or if one is superior or inferior to the other.

In the supine position, if one ischial tuberosity is higher and if the iliosacral joint test (while the athlete was standing) was positive (i.e., posterior superior iliac spine moved higher than opposite posterior superior iliac spine), there is a sacroiliac joint dysfunction (an upslip or an anterior iliac rotation). Other clinical findings of an upslip include a higher anterior superior iliac spine, higher posterior superior iliac spine, and higher pubic tubercle on one side while the athlete is supine and upright.

The sacrotuberous ligament on the high tubercle side will lack tonus.

Coccyx

Palpate the coccyx gently for point tenderness or deformity.

Direct trauma to the coccyx (coccydynia) will cause pain with palpation. A physician's rectal examination or x-ray may be necessary if a fracture is suspected.

Posterior Structures

Soft Tissue

Palpate for reactive muscle spasm, trigger points, a pilomotor reflex (goose flesh response), a sudomotor reflex (increased skin perspiration), or subcutaneous trophedema (thickened subcutaneous tissue; 'peau d'orange'). If the subcutaneous tissue appears thickened, the skin and tissue can be pinched and rolled between the thumb and forefingers to confirm the abnormal thickening and pain elicited in the thickened area—skin roll T12 to the top of the sacrum paraspinally.

A pilomotor or sudomotor response indicates signs of a facilitated segment that serves that area. Thickened tissue and muscle spasm in specific areas also can indicate a facilitated segment. A facilitated segment is an area of increased irritation in the skin, muscle, nerve, periosteum, ligament, or tendon that causes an afferent response. The efferent reaction to this can be sensory (pins and needles), motor (muscle spasm), and/or autonomic (increased sweating or piloerection). The facilitated segment can occur at any lumbar level, although L4, L5, and S1 are the most common. Further testing for disc herniation, joint hypermobility, a disease state, etc., determines the cause for the facilitated segment.

ASSESSMENT

INTERPRETATION

Interspinous Ligaments
   Firmly palpate the interspinous ligaments with the thumb or index finger for point tenderness.

Any rupture of the supraspinous or interspinous ligaments is not palpable but an increased gap between the processes involved may be apparent.

Paraspinal Muscles

Any trigger points or increased spasm in the erector spinae muscles should be noted.

ILIOCOSTALIS LUMBORUM

Myofascial trigger points in the iliocostalis lumborum muscle occur opposite to the level of the first lumbar vertebrae. These trigger points develop in the deep erector spinae muscles when they are strained in forward bending and rotation. The referred pain extends down from the trigger point to a sensitive area in the central buttock.

MULTIFIDUS AND ROTATORES

Myofascial trigger points in the multifidus and rotatores occur over the upper sacrum (S1) and over the lower sacral foramen. Pain is referred into the sacrum and the medial edge of the central gluteal crease. Myofascial trigger points can be found opposite the first lumbar vertebra—these refer pain to the iliac crest and to the anterior abdominal wall.

Thoracolumbar Fascia

This tissue has three layers that influence the lumbar spine. The anterior layer arises from the lumbar transverse processes and covers the quadratus lumborum. The middle layer arises from the tips of the lumbar transverse processes. The posterior layer arises from the midline and covers the back muscles and serves as the attachment for latissimus dorsi and serratus posterior. All three layers join at the lateral border of the erector spinae muscles, which gives origin to the transversus abdominis and internal obliques.
   This fascia may assist with lumbosacral extension and support the fixed vertebral column and the posterior longitudinal ligament. Any disruption in the fascia may be palpable and can indicate an injury.

Pelvic Ligaments, Sacroiliac Joint Ligaments, Sacrotuberous Ligaments, Iliolumbar Ligaments (See Hip and Pelvis Assessment, Chapter 2)

Quadratus Lumborum

According to Simons and Travell, the quadratus lumborum is an often overlooked source of myofascial low back pain. The trigger points are located in both the superficial and deep portions of the muscle. The superficial portion's trigger points are just below the twelfth rib and just above the iliac crest and pro-

ASSESSMENT

INTERPRETATION

ject pain under the iliac crest and over the greater trochanter area of the hip. The deep portion's trigger points are opposite the L3 transverse process and just above the iliac crest and the L5 transverse process. Pain from the deep fibers spreads into the sacrum and the outer aspect of the lower buttock.

Glutei
  • Gluteus Maximus
  • Gluteus Medius
  • Gluteus Minimus

Tenderness and spasm can occur in the glutei muscles when they are locally injured or secondary to a herniated disc with referred pain. Glutei muscle tone and shape can be lost with nerve root involvement following a lumbar disc herniation. Fibrofatty nodules may be present under the iliac crest and may be point tender. Neuroma of the cluneal nerves, which supply the posterior iliac spine and the iliac tubercles, can cause discomfort on palpation under the crest. If an iliac bone graft has been taken or the area is traumatized, neuromas can develop, causing pain or tingling on palpation.

The myofascial trigger points in gluteus maximus are in the midbelly of the upper, middle, and lower fibers. Pain is referred from the trigger points into the periphery of the muscle and on to the lower part of the sacrum.

The myofascial trigger point in gluteus medius is in the muscle next to the sacrum and the pain is referred into the gluteal area and down the posterior thigh with the concentration of discomfort along the edge of the iliac crest and sacrum.

Another myofascial trigger point for gluteus minimus is in the center of the muscle posteriorly. Pain is referred down the posterior thigh and calf with a pain pattern similar to sciatic pain or referred pain from a L5-S1 disc herniation. A myofascial trigger point for gluteus minimus is in the anterolateral section of the muscle also. Pain is referred down the lateral thigh and lower leg, with a pain pattern similar to the lateral leg pain experienced by a disc herniation at L5-S1.

Piriformis

The piriformis muscle, through overuse or spasm, can compress the sciatic nerve and cause pain down the course of the nerve. The myofascial trigger point in this muscle is midbelly and can cause pain localized in the lateral gluteal area and down the posterior aspect of the thigh, calf, and sole of the foot.

Sciatic Nerve (Fig. 1-64)
Palpate midway between the greater trochanter and the ischial tuberosity over the sciatic nerve for spasm or referred pain. If palpation of the sciatic nerve elicits pain, a side-lying palpation of the nerve can also be done. The athlete lies on his or her side with the hip

Tenderness on local palpation of the sciatic nerve can be caused by the following:
  • herniated disc in the lumbar spine
  • piriformis muscle spasm from overuse (occasionally occurs especially in athletes with coxa retroversion)
  • contused or injured sciatic nerve (rare)
  • dural sleeve adhesions or tightness in the low back area

ASSESSMENT   INTERPRETATION

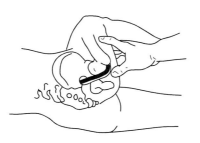

Fig. 1-64 Sciatic nerve palpation (side lying).

and knee flexed to an angle of 90°—palpate the sciatic notch, midway between the ischial tuberosity and the greater trochanter, and then palpate the upper section of the sciatic nerve.

Hamstrings

The hamstrings can go into protective muscle spasm with significant lumbar spine dysfunction.

Specific trigger points in the midbelly of the hamstrings are common. Often, these trigger points are very tender on palpation and are related to significant lumbar conditions (i.e., a disc herniation or spondylolisthesis).

The myofascial trigger point for biceps femoris is midbelly and pain is referred down the posterior thigh and to the upper half of the calf (the locus of pain is in the popliteal space).

The myofascial trigger points for semimembranosus and semitendinosus are at the junction of the posterior thigh and buttock, with referred pain running down to the midleg.

Gastrocnemii

The myofascial trigger point for the gastrocnemius muscle is in the upper section of the muscle, with referred pain extending down the posterior calf and into the sole and particularly the arch of the foot.

Anterior Structures (Supine Position)

Boney
Iliac Crest and Anterior Superior Iliac Spines (Fig. 1-65)
Palpate the crests and spines for level and pelvic asymmetry.

If the crests or spines are not level, palpate the pelvis for obliquity, or determine if muscle spasm may be altering the pelvic position.

Pubic Tubercles (see Fig. 1-65)
Gently palpate the tubercles, then position each thumb on them to deter-

If right posterior iliac rotation exists, the right pubic tubercle will appear higher (superior). If a right sacroiliac upslip is present, the right pubic tubercle will also be higher.

ASSESSMENT

INTERPRETATION

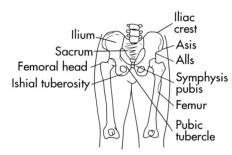

Ilium
Sacrum
Femoral head
Ishial tuberosity

Iliac crest
Asis
Alls
Symphysis pubis
Femur
Pubic tubercle

Fig. 1-65 Anterior structures (boney).

mine if one side is more superior, inferior, anterior, or posterior than the other.

If there is tenderness or asymmetry here, there may be iliosacral dysfunction, symphysis pubis dysfunction, or an adductor strain. Excessive mobility in the sacroiliac joints or sacroiliac joint dysfunction often leads to symphysis pubis point tenderness or dysfunction.

Dysfunction of symphysis pubis can also be primary.

Soft Tissue
Abdominals

Ask the athlete to contract the abdominals while you observe the muscle for symmetry.

Observe the umbilicus for deviation to either side.

Asymmetry in muscle development of the abdominals can result from structural problems (such as scoliosis or leg-length discrepancy) or muscle imbalances caused by injury.

It is important to have symmetry in abdominal strength and good muscle tone to protect the lumbar spine.

Rectus Abdominis

Myofascial trigger points in the rectus abdominis muscle occur at its upper and lower attachments. Pain referred from the upper attachment trigger point causes lower thoracic pain in the back. Pain referred from the lower attachment trigger point causes pain across the sacrum, iliac crest, and upper gluteal area.

Iliopsoas

Iliopsoas myofascial trigger points are common and usually occur with quadratus lumborum trigger points. These trigger points can be felt on deep-pressure palpation lateral to the rectus abdominis. The trigger points are located in the psoas major midbelly, on the inside edge of the iliac crest behind the ASIS, and at the muscle's insertion along the medial wall of the femoral triangle. Pain is referred down the anterior thigh, along the length of the lumbar and sacral spines, and into the sacroiliac joint. This is a pain pattern that is similar to pain that can arise from L2-L3 lumbar problems or femoral nerve pathology.

ASSESSMENT

INTERPRETATION

Adductors
- Adductor longus and brevis
- Adductor magnus

The adductor myofascial trigger points should be palpated because anterior and anteromedial leg pain can also be referred here from the L2-L4 lumbar spine. The adductor longus and brevis have myofascial trigger points in the upper anteromedial aspect of the muscles. Pain is referred down the inner thigh (especially medially above the patella) and down the medial lower leg (i.e., L4 dermatome).

The adductor magnus myofascial trigger point is midbelly with pain referred down the upper anteromedial thigh and over the pelvis.

REFERENCES

Adams MA, Hutton WC, and Stott JRR: The resistance to flexion of the lumbar intervertebral joint, Spine 5:245-253, 1980.

Adams MA and Hutton WC: The mechanical function of the lumbar apophyseal joints, Spine 8 (3):327-330, 1983.

Aggrawal ND et al.: A study of changes in the spine in weight lifters and other athletes, Br J Sports Med 13:58-61, 1979.

Ahmed A, Duncan N, and Burke D: The effect of facet geometry on the axial torque-rotation response of lumbar motion segments, Spine 15 (5):392, 1990.

Alderink GJ: The sacroiliac joint: review of anatomy, mechanics, and function, JOSPT 13(2):71 February 1991.

Anderson JE: Grant's Atlas of anatomy, ed 7, Baltimore, 1980, Williams & Wilkins.

Bemis T and Daniel M: Variation of the long sitting test on subjects with iliosacral dysfunction, J Orthop Sports Phys Ther 8 (7):336, 1987.

Bogduk N and Twomey L: Clinical anatomy of the lumbar spine, New York, 1987, Churchill Livingstone.

Bogduk N and MacIntosh JE: The applied anatomy of the thoracolumbar fascia, Spine 9(2):164, 1984.

Booher JM and Thibodeau GA: Athletic injury assessment, Toronto, 1985, Times Mirror/Mosby College Publishing.

Butler D et al.: Discs degenerate before facets, Spine 15(2):111, 1990.

Butler DS: Mobilization of the nervous system, New York: 1991, Churchill Livingstone.

Cailliet R: Low back pain syndrome, Philadelphia, 1986, FA Davis.

Chan KH: Common low back pain, Univ Toronto Med J 5:91, 1978.

Cyriax J: Textbook of orthopedic medicine—diagnosis of soft tissue lesions, vol 1, London, 1978, Bailliere Tindall.

Cyron BM and Hutton WC: The fatigue strength of the lumbar neural arch in spondylolysis, J Bone Joint Surg 60 (B):234, 1978.

Dangles C and Spencer D: Spondylolysis in competitive weight-lifters, Am J Sports Med 15(6):624, 1987.

Daniels L and Worthingham C: Muscle testing, techniques of manual examination, Toronto, 1980, WB Saunders.

Day A, Friedman W, and Indelicato P: Observations on the treatment of lumbar disk disease in college football players, Am J Sports Med 15(1):72, 1987.

Depodesta M: Lower back, Unpublished paper, 1979.

DeRosa C and Portefield J: Review for advanced orthopedic competencies: the low back and the sacroiliac joint and hip, Chicago, 1989, APTA.

Donatelli R: Physical therapy of the shoulder, New York, 1987, Churchill Livingstone.

Donelson R, Silva G, and Murphy K: Centralization phenomenon, its usefulness in evaluating and treating referred pain, Spine 153:211-213, 1990.

Edwards BC: Manual of combined movements, New York: 1992, Churchill Livingstone.

Elam B and Stanhope W: Segmental instability of the lumbar spine and its management, J Orthop Sports Phys Ther 4(1):3, 1982.

Farfan HF: Mechanical disorders of the low back, Philadelphia, 1973, Lea and Febiger.

Farfan HF et al.: The effects of torsion on the lumbar intervertebral joints: the role of torsion in the production of disc degeneration, J Bone Joint Surgery 52(A):468, 1970.

Fisk James W: The painful neck and back, Illinois, 1977, Charles C Thomas, Publisher.

Freer D: Muscle energy—a therapeutic tool, Unpublished paper presented at CATA conference, May 7, 1987.

Gainor B and others: Biomechanics of the spine in the polevaulter as related to spondylolysis, Am J Sports Med 2(vol II):53, 1983.

Giles LGF and Taylor JR: Low back pain associated with leg length inequality, Spine 6(5):510, 1981.

Goodman C: Low back pain in the cosmetic athlete, Physician Sports Med, 15(8):97, 1987.

Goodman C and Snyder T: Differential diagnosis in physical therapy, Toronto: 1990, W.B. Saunders.

Gould JA and Davies GJ: Orthopaedic and sports physical therapy, Toronto, 1985, Mosby.

Grieve GP: Modern manual therapy of the vertebral column, Edinburgh, 1986, Churchill Livingstone.

Grieve GP: Common vertebral joint problems, ed 2, New York, 1988, Churchill Livingstone.

Gunn Chan C: Reprints on pain, acupuncture, and related subjects, Vancouver, 1979.

Hansson T et al.: The lumbar lordosis in acute and chronic low back pain, Spine 10:154, 1985.

Hensinger R: Current concepts review: spondylolysis and spondylolisthesis in children and adolescents, J Bone Joint Surg 71(A):1098, 1989.

Hesch J: Personal communications: sacroiliac testing, 1989-1990, Unpublished manuscript, 1987.

Hoppenfeld S: Physical examination of the spine and extremities, New York, 1976, Appleton-Century-Crofts.

Inman VT and Saunders JB: Referred pain from skeletal structures, J Nerve Ment Dis 99:660, 1944.

Jackson D and Wiltse L: Low back pain in young athletes, Physician and Sport Med, 11:53, 1974.

Jackson D et al.: Stress reactions involving the pars interarticularis in young athletes, Am J Sports Med 9(5):304, 1981.

Kapandji IA: The physiology of the joints, vol III, The trunk and the vertebral column , New York, 1983, Churchill Livingstone.

Kellgren JH: Observations of referred pain arising from muscle, Clin Sci 3:175, 1938.

Kellgren JH: On the distribution of pain arising from deep somatic structures with charts of segmental pain areas, Clin Sci 4:35, 1939.

Kendall FP and McCreary EK: Muscles testing and function, Baltimore, 1983, Williams & Wilkins.

Kessler RM and Hertling D: Management of common musculoskeletal disorders—physical therapy principles and methods, New York, 1983, Harper & Row.

Klafs CE and Arnheim DD: Modern principles of athletic training, St Louis, 1981, Mosby.

Kornberg C and Lew P: The effect of stretching neural structures on grade one hamstring injuries, J Orthop Sports Phys Ther 6:481, 1989.

Kraus H: Clinical treatment of back and neck pain, New York, 1970, McGraw-Hill.

Kulund DN: The injured athlete, Toronto, 1982, JB Lippincott.

Laban MM et al.: Lumbosacral-anterior pelvic pain associated with pubic symphysis instability, Arch Phys Med Rehabil 56:548, 1975.

Lee D: The pelvic girdle, New York, 1989, Churchill Livingstone.

Loeser JD: Pain due to nerve injury, Spine 10:232, 1985.

Luk KDK et al.: The iliolumbar ligament: a study of its anatomy, development, and clinical significance, J Bone Joint Surg 68:197, 1986.

Magee DJ: Orthopaedics conditions, assessments and treatment, vol II, Alberta, 1979, University of Alberta Publishing.

Magee D: Orthopaedic physical assessment, Toronto, 1987, W. B. Saunders.

Mayer TG and Gatchel RJ: Functional restoration for spinal disorders: the sports medicine approach, Philadelphia, 1988, Lea & Febiger.

McCarroll JR, Miller JM, and Ritter M: Lumbar spondylolysis and spondylolisthesis in college football players, a prospective study, Am J Sports Med 14(5):404, 1986.

McNab I: Backache, Baltimore, 1977, Williams & Wilkins.

McLeod C: A diversified approach for the evaluation and treatment of somatic dysfunction, Course, April 1989, Hamilton, Ontario, Canada.

Mitchell F, Moran P, and Pruzzo N: Evaluation and treatment manual of osteopathic muscle energy procedures, 1979. (Available from Mitchell, Moran, and Pruzzo, 911 Hazel Falls Dr., Manchester, Mo. 63011).

Mooney V and Robertson J: The facet syndrome, Clin Orthop 115:149, 1976.

O'Donaghue D: Treatment of injuries to athletes, Toronto, 1984, W.B. Saunders Co.

O'Neill D and Mitcheli LJ: Postoperative radiographic evidence for fatigue fracture as the etiology in spondylolysis, Spine 14(12):1343, 1989.

Panjabi M, Krag M, and Chung T: Effects of disc injury on mechanical behavior of the human spine, Spine 9(7):707, 1984.

Peterson L and Renstrom P: Sports injuries, their prevention and treatment, Chicago, 1986, Year Book Medical Pub, Inc.

Pope M: Bioengineering—the bond between basic scientists, clinicians and engineers—The 1989 Presidential Address, Spine 15(3):214, 1990.

Porterfield JA: Dynamic stabilization of the trunk, J Orthop Sports Phys Ther 6(5):271, 1985.

Porterfield JA and DeRosa C: Mechanical low back pain, Toronto, 1991, W.B. Saunders.

Reid DC: Functional anatomy and joint mobilization, Alberta, 1970, University of Alberta Publishing.

Reid DC: Sports Injury Assessments and Rehabilitation, New York, 1992, Churchill Livingstone.

Revere G: Low back pain in athletes, Physician Sports Med 15(1):105, 1987.

Roy S and Irvin R: Sports medicine, prevention, evaluation, management and rehabilitation, Englewood Cliffs, NJ, 1983, Prentice-Hall.

Ruge D and Wiltse LL: Spinal disorder diagnosis and treatment, Philadelphia, 1977, Lea & Febiger.

Saunders D: Classification of musculoskeletal spinal conditions, J Orthop Sports Phys Ther 1(1), 1979.

Shiquing X, Quanzhi Z, and Dehao F: Significance of the straight-leg raise test in the diagnosis and clinical evaluation of lower lumbar intervertebral disc protrusion, J Bone Joint Surg 69A(4):517, 1987.

Simons DG: Myofascial pain syndromes. In Basmajan V and Kirby C (eds): Medical rehabilitation, Baltimore, 1984, Williams and Wilkins.

Simons DG: Myofascial pain syndromes due to trigger points, Manual Med 1:72, 1985.

Simons DG and Travell JG: Myofascial origins of low back pain. 1: Principles of diagnosis and treatment. 2: Torso muscles. 3: Pelvic and lower extremity muscles, Post grad Med 73(2):81, 1983.

Smyth MJ and Wright V: Sciatica and the intervertebral disc. An experimental study, J Bone Joint Surg 40(A):1401, 1959.

Stanitski C: Low back pain in young athletes, Physician Sports Med 10(10):77, 1982.

Taylor JR and Twomey LT: Age changes in lumbar zygaphophyseal joints—observations on structure and function, Spine 11(7):739, 1986.

Torgerson WR and Dotter WE: Comparative roentgenographic study of the asymptomatic and symptomatic lumbar spine, J Bone Joint Surg 58(A):850, 1976.

Travell JG and Simons DG: Myofascial pain and dysfunction—the trigger point manual, Baltimore, 1983, Williams & Wilkins.

Twomey L and Taylor JR (eds): Physical therapy of the low back. Clinics in physical therapy, New York, 1987, Churchill Livingstone.

Vleeming A et al.: Relation between form and function in the sacroiliac joint. Part 1: Clinical anatomical aspects, Spine 15(2):130, 1990.

Vleeming A et al.: Relation between form and function in the sacroiliac joint. Part 2: Biomechanical aspects, Spine 15(2):133, 1990.

Urban LM: The straight leg raising test—a review, J Orthop Sports Phys Ther 2(3):117, 1981.

Walker J: Age-related difference in the human sacroiliac joint: a histological study; implications for therapy, J Orthop Sports Med 7(6):325, 1986.

Warwick R and Williams PL: Gray's Anatomy, ed 35, London, 1978, Longman Inc.

White AA and Panjabi MM: Clinical biomechanics of the spine, Toronto, 1978, JB Lippincott.

Wilder DG et al.: The functional topography of the sacroiliac joint, 1980, Spine 5:575.

Wiley J, McNab I, and Wortzman G: Lumbar discography and its clinical applications, Can J Surg 11:280, 1968.

Williams P and Warenick R: Gray's anatomy, New York, 1980, Churchill Livingstone.

Wiltse L, Widell E, and Jackson D: Fatigue fracture—the basic lesion in isthmic spondylolisthesis, J Bone Joint Surg 57A(1):17, 1975.

Wooden Michael J: Preseason screening of the lumbar spine, J Orthop Sports Phys Ther 3:6, 1981.

Workshop—The low-back dilemma: an eclectic approach to evaluation and treatment, Williamsburg, Virginia, Nov, 1989, Faculty included Carl DeRosa, James Gould, Florence Kendall, Michael MacQueen, Stanley Paris, Walter Personius, and Philip Tehan.

Yamamoto I et al: Three-dimensional movements of the whole lumbar spine and lumbosacral joint, Spine, 14(11):1256, 1989.

Yasuma T: Histological development of intervertebral disc herniation, J Bone Joint Surg 68A(7):1066, 1986.

Zohn DA: Musculoskeletal pain diagnosis and physical treatment, ed 2, Toronto, 1988, Little, Brown and Co.

CHAPTER 2

Hip and Pelvis assessment

The pelvic girdle is the link between the lower extremities and the spine. The lumbar spine, sacrum, ilia, and lower extremities all influence one another. Dysfunction in one of these structures leads to dysfunction in the others. Any problems in the pelvis, spine, or hip will directly affect the athlete's upper quadrant also. Any athlete who uses the upper quadrant for their sport will also be severely hampered by a lower quadrant injury (e.g., pitcher, tennis, basketball, etc.). This concept is important to remember when assessing and rehabilitating any segment.

During normal ambulation or sporting activities, several muscles link the lumbar spine, sacrum, pelvis, femur, patella, tibia, and fibula into one kinetic chain. Any muscle imbalance or injury can therefore influence the entire kinetic chain and athletic performance will be affected. Some of the key muscles include:

- Psoas major—influences the lumbar spine, pelvis, and femur
- Rectus femoris—influences the pelvis and patella
- Biceps femoris—influences the pelvis and fibula
- Piriformis—influences the sacrum and femur
- Iliacus—influences the pelvis and femur
- Tensor fascia lata and iliotibial band—influence the pelvis and femur
- Semitendinosus and semimembranosus—influence the pelvis and tibia
- Sartorius—influences the pelvis and tibia
- Gluteus medius—influences the pelvis and femur
- Gluteus maximus—influences the pelvis and femur

The coordination and synchronization of these muscles has an influence on all locomotor actions. Consequently, all these muscles should be tested when the function of the hip and pelvis is being assessed. Ligaments and fascia also connect the lumbar spine, pelvis, and femur and should be tested when this area is being assessed. Important ligaments and fascia include:

- lumbodorsal fascia
- iliolumbar ligament
- iliofemoral ligament
- lateral fascia of the thigh
- sacroiliac ligament
- sacrotuberous ligament
- sacrospinous ligament
- ischiofemoral ligament
- pubofemoral ligament
- iliotibial band

The hip joint's fibrous capsule can also influence the lower limb kinetic chain: restrictions, contractures, or laxity in the capsule can result in hip joint dysfunction and quadrant mechanical problems. The joints that directly influence one another in this region include:

- hip joint
- sacroiliac joint
- symphysis pubis
- L5-S1 facet joints

It is important that the boney structure and muscle groups be symmetrically balanced in each plane surrounding the pelvic girdle. If the pelvis is not symmetric, muscle imbalances occur, and with time some muscles will develop tightness while their antagonists will develop stretch weakness.

SAGITTAL PLANE

Anterior or Posterior Pelvic Tilt

The pelvis should not be in an excessive anterior or posterior pelvic tilt.

If an anterior pelvic tilt exists, the lumbar spine moves into excessive lordosis, the hip flexors and lumbar erector spinae shorten and become tight, and the abdominals, glutei, and hamstrings become stretched and weakened.

If a posterior pelvic tilt exists, the lumbar spine moves into a flat-back position (extends), the hip flexors and erector spinae become weak, and the hamstrings, adductor magnus, and glutei become tight.

This anterior or posterior pelvic tilt can lead to

the muscle imbalances indicated and can also subject the hip joint, the sacroiliac joint, and the lumbar spine to abnormal forces and loads.

Anterior or Posterior Ilium Rotation

Each ilium can also become rotated independently into a position of anterior or posterior ilium (or innominate) rotation. If a unilateral posterior iliac rotation exists, the gluteus muscles, hamstrings, and adductor magnus on that side become shortened and tight. The hip flexors, sartorius, and remaining adductors become stretched and weak on the affected side. If unilateral anterior iliac rotation exists, the hip flexors, adductors, and tensor fascia lata become tight on that side while the hamstrings, glutei, and abdominals become stretched and weak. Anterior or posterior iliac rotation can cause these muscle imbalances or these rotations can be the result of muscle imbalances. These rotations can cause sacroiliac joint dysfunction and eventual hip and lumbar spine problems.

FRONTAL PLANE

The structures and muscles in this plane must also be balanced and symmetric.

If one leg is longer, the ilium on that side is elevated, which causes unbalanced forces through the sacroiliac joint, hip joint, pubic symphysis, sacrum, lumbar spine, and the entire lower limb. Altered weight-bearing forces also go through the opposite side.

On the elevated side the quadratus lumborum, iliocostalis lumborum, iliopsoas, obliques, and rectus abdominus become tight while the hamstrings, adductors, rectus femoris, sartorius, and tensor fascia lata become stretched and weak—the opposite muscle imbalances occur on the side of the shorter leg. The lumbar spine laterally tilts and rotates with this asymmetry.

This lateral pelvic tilt can also occur with weakness in the abductors on the opposite hip (especially gluteus medius). This becomes particularly noticeable when the athlete stands on one leg, during ambulation, or when the abductor is eccentrically loaded.

TRANSVERSE PLANE

Either ilium can be inflared (one ilium ASIS is closer to the midline than the opposite ASIS) or outflared (one ilium ASIS is farther from the midline than the opposite ASIS), which with time will lead to muscle imbalances.

On the inflare side the adductors, obliques, and sartorius become tight while the gluteus medius, minimus, and tensor fascia lata become stretched and weak.

On the outflare side the gluteus medius, minimus, and tensor fascia lata become tight while the adductors, obliques, and sartorius become stretched and weak.

These muscle imbalances twist the pelvic girdle and cause excessive rotational forces through the lumbar spine and the entire lower limb on the involved side. The hip joint becomes rotated and the symphysis pubis, sacroiliac joint, or lumbar spine may develop dysfunction.

HIP JOINT

The hip joint is very stable yet mobile. It is stable because of its deep cuplike acetabulum, strong capsule and capsular ligaments, and its surrounding powerful musculature. The multiaxial ball and socket design gives it mobility.

It is part of the closed kinetic chain of the lower limb and trunk; therefore any problem in the foot, knee, or ankle is transmitted superiorly to the hip, whereas any pelvis or lumbar dysfunction is transmitted inferiorly to the hip joint. Conversely, hip dysfunction can cause problems in the lower limb or upper body, especially during weight bearing. Any hip problem will affect gait, lifting, and any daily activity that involves forward bending.

The position of the pelvis is very important when observing and testing the hip joint. Most of the hip muscles originate on the pelvis, so the pelvis must be fixed when the hip joint is tested. The position of the lumbar spine influences the pelvis and hip joint; therefore the athlete may need to do a pelvic tilt before testing is carried out to stabilize and eliminate spinal involvement.

The capsular pattern for the hip joint is the greatest limitation in medial (internal) rotation and abduction, slightly limited flexion and extension, and full lateral (external) rotation. (Kaltenborn includes a limitation of external rotation.)

The resting position or loose-packed position of the hip joint is 30° of hip flexion and 30° abduction with slight lateral rotation.

The close-packed position of the hip joint is full extension and medial rotation. (Kaltenborn includes abduction.)

PELVIS

The pelvis acts as a base for the lower extremities and is in turn affected by lower-limb imbalances or leg-length discrepancy. Forces reaching the pelvis that are asymmetric can result in joint adaptations above or below the pelvis; e.g., a leg-length discrepancy can cause scoliosis. The primary function of the pelvis (including the muscles, joints, ligaments, and bones) is the mechanical transfer of weight, and secondarily, protection of the viscera (genitals, uterus, ovaries, prostate, lower intestine, bladder, rectum, blood vessels, and nerves). The pelvis has a significant role in supporting the spinal column and therefore can affect the vertebral joints, the upper extremity, and even the position of the skull. When the pelvis is fixed, the hip and spine are free to move. When the spine is fixed, the pelvis and hip are free to move. If dysfunction causes hypo- or hyper-mobility in any of these areas (spine, pelvis, or hip), all three areas will be affected.

SYMPHYSIS PUBIS

The symphysis pubis moves very little (approximately 2 mm) and is rarely injured. Hypermobility problems that develop in the sacroiliac joints can cause symptoms at the symphysis pubis and adductor muscles. Conversely, problems with the adductor muscles or symphysis pubis can also cause discomfort at the sacroiliac joint.

SACROILIAC JOINT

The sacrum is often described as the keystone of the arch of the pelvis. The sacroiliac joints on either side are synovial joints. The sacroiliac joint has only a little joint play and is commonly injured because of overuse mechanisms, especially if a leg-length discrepancy exists. It is a very stable joint that is more mobile in youth and decreases in mobility as the athlete ages. It can become less stable with trauma, overuse, or multiple pregnancies. When equal amounts of force are experienced from the extremities to the pelvis, mobility of the ilium on the sacrum is symmetric. When uneven forces (caused by a leg-length difference or abnormal lower limb mechanics) are experienced, then the sacroiliac joint may adapt by becoming dysfunctional.

L5-S1 APOPHYSEAL OR FACET JOINTS

The body and facet joints of S1 articulate with the body and facets of L5.

Forces from the trunk are transferred through these joints to the pelvis. If there is frontal plane pelvic asymmetry, the L5-S1 facet on the lower side will be distracted while on the elevated side it will be compressed. In time, this can lead to facet joint degeneration. Rotational forces from the pelvis or hip also cause excess shearing forces through the facet joints.

ASSESSMENT

INTERPRETATION

HISTORY

Mechanism of Injury
Direct Trauma
   Was it direct trauma?

Contusion

Contusions are fairly common to the boney prominences like the iliac crest, greater trochanter, ischial tuberosity, pubic bone, and the posterior superior iliac spine. These injuries usually occur in contact sports. For example, when a football player is tackled (Fig. 2-1) or when a hockey player is checked into the boards.

ASSESSMENT   INTERPRETATION

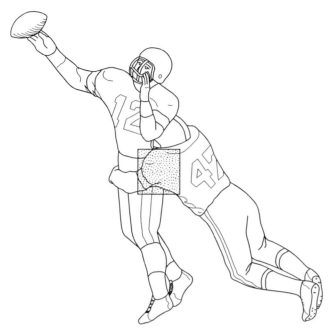

Fig. 2-1 Direct trauma— mechanism of iliac crest contusion.

Iliac Crest

Iliac crest contusions (hip pointer) can be very painful and disabling especially if the periosteum is involved. A hematoma develops along the periosteum of the crest where the boney tissue is very pain sensitive (Fig. 2-2). This should be differentiated from a muscle avulsion or tear. The muscles in the area go into spasm and walking can be painful.

Sacrum

Sacral contusions can occur because the sacrum is so vulnerable and superficial. Football and hockey players wear sacral pads to help protect or minimize these injuries. Fracture may need to be ruled out.

Buttock

Buttock contusions are frequent and usually involve injury to the musculature. A blow to the ischial tuberosity area may cause severe pain and local tenderness.

Sciatic nerve

Sciatic nerve contusions can cause pain along the nerve but the possibility of referred pain from a lower back problem needs to be ruled out.

Pubis

Contusions of the descending ramus of the pubis occasionally occur when a split-legged fall occurs (e.g., over a bar during gymnastics), or from a saddle injury while horseback riding.

ASSESSMENT

INTERPRETATION

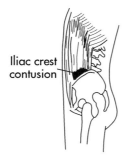

Iliac crest
contusion

Fig. 2-2 Iliac crest contusion (hip pointer).

Scrotum

Scrotum contusions can occur frequently during sports, but protection with athletic supports can help prevent or lessen the severity of the injury.

Femoral Triangle

Femoral triangle area contusions are uncommon but can occur with possible damage to the femoral nerve, artery, or vein. The major effect of injury to the femoral nerve can be paralysis of the quadriceps and decreased cutaneous sensation on the anterior medial thigh.

Obturator Nerve

Irritation of the obturator nerve causes referred pain to the medial thigh or knee joint.

Greater Trochanter

The greater trochanter can be contused easily from falls on the side (e.g., sliding during baseball), and if the force is significant, trochanteric bursitis can result.

Fractures

Fractures of the hip and pelvis are rare because of the protective musculature and the use of protective athletic equipment. Generally, forces greater than sporting forces are necessary to cause a pelvic ring or hip fracture. Some have been reported in cycling, horseback riding, hang gliding and snowmobiling. Fractures that do occur are listed below.

Intertrochanteric

Intertrochanteric fractures occur as a result of a fall, with both direct and indirect forces being responsible—the indirect forces are the pull of the iliopsoas and the abductor muscles on the lesser and greater trochanters; the direct forces act down the axis of the femur, causing the fracture.

Subtrochanteric

Subtrochanteric fractures are extremely rare, but can occur in younger athletes from direct trauma of considerable force.

ASSESSMENT	INTERPRETATION

Sacrum

Sacral fractures are rare; when they do occur they are usually transverse or stellate (star shaped). They are acutely painful. If the fracture is displaced, there is the possibility of rectal damage.

Ischial Tuberosity

Ischial tuberosity fractures can occur, but more commonly the blow causes periosteitis on the boney surface. Ischial tuberosity bursitis can also develop here from trauma.

Acetabulum

Fracture of the acetabulum is infrequent in athletes. If it does occur, the fracture is usually along the margin of the acetabulum. The acetabulum labrum may be torn from a twisting mechanism.

Femoral Neck (Fig. 2-3)

A femoral neck fracture is more common in the older athlete who has osteoporosis. In a young person, considerable force is needed to fracture the neck of the femur. The fracture can occur as a result of a direct blow along the femoral shaft or over the trochanter, or a rotational force through the femur. The injured limb is held in lateral rotation and the leg appears shortened.

Epiphyses

Fractures of the epiphysis in the adolescent athlete can occur to the proximal femur, the greater trochanter, or the capital femoral epiphysis (Fig. 2-4).

Dislocation

Hip joint dislocations are rarely sustained by athletes, although they are more common than fractures in the adolescent group. Hip joint dislocations usually occur only when a violent force is exerted on a flexed hip and knee joint or a force is transmitted along the femur in an abducted hip position. Dislocations are a medical emergency and must be x-rayed and treated as

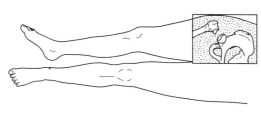

Fig. 2-3 Femoral neck fracture. The injured limb is laterally rotated with a shortened limb length on that side.

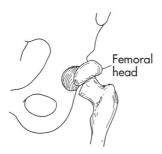

Fig. 2-4 Fractured capital femoral epiphysis.

ASSESSMENT   INTERPRETATION

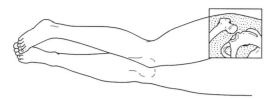

Fig. 2-5 Hip joint dislocation. The hip joint is flexed, adducted, and internally rotated.

soon as possible. The femoral head blood supply can be disturbed, resulting in avascular necrosis of the femoral head. A delay in reduction compromises the blood supply.

Posterior Hip Dislocation

The greater trochanter is prominent and the hip stays flexed, adducted, and internally rotated as a result of a posterior dislocation (Fig. 2-5). An associated posterior ring fracture can occur with this dislocation in the adolescent athlete. On occasion, the sciatic nerve can also be damaged.

Anterior Hip Joint Dislocation

With an anterior dislocation, the hip is held abducted, externally rotated, and in slight flexion. The femoral head is palpable and, on occasion, the femoral nerve can be damaged as well.

Slipped Capital Femoral Epiphysis

In the young athlete, a slipped capital femoral epiphysis (see Fig. 2-4) can occur as a result of relatively minor trauma. Pain is usually in the groin and anteromedial aspect of the thigh and often can be referred to the knee. This injury is often sustained by preadolescent or adolescent male athletes (ages 10 to 15) who are endomorphic in build and in whom the development of secondary sex characteristics is delayed. The athlete develops an antalgic gait and limb external rotation. The slip may be from an acute injury (fall on one leg) or chronic condition (progressive slip). The chronic slip may have an insidious onset and this slippage shows a correlation to a hormonal imbalance. There is an increase in the ratio of growth hormones to sex hormones. The capital epiphysis becomes displaced posteriorly and inferiorly, while the femoral neck moves anteriorly and superiorly on the capital epiphysis. As the slippage progresses the hip loses its ability to internally rotate and the hip tends to abduct and externally rotate during hip flexion.

Bursitis (Fig. 2-6)
Greater Trochanter Bursa

The greater trochanter bursa is the most commonly injured bursa around the hip. Bursitis can develop from a direct blow, but it more commonly develops because of overuse. Other caus-

ASSESSMENT   INTERPRETATION

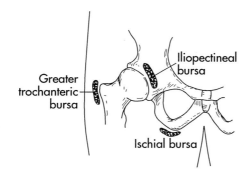

Fig. 2-6 Hip bursae locations.

es include weakness of gluteus medius on the opposite side, a leg-length difference, or incorrect running mechanics.

Ischial Bursa

Ischial bursitis is most often caused by prolonged sitting or occasionally from a direct blow to the ischial bursa as a result of a fall.

Iliopectineal Bursa

Iliopectineal (iliopsoas) bursitis is usually caused by overuse of the iliopsoas muscle, but it can develop because of direct trauma. The hip assumes a position of flexion and external rotation.

Overstretch
Was it an overstretch?

A number of muscles that attach to the pelvis and lower limb are strained or avulsed. The primary reason is that many of the muscles cross two joints and can be easily overstretched. Strains also occur when a muscle is on stretch and is contracting eccentrically. In kicking and contact sports the leg is often forced into a flexed, extended, or abducted position, leading to strains or avulsions, depending on the age of the athlete.

Hip Flexion with Knee Extension

Hip flexion and forced knee extension can cause a hamstring muscle strain, tear, or avulsion as it contracts eccentrically. Injury to the hamstrings can occur at the point of origin, insertion, or at the midbelly location. Some researchers now believe that muscles only tear at their weakest point, which is the musculotendinous junction.

An avulsion fracture of the ischial tuberosity can occur, particularly in the adolescent whose epiphyses are not yet closed (Fig. 2-7). It can also occur in the dancer, gymnast, or cheerleader who performs anterior-posterior splits.

A strain or tear of the long head of the biceps femoris muscle at its point of origin is most common. This injury occurs in football punters, gymnasts, soccer kickers, and divers. A muscle imbalance between the quadriceps and hamstrings is often sug-

ASSESSMENT   INTERPRETATION

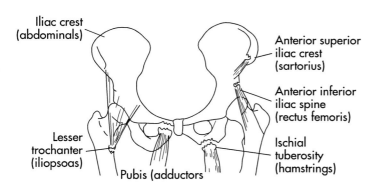

Iliac crest
(abdominals)

Anterior superior
iliac crest
(sartorius)

Anterior inferior
iliac spine
(rectus femoris)

Lesser
trochanter
(iliopsoas)

Ischial
tuberosity
(hamstrings)

Pubis (adductors)

Fig. 2-7 Avulsion fractures to the epiphyseal growth plates.

gested as the reason for this injury—the hamstrings should have at least 60% to 70% of the strength of the quadriceps. Poor hamstring and/or low back flexibility, an inadequate warmup, and overtraining or fatigue are other causes of this injury. Also, hamstring strains and tears occur more frequently with a hip joint injury, superior tibiofibular joint hypermobility or hypomobility, and lumbar or sacroiliac dysfunction.

Hip Extension with Knee Extension (Fig. 2-8)

Hip extension with forced knee extension can cause an iliopsoas strain or tear at its point of attachment to the lesser trochanter of the femur or in the musculotendinous junction as it contracts eccentrically. It can also cause an avulsion fracture that can pull the lesser trochanter off. The hip ligaments can sprain, especially the inferior band of the iliofemoral ligament, which is tautest. Additionally, the abdominal muscles can become damaged at their point of attachment near the inguinal ligament or on the pubis.

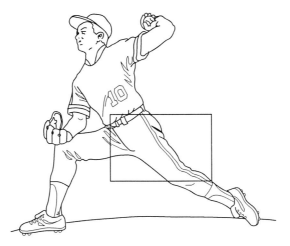

Fig. 2-8 Overstretch in hip extension with knee extension.

ASSESSMENT   INTERPRETATION

Hip Extension with Knee Flexion

Hip extension with forced knee flexion can cause damage to all the structures above, but the rectus femoris muscle is most susceptible to a strain or tear because it is stretched over the hip and knee joint.

Hip Abduction (Fig. 2-9)

Forced hip abduction can cause the following:
- strain of a hip adductor muscle
- tear or avulsion of the adductor longus, brevis, magnus, gracilis, and pectineus
- avulsion fracture of one of the adductors, usually adductor longus—the adductors at the ischiopubic rami seem to be the most vulnerable to injury
- avulsion fracture of the lesser trochanter.

Forceful bilateral abduction (straddle) can sprain the pubic ligaments joining the pubic symphysis, especially in the adolescent (according to Hanson et al. and Liebert et al.)—the pubofemoral and ischiofemoral ligaments can spain or tear.

Hip Medial Rotation

Forced hip medial rotation can cause the following:
- hip lateral rotator strain or tear of the piriformis, obturator internus, obturator externus, gluteus medius, gluteus maximus, quadratus femoris, and gemelli
- posterior ischiofemoral ligament sprain or tear
- lateral hip capsule sprain or tear

Hip Lateral Rotation

Forced hip lateral rotation can cause the following:
- hip medial rotator strain or tear (the tensor fascia lata, gluteus medius, or gluteus minimus [anterior fibers])
- iliofemoral ligament sprain or tear
- pubofemoral ligament sprain or tear
- medial hip capsule sprain or tear

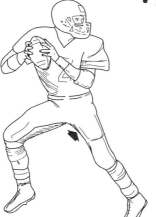

Fig. 2-9 Overstretch in hip abduction.

ASSESSMENT   INTERPRETATION

Trunk Lateral Flexion

Trunk lateral flexion can cause the hip and abdominal muscles to be strained or avulsed (hip pointer) if the trunk is forced into lateral flexion while these muscles are contracting.

Overuse
Was it an overuse repetitive mechanism?

Trunk Rotation
Trunk rotation over a fixed hip or foot (i.e., a position assumed during paddling, baseball pitching, and javelin throwing). Repeated hip rotation over a fixed pelvis, (i.e., during ballet, gymnastics; by assuming a poor form while posing, or running with poor mechanical form).

Repeated trunk rotation over a fixed hip or repeated hip rotation with a fixed pelvis can put stress on the lateral or medial rotators.

Hip Lateral Rotation

Repeated stress to the hip lateral rotators can lead to the following:
- piriformis syndrome, or activation of piriformis myofascial trigger points
- hip joint capsulitis
- hip joint synovitis

Hip Medial Rotation

Repeated stress to the hip medial rotators can lead to the following:
- gluteus medius tendonitis or activation of gluteus medius myofascial trigger points
- hip joint capsulitis
- hip joint synovitis

Hip Flexion
For example, during football punting and gymnastics posing.

Repeated hip flexion can lead to the following:
- rectus femoris tendonitis or activation of rectus femoris myofascial trigger points
- sartorius tendonitis or activation of sartorius myofascial trigger points
- iliopsoas tendonitis or activation of iliopsoas myofascial trigger points
- iliopectineal bursitis

Hip Extension and Knee Extension
For example, while weight lifting, volleyball setting, basketball shooting.

Repeated hip extension and knee extension in the standing position can lead to the following:
- greater trochanteric bursitis

ASSESSMENT

INTERPRETATION

- iliopsoas tendonitis or activation of iliopsoas myofascial trigger points
- rectus femoris, sartorius or tensor fascia lata strain, or activation of the muscles' myofascial trigger points

Hip and Knee Flexion and Extension

For example, doing repeated sit ups, rowing, running, high-jumping, hurdling, and long-jumping.

Repeated hip and knee flexion and extension can lead to iliopsoas tendonitis or bursitis.

Vertical Shearing Forces (Fig. 2-10)

Vertical shearing forces exerted on an asymmetric pelvis (e.g., during running, jumping, and kicking).

Repeated vertical shearing forces to an asymmetric pelvis or to an athlete who has a leg-length difference can lead to the following:

- sacroiliitis
- osteitis pubis
- adductor tendonitis, strain or activation of adductor myofascial trigger points
- gluteus medius tendonitis or activation of gluteus medius myofascial trigger points
- quadratus lumborum tendonitis, strain or activation of myofascial trigger points

Hip adduction

For example, during soccerball passing and swimming whipkick.

Repeated adduction can lead to the following:
- adductor tendonitis (especially to the adductor longus) or activation of the adductor myofascial trigger points
- osteitis pubis—repeated contraction of the adductors pulls one side of the pubis inferiorly, causing a shearing force at the symphysis pubis

Greater Trochanteric Bursitis

Running can cause a greater trochanteric bursitis, which can develop in a runner when the iliotibial band irritates the bursa. This irritation occurs when the iliotibial band moves anterior to the greater trochanter with hip flexion and posterior during hip

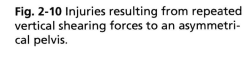

Sacroiliitis (shearing action on the sacroiliac joint)

Adductor tendonitis

Osteitis pubis (shearing action on the pubic symphysis)

Fig. 2-10 Injuries resulting from repeated vertical shearing forces to an asymmetrical pelvis.

ASSESSMENT

INTERPRETATION

extension. This occurs in the runner who has any of the following:

- a wide pelvis
- lack of flexibility in the iliotibial band and/or quadratus lumborum
- increased supination at the subtalar joint
- excessive wear on the posterolateral heel of the running shoe
- a leg-length difference
- muscle imbalance between hip adductors and abductors
- weakness of gluteus medius
- abnormal running mechanics (especially crossover running gait)
- running on a banked or slippery surface

Ischial Bursitis

Ischial bursitis, chronic hamstring strains, and hamstring syndrome* can develop in the adolescent runner doing hill or speed work.

*Hamstring syndrome—a tendinous fibrotic band of the biceps femoris muscle at its point of insertion that irritates the sciatic nerve (according to Puranen and Orava).

Stress Fractures

Stress fractures of the hip and pelvis are relatively uncommon. These usually occur in the long-distance runner who overtrains.

Pelvis stress fractures are seen in the ischial pubic ramus and are more common in women. The site depends on the muscle that is overused; the adductors medially or the hamstrings laterally will cause the ramus breakdown.

Stress fractures of the iliac crest or epiphysis of the anterior iliac crest can occur in the adolescent runner who swings his or her arms across the body.

Stress fractures can occur in the lesser trochanter, femoral neck, or proximal femur. Deep anterior groin pain and an antalgic gait with pain at the extremes of hip motion are key signs.

A femoral neck stress fracture, if complete, can cause displacement of the femoral head and severe complications.

Others

Runners with functional or structural leg-length discrepancies can develop sacroiliitis, osteitis pubis, and/or adductor tendonitis.

Explosive Muscle Contraction

Was it a single explosive muscle contraction (e.g., sprinter, jumper)?

One explosive muscle concentric or eccentric contraction can cause muscle strains, tears, or avulsions. These injuries usually

ASSESSMENT

INTERPRETATION

Were there repeated contractions of a strained muscle?

Was an explosive contraction sustained by an adolescent athlete?

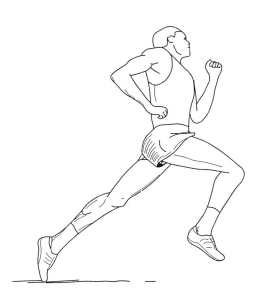

Fig. 2-11 Sprinter—frequent hamstring strains.

occur with a powerful contraction that accelerates or decelerates the body. Often a hamstring muscle strain occurs at the start of a sprinter's race or at the time the jumper takes off for a jump (Fig. 2-11). The muscle can strain if it is fatigued, inflexible, or if a muscle imbalance exists between the muscle groups. The hamstring strain is the most common injury, but a rectus femoris, iliopsoas, or an adductor muscle strain can also occur.

Repeated contractions of the strained muscle can lead to a chronic lesion with scar tissue developing at the lesion site. This can occur in the hamstrings, adductors (especially longus), iliopsoas, or rectus femoris muscles.

In the teenage athlete (usually between the ages of 13 to 17 years) whose epiphyseal growth plates are not completely closed, the following structures can be avulsed (see Fig. 2-7):

- The anterior superior iliac crest or spine can be avulsed by a forceful contraction of the sartorius muscle during sprinting, jumping, or hyperextension of the trunk.
- The anterior inferior iliac spine can be avulsed by the rectus femoris during a violent hip-flexion contraction, usually in the sprinter who is leaving the starting blocks (also long jumpers, football players, cross-country runners).
- The ischial tuberosity can be avulsed by the hamstrings from a violent hip extension with the pelvis fixed in an anterior pelvic tilt and the knee in extension (i.e., hurdling, gymnastics, running, football, dance).
- The lesser trochanter can be avulsed by the iliopsoas muscle during vigorous running, but this is rare.
- The iliac crest can be avulsed by the abdominal muscles (usually the external oblique muscles) from a sudden contraction of the abdominal muscles with an abrupt change in direction while running (Godsall and Hansen).

Reenacting the Mechanism

Demonstrate the mechanism with the opposite limb or by the repetitive movement that aggravates the injury.

Demonstrating the injury mechanism or the movement that aggravates the lesion often clarifies the athlete's verbal description. Note if the athlete was weight bearing at the time of a direct blow because if the leg or body is hit while the foot is fixed, the injury sustained is more serious (i.e., ligaments can be sprained more severely or can be torn and contusions are more severe—even a fracture can occur).

Nature and Forces of the Sport

Determine the nature and forces of the sport.

Determining the nature and mechanics of the sport helps you understand the degree of injury. Understanding the mechanics is particularly important when you are dealing with an overuse injury.

Insidious Onset

Slipped Capital Femoral Epiphysis

Pain in the groin or medial part of the thigh or knee may be present for months or years in the chronic case. Weakness and

ASSESSMENT	INTERPRETATION

loss of hip medial rotation especially with knee extension (leg-roll test) are usually present. The cause is unclear but a hormonal imbalance is suspected. This occurs more frequently in boys than girls. The slip may be small initially but the femoral cap can progress inferiorly and posteriorly with time (for more details see Dislocation).

Pain

Location (Fig. 2-12, A and B)
  Where is the pain located?

Local

Local point tenderness usually indicates a more superficial lesion—local superficial pain is caused by injury to the following:
  • skin and superficial fascia
  • superficial muscles and tendons (e.g., hamstring muscle strain or tendonitis, rectus femoris muscle strain or tendonitis, adductor muscle strain or tendonitis, sartorius muscle strain or tendonitis, and gluteus maximus muscle strain)
  • superficial ligaments—most ligaments are deep and do not give a localized pain (e.g., symphysis pubis ligaments)
  • bursae (e.g., greater trochanteric and iliopectineal)
  • periosteum (e.g., iliac crest contusions and avulsions; pubis contusions, avulsions, and osteitis pubis; ischial tuberosity contusions and avulsions; and anterior superior or anterior inferior iliac spine avulsions)
  • nerves (e.g., femoral nerve contusion or impingement, sciatic nerve contusion or impingement, and anterior or lateral cutaneous nerve impingement)

Diffuse

Diffuse pain, which is pain that is not well localized, is often caused by an injury to a deep somatic or neural structure.

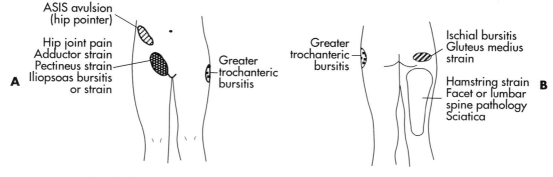

Fig. 2-12 A, Local pain sites, anterior view. **B,** Local and referred pain sites, posterior view.

ASSESSMENT

INTERPRETATION

Referred (see Fig. 2-12, B)

Since the hip joint is formed mainly from the third lumbar segment, true hip joint pain is referred to the groin, the front of the thigh, and occasionally down the front of the leg along the dermatome. It is a very deep pain that can extend to the knee but rarely any further.

MYOTOME

A deep muscle injury can refer pain segmentally to that myotome or along the length of the muscle. Such pain can be caused by:
- gluteus medius strain or tendonitis
- lateral rotators, especially piriformis tendonitis
- deep adductors strain or tendonitis
- pectineus strain

SCLEROTOME

A deep capsular ligamentous injury can refer pain segmentally to the involved sclerotome. The fibrous capsule of the hip or the hip joint itself can refer pain along the myotome or sclerotome. A fracture can cause radiating pain along the length of the bone and in that sclerotome.

The genitofemoral pain of hip osteoarthritis also is referred into the thigh, and eventually even the knee may experience stiffness in the morning.

DEEP AND CUTANEOUS NERVES (FIG. 2-13)

Deep and cutaneous nerves can refer pain along a nerve, usually distally from the traumatized or impinged area. These deep nerves include the following:
- sciatic
- femoral
- obturator

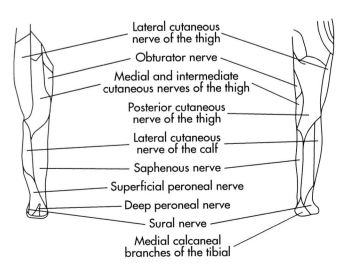

Lateral cutaneous nerve of the thigh
Obturator nerve
Medial and intermediate cutaneous nerves of the thigh
Posterior cutaneous nerve of the thigh
Lateral cutaneous nerve of the calf
Saphenous nerve
Superficial peroneal nerve
Deep peroneal nerve
Sural nerve
Medial calcaneal branches of the tibial

Fig. 2-13 Cutaneous nerve supply of the lower limb.

ASSESSMENT

INTERPRETATION

The cutaneous nerves of the upper leg include the following:
- lateral
- medial
- posterior
- obturator
- anterior
- cluneal
- ilio-inguinal

GROIN, MEDIAL THIGH, HIP, OR KNEE PAIN

Pain caused by other conditions can radiate to the hip or groin area.

These conditions include:
- inguinal or femoral hernia
- inflammation or infection of the abdominal organs (i.e., appendicitis, urinary tract infection, Crohn disease)
- gynecological or urinary infection or disease (i.e., prostatitis, ovarian cyst, ureteral dysfunction)
- tumors, osteoma, metastatic disease of the femur or lower pelvis
- sickle cell anemia that causes femoral head avascular necrosis
- enlarged lymphatic vessels in the femoral triangle area (i.e., infection, Hodgkin's disease)
- inflammatory conditions (i.e., ankylosing spondylitis [later in the disease process the hip joints can become involved], Reiter syndrome, rheumatoid arthritis)
- circulatory problems of the femoral artery (i.e., arteriosclerosis)
- iliopsoas abcess
- tubercular disease of the hip

Pain in the groin, medial thigh, hip, or knee in the adolescent can be attributed to a slipped capital femoral epiphysis (the femoral neck actually tends to swing superiorly and laterally while the head rotates inferiorly). According to Kelsey, a slipped capital epiphysis is the most common disorder of the hip in the adolescent, with an incidence of 2 per 100,000 people. The affected adolescent typically tends to be male, obese, and skeletally immature. This disorder usually affects the left hip and can have bilateral involvement of 20% to 30%, according to Bloom.

In the 4 to 6 year old, this pain can be caused by Legg-Calve'-Perthes disease, which is an articular osteochondrosis of the entire secondary ossification center of the femoral head (Pappas). The accompanying symptoms can be an antalgic gait, limitation of hip internal rotation abduction, and spasm in extension (flexion-adduction deformity) (see Mechanism of Injury, Dislocation, earlier in this chapter for more details).

Pain in the medial thigh, groin, and pubic area can be caused by:

ASSESSMENT   INTERPRETATION

- pubic symphysis instability (post-trauma)*
- osteitis pubis*
- pubic ramus stress fractures (overuse or traumatic)*

*In these cases there will also be exquisite boney point tenderness.

- femoral neck stress fracture. According to Fullerton and Snowdy, pain in the anterior groin (inguinal area) is the earliest and most frequent sign of a femoral neck stress fracture.
- adductor tendonitis

POSTERIOR BUTTOCK AND THIGH PAIN

Pain in the posterior buttock and thigh can be caused by:
- lumbar spine nerve root irritation; a facet; ligamentous, capsular lesion; or intervertebral disc herniation
- chronic posterior thigh compartment syndrome
- piriformis syndrome (according to Raether and Lutter)
- hamstring strain or partial tear
- hamstring syndrome (according to Puranen and Orava) that can cause ischial tuberosity pain as well as posterior thigh discomfort. It is caused by a tendinous fibrous band at the lateral proximal point of insertion of the biceps femoris muscle, which irritates the sciatic nerve.
- ischiogluteal bursitis
- sciatic nerve contusion

Type of Pain
Describe the pain.

Sharp

Sharp, local pain can be caused by injury to:
- skin, fascia
- ligaments (e.g., the iliofemoral ligaments)
- superficial muscle (e.g., iliotibial band)
- periosteum (e.g., the iliac crest)

Dull

Dull pain can be caused by injury to:
- joints (e.g., hip synovitis)
- deep muscles (e.g., the gluteus medius)
- chronic muscle (e.g., the hamstring)

Aching

Aching pain can be caused by injury to:
- deep muscles (e.g., the piriformis)
- deep bursa (e.g., the iliopectineal bursa)
- deep ligament (e.g., the sacrotuberous ligament)
- fibrous capsule
- ventral nerve root
- deep or peripheral nerve (e.g., the sciatic nerve)

ASSESSMENT	INTERPRETATION

Pins and Needles

The sensation of pins and needles can be caused by injury to:
- dorsal nerve root (e.g., L2, L3, L4, L5, S1)
- nerve trunk

Numbness

Numbness can be caused by injury to the dorsal nerve root (e.g., L2-S1).

Timing of Pain
How quickly did the pain begin?
Immediate pain that does not let up.
Immediate pain, then relief, then pain again after a few hours.

Pain that occurs suddenly and remains intense suggests a more severe injury than pain that eases and returns later. Pain that returns later is usually an indication of synovial swelling versus hemorrhagic swelling—the latter causes immediate pain. With a direct blow, often the pain remains intense if more than soft tissue is involved (e.g., pain persists if the periosteum or an internal organ is involved).

Pain that gradually builds without a mechanism and progressively gets worse even with rest suggests some underlying disease process and should be looked into further.

When the Pain Occurs
All the Time

Pain all the time usually indicates a severe injury, an active inflammatory state, or a disease process, and further evaluation is necessary.

Repeating Mechanism

Pain that occurs only when the mechanism is repeated suggests a local lesion, either ligamentous or muscular. Ligaments cause pain when they are stretched; muscles cause pain when they are stretched and contracted. Pain after repetitive movements suggests a bursitis or tendonitis. Bursitis can cause pain when the soft tissue around the bursa is overworked or if the bursa is compressed.

Morning

Pain in the morning accompanied by stiffness suggests intracapsular swelling that builds overnight—this is common with arthritic or degenerative joint pathology.

End of the Day

Pain that occurs only at the end of the day suggests inflammation due to too much stress on the injured structure during daily or sporting activities.

Weight-bearing

Pain only on weight-bearing suggests articular or muscular injury.

ASSESSMENT

INTERPRETATION

Degree of Pain
- Mild
- Moderate
- Severe

Usually, the worse the pain, the more severe the injury, but this is not always true—complete muscular or ligamentous tears can be painless. Usually, the further the pain radiates from the lesion site, the more damage there is. Every individual has a different pain threshold and what is mild pain for one athlete may be severe pain for another. The perception of pain can be influenced by physiological, cultural, emotional, and mental factors.

Swelling

Location
Where is the swelling?

Local

INTRACAPSULAR

Intracapsular swelling cannot be determined by your history-taking, observations, or palpations. Functional testing will indicate a capsular pattern.

INTRAMUSCULAR

Intramuscular swelling may be described by the athlete as a lump within the muscle. The midbelly of the hamstrings and adductors are common sites. The swelling will be observable locally. The muscle must be tested and palpated to ensure the muscle is not torn.

BURSAL

Bursal swelling is very local. The most common location for bursal swelling is in the greater trochanteric bursa. This bursa is very vulnerable to trauma or to irritation by the iliotibial band. The iliopectineal or ischial bursa can also develop bursitis from overuse or direct trauma.

Diffuse
INTERMUSCULAR

Bruising or tracking down the leg or up over the pelvis may be described by the athlete, indicating intermuscular swelling or a superficial hematoma. It is common to have tracking or swelling down the posterior thigh from a hamstring strain. The swelling tracks down the leg because of the gravitational force.

Tracking around the iliac crest is often found from a hip pointer with a contusion to the soft tissue surrounding the crest.

Time of Swelling
Did the swelling develop soon after the injury?

Immediate swelling indicates a more severe injury, including:
- hemarthrosis
- fracture
- local hemorrhage

ASSESSMENT

INTERPRETATION

Immediate local swelling in response to a direct blow to the greater trochanter can suggest a greater trochanteric bursitis.

Acute hip synovitis is not observable when viewing the joint and it is difficult to test for, yet it is fairly common. A painful hip that results in limping during weight bearing and that only settles down with rest are common signs of hip joint synovitis. In athletes, it usually develops after overtraining. Pain develops in the groin and thigh. Any young athlete who complains of hip pain should have a thorough evaluation for rheumatoid arthritis, Legg-Calve'-Perthes disease, and a slipped capital femoral epiphysis.

Function

Activities

Which activities make it worse?
- Standing
- Walking
- Running
- Sitting
- Forward Bending

Since the hip and pelvis carry and distribute the load from above and below, any injury to them will drastically affect the ability to weight-bear and the even distribution of weight bilaterally. Standing on one leg creates a force that is two to five times the body weight. Walking up stairs creates a force that is three times the body weight. Running creates a force that is four and one half to five times the body weight. The ability to sit and to forward bend depends on asymptomatic hip joints (and asymptomatic sacroiliac joints and lumbar spine).

Athlete's Function Post-injury

How well could the athlete function after the injury?

Could the athlete continue playing his or her sport?

Was the athlete able to weight-bear immediately or not?

Does the athlete limp?

Was the athlete carried off the court or field?

If the athlete was carried off the court or field because of an inability to weight-bear, in what position was he or she most comfortable?

The athlete's inability or lack of desire to continue a sport after a hip injury suggests a more significant injury.

If the athlete was transported because of an inability to weight-bear, it is a significant injury. It is important to determine what position was most comfortable during transport.

When a hip is dislocated posteriorly, the leg is shortened and the hip is internally rotated and adducted. There is a tendency to rest the affected foot on top of the opposite foot. When a hip is dislocated anteriorly, the hip is abducted, externally rotated, and flexed.

When the capital femoral epiphysis is fractured, there is shortening of the limb, external rotation, and abduction of the leg.

In case of an iliopsoas tendon strain the athlete holds the leg in a flexed, adducted position with slight external rotation.

Pain Alleviating and Aggravating Positions

What positions relieve the pain?
What positions aggravate the pain?

By determining what activities are painful and which positions are comfortable, you can help determine the muscles that are injured and the joint positions that aggravate or relieve the pain. This helps determine the best functional testing positions, the order of testing, the degree of disability, and the level of the athlete's daily functional ability. Knowing which positions relieve the pain is also helpful in designing the rehabilitation program.

ASSESSMENT

INTERPRETATION

Sensations

Describe the sensations felt at the time of injury and now.

Numbness or Hypersensitivity

See Dermatomes or Local Cutaneous Nerve Supply if numbness or hypersensitivity is in a specific segment or area.

Snapping or Clicking

Snapping at the lateral aspect of the hip joint is usually due to a thickening of the bursal walls so that the tensor fascia lata slides back and forth over the greater trochanter, resulting in an audible and palpable snap (according to Schaberg J et al.).

The gluteus maximus tendon can snap over the greater trochanter as well.

Other possible causes of anterior joint clicking or snapping are:
- psoas tendon slipping over the iliopectineal eminence of the pubis or lesser trochanter
- iliofemoral ligament slipping over the anterior hip capsule or femoral head
- hip joint subluxation, loose body, osteochondromatosis (rare)

Snapping or clicking in the symphysis pubis area can be from joint subluxation following trauma or postpartum.

Snapping or clicking in the posterior hip area can be caused by the biceps femoris tendon catching on the ischial tuberosity.

Popping Sensation

If the popping sensation was experienced after a sudden explosive contraction, a muscle strain or tear can exist.

Tightness or Tension

Tightness or tension may indicate the presence of swelling or protective muscle spasm.

Joint Stiffness

Stiffness of the joint can suggest osteoarthritic or rheumatoid arthritic changes in the joint.

Particulars

Has this happened before?
Has a physician or surgeon seen it?
Were x-rays taken and what were the results?
What was done for the injury?
PIER (pressure, ice, elevation, rest)
Heat

A previous history of injury should always be investigated because chronic muscle strains and chronic overuse injuries are common in the hip and pelvis area. Chronic recurring hip conditions include:
- hamstring strains
- adductor strains
- greater trochanteric bursitis

ASSESSMENT

INTERPRETATION

Did the athlete continue to play?
Any family history of problems?
Previous treatment, physiotherapy, and results.

- iliopsoas tendonitis
- iliopectineal bursitis

Any previous diagnosis, including the physician's name and location, should be obtained. X-ray results and where they were done should be recorded.

If the injury was treated conservatively with pressure, ice, elevation, and rest versus a heat modality, the inflammation may have been reduced. If the athlete continued to play, the inflammation may have progressed accordingly.

Any family history of leg-length discrepancy, Legg-Calve'-Perthes disease, anteversion, retroversion, coxa valgum or varum, or avascular necrosis of the femoral head should be recorded at this time.

Any previous treatment or rehabilitation for this problem should be recorded, as well as its results.

OBSERVATIONS

Standing
Anterior View
Anterior Superior Iliac Spines and Iliac Crests

The crests and spines should be level—if one spine or crest is higher than the other, there could be a leg-length difference. If such a difference is suspected, the leg should be measured from the anterior superior iliac spine to the floor bilaterally.

Leg-length Discrepancy

An anatomical or structural leg-length discrepancy will cause the anterior superior iliac spine and the posterior superior iliac spine on one side to be lower than on the other side.

With a functional leg-length discrepancy, the anterior superior iliac spine will be lower on one side and the posterior superior iliac spine will be higher on the same side.

Leg-length discrepancies can lead to problems with:
- sacroiliac joint
- symphysis pubis
- facet and intervertebral joints of the lumbar spine
- muscle imbalances (e.g., quadratus lumborum, iliopsoas, and adductors)
- facet joints of the thoracic or cervical spine if scoliosis occurs

Coxa Varum (Genu Valgum) (Fig 2-14, A and B)

The angle of inclination, with one axis through the head and neck of the femur and the other axis down the shaft of the femur, should be 125°. If the angle is less than this, coxa varum exists. Coxa varum can be caused by several factors, including a slipped capital femoral epiphysis, trauma, arthritis, and rickets, or it may be congenital. This condition causes increased bending of the neck of the femur and may predispose it to fracture. Coxa

ASSESSMENT   INTERPRETATION

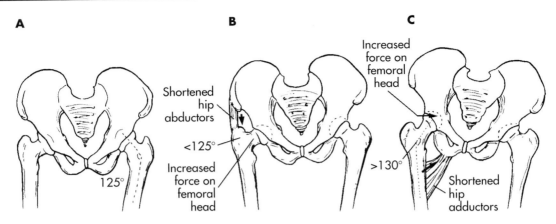

Fig. 2-14 A, Normal anterior view. **B,** Coxa varum. **C,** Coxa valgum.

varum is often bilateral. If it is unilateral, there will be a leg-length difference with the pelvis on the affected side being lower, which results in pelvis obliquity. This may cause back pain or sacroiliac dysfunction. An abductor contracture (shortened abductors) and develop because the pelvis is dropped toward that side. Coxa varum causes genu valgum, which leads to malalignment problems in the patellofemoral joint.

Coxa Valgum (Genu Varum) (Fig. 2-14, C)

The angle of inclination is greater than 130° with coxa valgum. This condition can be caused by previous hip dislocation, trauma, or spastic paralysis, or it may be congenital. As a result of coxa valgum more force is placed on the head of the femur and less force is placed on the femoral neck. This may lead to eventual osteoarthritic changes in the hip joint. The length of the limb is increased, which also causes upward pelvic obliquity on that side. The hip on the affected side is adducted and the adductor muscles are shortened, which may cause back pain or sacroiliac problems. The iliotibial band is stretched more, which increases susceptibility to trochanteric bursitis. Coxa valgum causes genu varum. This coxa valgum position predisposes the hip to dislocation because the adductors are tight and tend to pull the joint toward a position of dislocation.

Femoral Anteversion (Figs. 2-15, A and 2-16, B)

The angle formed by the transverse axis through the femoral neck and through the transverse axis of the femoral condyles (transcondylar axis). should be 12° to 15° (it can range from 8° to 25°). When femoral anteversion exists, this angle is greater than 15°. This femoral torsion may result in extra pressure through the femoral head, which may contribute to osteoarthritis in later life. There is also increased femoral head pressure against the superior and anterior acetabulum, dysplasia of the acetabulum, and a susceptibility to anterior femoral dislocation. Because of the increased femoral torsion, the knee

ASSESSMENT

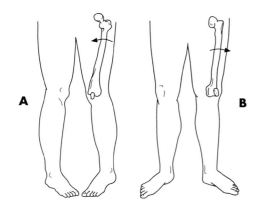

Fig. 2 -15 A, Femoral anteversion, toed-in gait. **B**, Femoral retroversion, toed-out gait

INTERPRETATION

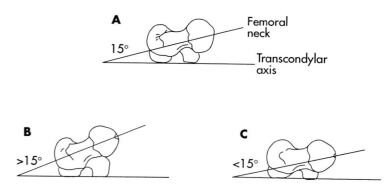

Fig. 2-16 A, Normal. **B**, Femoral anteversion. **C**, Femoral retroversion.

joint may suffer from malalignment syndromes or patellar dislocations; the subtalar joint is more susceptible to pronation problems if the femoral torsion is not compensated for by the tibia. Excessive lumbar lordosis may develop because of the anterior femoral head position—this can lead to lower back problems. A unilateral problem may cause a leg-length discrepancy. During testing the individual will have increased internal hip rotation and decreased external hip rotation and may have a toed-in gait. The body may compensate by increasing the external tibial torsion and/or pronating the feet.

Femoral Retroversion (Figs. 2-15, B, and 2-16, C)

In femoral retroversion, the angle between the femoral neck and the transcondylar axis is decreased to less than 15°. A toed-out gait often results and contributes to the body correcting the problem by internally rotating the tibia and/or supinating the feet. The retroverted hip promotes the stability of the joint. A unilateral problem may lead to a leg-length discrepancy, leading to low back or sacroiliac problems. During testing the individual may have a toed-out gait, increased external hip rotation, and decreased internal hip rotation.

Lateral View
Pelvic Position
  • Anterior tilt (Fig. 2-17)
  • Posterior tilt (Fig. 2-18)
  • Level ASIS, PSIS bilaterally

The anteriorly tilted pelvis is often associated with excessive lumbar lordosis and its related problems. This position also results in shortening of the hip flexors, lumbar extensors, and thoracolumbar fascia (see Fig. 2-17). If the pelvis has a posterior tilt it is often combined with the flat-back position and hyperextended hips, resulting in lax hip ligaments and weak hip flexors (see Fig. 2-18). When you place your hands on top of the iliac crests anteriorly and over the posterior superior iliac spines bilaterally, any tilting, twisting, or asymmetry can be seen and felt.

ASSESSMENT   INTERPRETATION

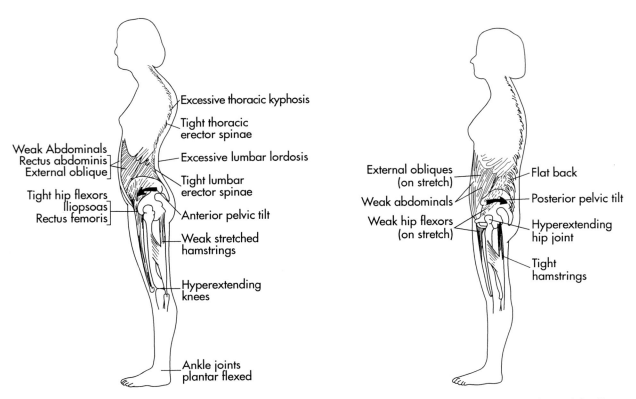

Fig. 2-17 Lateral view, anterior pelvic tilt.

Fig. 2-18 Lateral view, posterior pelvic tilt.

The position of three pelvic boney prominences—the crest, the anterior superior iliac spine, and the posterior superior iliac spine—will indicate the status of the ilia. What is frequently found is that all three points are higher on one side, indicating that the leg is longer. If the right iliac crest is higher than the left while the right posterior iliac spine is lower and the right anterior iliac spine is higher, this indicates a right posterior iliac rotation. Any asymmetries, whether from a leg-length difference, muscle spasm (especially in quadratus lumborum), scoliosis, or pelvic asymmetry, can cause problems to the lower limb or to the trunk or spine above.

Lateral tilting of the pelvis causes a compensatory lateral flexion and rotation of the lumbar spine and slight adduction of one hip and abduction of the other. The lateral tilt is controlled by the contralateral abductors. Weakness in the adductors (often gluteus medius) can also cause a lateral tilt. Conversely, a boney cause of the tilt can result in abductor weakness on the contralateral side.

Excessive Lumbar Lordosis (Anterior Pelvic Tilt) (see Fig. 2-17)

Excessive lordosis of the lumbar spine can be caused by or result in:

ASSESSMENT

INTERPRETATION

- tight hip flexors
- tight low back musculature
- weak abdominals
- weak hamstrings and glutei

This posture can lead to several lower back disorders that may refer pain to the lower limb.

Flat Back with Hip Joints Hyperextended (Posterior Pelvic Tilt) (see Fig. 2-18)

This is usually associated with a flat back and a posterior tilt of the pelvis. According to Kendall and McCreary, this position puts a stretch on:
- anterior hip joint ligaments
- iliopsoas muscles
- external oblique muscles

Iliopsoas and the external oblique muscles will develop stretch weakness and the low hamstrings often are tight and shortened. This posture can lead to problems in the weak muscle groups, and if the hip joint is forced into further extension, injury to the stretched and weakened structures can result.

A posterior pelvic tilt for a prolonged period of time leads to facet degeneration and uneven pressure through the intervertebral discs. A kyphotic spine puts increased pressure through the intervertebral discs.

Tight Hip Flexors

The pelvis will assume an anterior tilt if the hip flexors are tight bilaterally. This can lead to an excessive lordotic lumbar spine, which can make the athlete susceptible to low back or hamstring problems. Anterior hip capsule tightness, which results from prolonged tight hip flexors, will accelerate the progression of degenerative hip joint disease.

Tight Hamstrings

With the pelvis tilted anteriorly the hamstrings are usually stretched and are susceptible to a strain or tear, especially if the low back muscles are also tight.

Abdominal Muscle Weakness

If the abdominals are weak, an anterior pelvic tilt will result, which in turn can add to the tightness in the hip flexor and hip anterior capsule.

Weight Distribution

Determine if the center of gravity falls through one leg more than the other. The body will lean to the weight-bearing side. This can be tested with the one leg standing test.

Any hip problems or pelvic injury can cause less weight to be placed on the injured side.

ASSESSMENT

INTERPRETATION

Posterior View
Spinous Processes

Palpate or mark the spinous process-es to determine their alignment and record if there is any scoliosis or steps.

A scoliosis can indicate a functional or structural leg-length difference. Leg-length differences will affect the mechanics of the lumbar spine, sacroiliac joint, and symphysis pubis. A step or a prominent spinous process at L5 can indicate a spondylolis-thesis, which can refer pain into the back, hips, or legs.

Posterior Superior Iliac Spines

The posterior superior iliac spines should be level.

If one posterior superior iliac spine, iliac crest, and anterior superior iliac spine is higher or lower on one side, there is a structural leg-length difference or an upslip or downslip of the ilium.

A quadratus lumborum muscle spasm or a weak gluteus medius on the opposite side can also raise an iliac crest. Leg-length differences are often associated with sacroiliac, facet joint, and disc dysfunction.

If one posterior superior iliac spine is higher than the other and the anterior superior iliac spine on that side is lower than the other, there is a functional leg-length difference or an anteri-or iliac rotation. The athlete with the anterior iliac rotation will stand with the painful side in more flexion than the uninvolved side.

The athlete with a posterior iliac rotation (backward rotation of the ilium on the sacrum) may tend to stand with the hip, knee, and low back slightly extended on the injured side. The posterior superior iliac spine and iliac crest will be lower on the involved side but the anterior superior iliac spine on the involved side will be higher. These rotational problems can lead primarily to sacroiliac joint pathology and sometimes to lumbar spine dysfunction.

If the iliac crest is low on one side but the posterior spines or greater trochanter are level, there is a boney abnormality of the pelvis, a positional fault of the sacroiliac joint, an abnormality of the femoral neck, or even a slipped capital femoral epiphysis. The position of the greater trochanter can also be altered by lower-limb biomechanical faults.

Gluteal Folds

The gluteal folds should be level and the gluteal muscle tone should be equal. A sag of one buttock can be caused by an L5 or S1 nerve root impingement or lesion, or a previous gluteus or hip joint injury.

Damage to the inferior gluteal nerve can also cause this.

Hamstring Development

Atrophy of the hamstrings and gastrocnemii on one side is a sign of chronic S1 or S2 radioculopathy.

ASSESSMENT

INTERPRETATION

Atrophy of the buttock and hamstring can also develop from a hip arthritis or previous hamstring strain or tear.

Popliteal Creases

Popliteal creases should be level—uneven creases can be caused by a functional or structural lower leg difference.

Gastrocnemii Development

Atrophy of either gastrocnemius may also be a sign of S1 or S2 nerve root impingement irritation, polio, or other neurological disorder. Ankle joint, Achilles tendon, or gastrocnemius muscle injuries can also cause atrophy.

Calcaneal Alignment

A unilateral calcaneal valgus will cause a slight functional leg-length difference because of the loss of the longitudinal arch. If one calcaneus is in valgus and the other in varus, the leg-length difference may be significant.

Unilateral or bilateral calcaneal valgus can cause prolonged pronation during gait and sporting activities. Repeated prolonged pronation can cause lower quadrant problems and uneven forces through the limb. (See Foot and Ankle Assessment chapter on prolonged pronation biomechanics.)

One Leg Standing (Stork Stand) (Fig. 2-19)

One knee is flexed and the level of the ASIS observed.

Look for the following:
• weakness of the gluteus medius, the gluteus minimus, and the tensor fascia lata muscles

Normally, the pelvis remains level or may even rise slightly on the flexed knee side. If the pelvis drops on the unsupported side, a gluteus medius weakness or inhibition exists in the supporting hip and the test is positive. As the athlete balances, the abductors must contract strongly on the side of the standing leg to stabilize the pelvis. A weakness in the gluteus medius (glu-

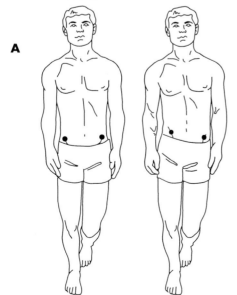

Fig. 2-19 One leg standing (stork stand) pelvis drops on unsupported side. **A,** Normal. **B,** Pelvis drops on left.

ASSESSMENT

- balance
- integrity of the joint
- athlete's willingness to bear weight

Repeat this test bilaterally.

Local Observations of the Lesion Site

Look for the following:

- swelling, bruising, scars, and atrophy
- asymmetry in muscle and boney development

Gait

What to look for while the athlete is walking if weight bearing is possible: watch the trunk, pelvis, and entire lower limb.

The athlete should have the limb and trunk well exposed—he or she should be wearing shorts, a halter top, or a swim suit with no shirt.

Stance Phase

Particularly watch the limb and pelvis during the stance phase.

Heel Strike and Foot Flat

INTERPRETATION

teus minimus and tensor fascia lata also assist) will allow the pelvis to drop on the unsupported side.

Neurological problems from nerve root irritation (L4, L5, S1) or damage to the superior gluteal nerve can also cause gluteus medius weakness or inhibition. A gluteus medius tendonitis, strain, or contusion can also cause a positive sign.

This also tests the strength of the limb and the integrity of the limb's joints.

Proprioception and balance in general can also be assessed. The athlete's willingness to perform this test or the length of time that elapses before discomfort is experienced helps determine the nature of the problem.

A pubic ramus or femoral neck stress fracture prevents one leg standing because of pain and inhibition around the hip and pelvis. Instability in the pubic symphysis or sacroiliac joint may cause pain during this test.

Swelling, bruising, scars, and atrophy all help to determine the severity and nature of the injury. Note and compare boney and soft tissue contours. Asymmetry in muscle development in the gluteals, thighs, and calves should be documented and measured whenever possible. Gaps in muscles or their tendons can indicate partial or complete tears.

Hip stiffness or pain causes an antalgic gait. Hip stiffness may force the athlete to move the entire trunk and the affected leg forward as a unit during the swing phase—this is called compass gait.

Particularly watch the limb and pelvis during the stance phase.

During heel strike and foot flat, the lateral rotators and abdominals contract to stabilize the hip and pelvis. Hip extension begins and will continue until heel off.

At heel strike, the center of gravity is shifted over the weight-bearing leg and pelvis. This lateral shift produces a closed chain hip adduction motion during heel strike and at the beginning of midstance.

Hip internal rotation occurs at heel strike and foot flat and the rotation is transferred down the limb.

ASSESSMENT	INTERPRETATION

Any hip extensor injury will limit the force of both hip extension and push off on that side. A hip adductor or internal rotator muscle injury may elicit pain on the weight-bearing side at heel strike and foot flat.

Midstance

During midstance the body weight is shifted over the hip joint. The hip adduction motion changes to hip abduction for the rest of the stance phase to control the weight transfer and then move the line of gravity to the opposite limb.

The internal motion at the hip changes to external rotation during midstance and push off.

A weak gluteus medius will cause the athlete to lurch over to the involved side—this is called gluteus medius lurch or Trendelenburg gait (Fig. 2-20). A weak gluteus maximus will cause the athlete's upper body to lurch backward to maintain hip extension—this is called gluteus maximus lurch. The side with the hip dysfunction is only able to weight bear for a short period of time.

Push-Off (Heel Off–Toe Off)

Abduction and external rotation continues until toe off. Any problem with the hip extensors, abductors, or lateral rotators will cause a weak, unstable push-off.

Swing Phase

Watch length of stride and rhythm of gait.

Is there less weight on the affected leg?

Hip flexors and internal rotators contract to bring the leg forward—if the hamstrings are injured, the time spent in the swing phase will be reduced.

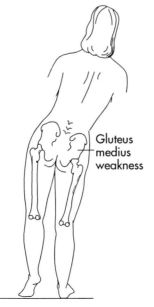

Gluteus medius weakness

Fig. 2-20 Gluteus medius gait (Trendelenburg gait). The body swings over the weaker hip.

ASSESSMENT

INTERPRETATION

Toed-in Gait

Toed-in gait is a sign of anteversion or internal tibial torsion.

Toed-in gait can be caused by internal tibial torsion or anteversion at the hip joint (see discussion of Hip Anteversion under Observations, Standing).

Toed-out Gait

Toed-out gait is a sign of retroversion or external tibial torsion.

Toed-out gait can by caused be external tibial torsion if it occurs only below the knee, or by hip retroversion (see discussion of Hip Retroversion under Observations, Standing).

Slipped Capital Femoral Epiphysis

Is one leg externally rotated (slipped femoral capital epiphysis)?

An athlete with a slipped capital epiphysis may prefer to walk with the leg externally rotated.

Antalgic Gait

Is the gait antalgic (limp)?

An antalgic gait or limp may be caused by:
- injury to a muscle, ligament, or joint in the lower extremity
- congenital dysplasia or hip dislocation
- coxa valgum or coxa varum
- hip joint osteoarthritis
- leg-length discrepancy
- slipped capital femoral epiphysis
- acute sacroiliac sprain
- Legg-Calve'-Perthes disease*
- anterior superior iliac spine epiphysitis (antalgic gait with listing toward the involved side)

*An avascularity of the femoral head (unknown etiology) that affects boys between the ages of 5 and 12. It leads to hip and groin pain with limitation of abduction and medial rotation.

Gluteus Medius Gait (Trendelenburg gait)

This is caused by:
- weakness or inhibition of the gluteus medius and a resulting positive Trendelenburg sign (see Fig. 2-20)
- congenital hip dislocation
- neurological problem (poliomyelitis, meningomyelocele, nerve root lesion)
- any occurrence that has caused the origin of the muscle to move closer to its insertion (i.e., coxa valga, a fractured greater trochanter, a slipped capital femoral epiphysis)

Gluteus Maximus Gait

This is caused by:
- weakness or inhibition of gluteus maximus
- nerve root L5, S1 problem
- muscle injury to gluteus maximus
- damage to inferior gluteal nerve

ASSESSMENT	INTERPRETATION

Weak Psoas Gait (Injured)

The athlete must exaggerate the movement of the pelvis and trunk to help move the thigh into flexion.

Weak psoas gait is caused by:
- iliopsoas muscle injury
- psoas injury or abscess
- iliopsoas bursitis
- L2 nerve root irritation (rare)

Weak adductor Gait (Injured)

The athlete walks with a wide stance and an unstable pelvis.

Weak adductor gait is caused by:
- adductor muscle injury
- osteitis pubis
- neurological problems at L2, L3, or L4 nerve roots

Hip Flexor Tightness or Contracture

This is compensated for by walking with an anterior pelvic tilt and an excessive lumbar lordosis.

Upper, Shoulder, and Arm Movements

Excessive upper body movements with the arms swinging across the body may be caused by faulty hip or lower limb mechanics.

Lumbar Spine

Stiffness in the lower back or trunk may cause a reluctance to move the pelvis during gait due to pain or muscle spasm. Hip pain causes a reflex hip flexion.

Painful Hip Joint

A painful hip joint is commonly held in slight flexion, abduction, and external rotation because this puts the least stress on the capsule or the inflamed synovial membrane (resting position for the hip joint). Walking speed is reduced and the time spent on each leg will be reduced.

Pelvic Movements

Normal pelvic movements include horizontal displacement, pelvic drop, and pelvic rotation.

Horizontal Displacement (Fig. 2-21)

A horizontal displacement consists of approximately 1 inch of displacement on either side of the midline. The pelvis moves toward the weight-bearing side. Excessive side-to-side sway indicates that the balance between the adductors and abductors is upset; this can be caused by an adductor or abductor muscle strain, tendonitis, or an adductor contracture (coxa valga).

Pelvic Drop (Fig. 2-22, A)

The pelvis drops slightly on the swing leg side. Additionally, an injury to the contralateral abductors (especially the gluteus

ASSESSMENT

INTERPRETATION

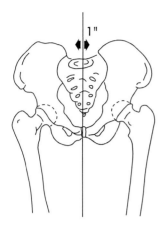

Fig. 2-21 Horizontal displacement (1 inch from vertical).

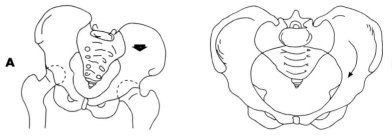

Fig. 2-22 A, Pelvic drop on swing leg side during gait. **B,** Pelvic rotation.

medius) or the same sided quadratus lumborum will cause an excessive drop.

Pelvic Rotation (Fig. 2-22, B)

There is a forward pelvic rotation approximately 40° on the swing leg side. An imbalance or an injury in the medial or lateral rotators can cause an abnormal rotation here, either excessive or limited. A hip extensor or flexor muscle injury can also affect this.

SUMMARY OF TESTS

FUNCTIONAL TESTING

Rule out
  Lumbar spine
  Knee
  Internal organ problems
  Inflammatory disorders
  Tumors or metastatic disease

FUNCTIONAL TESTS

Tests in Supine Position
  Active hip flexion
  Passive hip flexion
  Active hip abduction
  Passive hip abduction
  Resisted hip abduction
  Active hip adduction
  Passive hip adduction
  Resisted hip adduction

ASSESSMENT   INTERPRETATION

Tests in Sitting Position
    Resisted hip flexion
    Active hip medial rotation
    Passive hip medial rotation
    Resisted hip medial rotation
    Active hip lateral rotation
    Passive hip lateral rotation
    Resisted hip lateral rotation
    Active knee extension
    Resisted knee extension
Tests in Prone Position
    Active knee flexion
    Passive knee flexion
    Resisted knee flexion
    Active hip extension with knee extension
    Passive hip extension with knee extension
    Resisted hip extension with knee extension
    Active hip extension with knee flexion
    Passive hip extension with knee flexion
    Ely's test
    Resisted hip extension with knee flexion

SPECIAL TESTS

Thomas test
Ober's test
Piriformis test
Trendelenburg test
Scouring test (Quadrant test)
Sacroiliac joint tests
    Pelvic rocking test
    Gapping test
    Hip flexion and adduction test
    Gaenslen's test
    Sacroiliac joint test (Side lying Gaenslen's test)
    Patrick's or Faber test (Flexion, Abduction, External Rotation)
    Pelvic compression test
    Sit up test for iliosacral dysfunction
Leg-Length discrepancy tests
Dermatome and cutaneous nerve testing
Circulatory tests
Specific hip pointer test

ACCESSORY TESTS

Inferior glide
Posterior glide
Anterior glide

ASSESSMENT

INTERPRETATION

Rule out

Lumbar Spine

Through the history-taking and observations the possibility of the involvement of the lumbar spine should be ruled out. The athlete attempts active lumbar forward bending, back bending, side bending, and rotation. The straight-leg raise (Lasègue's sign), if necessary, should be performed. A slump test can be done to separate lumbar spine problems from a chronic hamstring injury (see Lumbar Spine, Special Tests).

Low back problems can cause referred hip pain or may mimic hip disorders. The keys to lumbar spine pathologic conditions include evidence obtained from the history, observations, and while the athlete performs active lumbar movements. The history of a lumbar spine problem can have:
- referred pain or numbness in the lower limb from L4, L5, or S1 dermatomes
- history of chronic low back pain
- problems after low back trauma or incorrect lifting
- dull, aching, tingling pain

The observations may uncover the presence of:
- excessive lumbar lordosis
- lumbar paraspinal muscle spasm
- scoliosis

Asking the athlete to perform active lumbar movements will reveal pain and/or limitation of range of motion, if a lumbar problem is present. If lumbar spine disc involvement is suspected, the straight-leg test to stretch the sciatic nerve over the disc may help to confirm this. The slump test helps to determine if the spinal nerve roots or dura are involved and can help to rule out chronic hamstring injuries. If any of these tests indicate problems in the lumbar spine, a full lumbar spine assessment should be done (see Lumbar Spine chapter).

Knee

The athlete, lying supine, flexes his or her knee to the end of range (heel to buttock position). Apply an overpressure. In this close-packed position any pain or limitation in the knee will indicate knee joint dysfunction. With the athlete lying supine as above, the athlete extends the knee to the end of range of motion; then apply an overpressure to the extended knee. Pain or limitation of movement in the knee indicates a knee joint dysfunction.

If problems suggest that the pain radiates to the knee or if there are knee symptoms in the history, it is necessary to clear the knee. If any knee limitation or pain occurs during these tests, a full knee assessment is necessary (see Knee Assessment chapter).

Internal Organ Problems

Internal organ problems should be ruled out during the history-taking.

Internal organ problems that can cause pain in the hip region include the following:
- gynecological problems (i.e., ovarian cysts or menstrual problems)
- inguinal or femoral hernia
- prostrate problems (i.e., prostatitis)
- bladder or urinary tract infections

ASSESSMENT   INTERPRETATION

- kidney infections
- appendicitis
- pelvic floor myalgia (Nicholas and Hershman)

Inflammatory Disorders

- ankylosing spondylitis
- Reiter syndrome
- rheumatoid arthritis

Tumors or Metastatic Disease

- malignant or benign cancers

Tests in Supine Position

Active Hip Flexion (110° to 120°) (Fig. 2-23)

The athlete is supine lying. With the knee flexed, the athlete attempts to flex his or her hip so that the knee comes toward the chest, keeping the opposite limb in neutral.

Pain, limitation of range of motion, or weakness can be due to injury to the muscles or their nerve supply. The prime movers are:
- Iliacus—femoral N (L2, L3)
- Psoas Major—femoral N (L1, L2, L3, L4)

The accessory movers are:
- Tensor fascia lata—superior gluteal N (L4, L5)
- Rectus femoris—femoral N (L2, L3, L4)
- Sartorius—femoral N (L2, L3)
- Pectineus—femoral N (L2, L3, L4)
- Adductor magnus or longus—obturator N (L2, L3, L4)

Pain can also come from the hamstring stretch if there is a hamstring problem or if a gluteus maximus strain exists.

Passive Hip Flexion (120°)
Knee Flexed (120° to 140°)

With the athlete's knee still flexed, flex the hip passively with one hand on the distal posterior thigh while your other hand stabilizes the pelvis at the anterior superior iliac spine.

Passively flex the hip until an end feel is reached. The opposite leg is in neutral.

Pain can arise at the gluteus maximus or at the origin of the hamstring if a lesion exists at either of these locations. Pain at the end of range of motion can also come from the hamstrings compressing the ischial bursa if bursitis exists.

A soft end feel can suggest bursitis or a loose body and a hard end feel can indicate arthrosis—the normal end feel is tissue approximation.

An overpressure causes a posterior rotation of the ilium on that side and then lumbar flexion. Any sacroiliac or lumbar pain with overpressure indicates pathology at these sites.

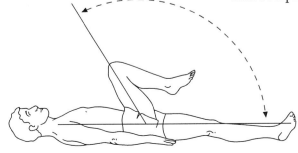

Fig. 2-23 Active hip joint flexion with knee flexed, 120°.

ASSESSMENT

INTERPRETATION

An overpressure can be done if the end of range is pain free. This overpressure stresses the sacroiliac joint and lumbar spine on this side.

Knee Extended (90° to 120°)

Have the athlete do a pelvic tilt first to fix the pelvis and limit lumbar spine involvement at the end of range.

As above but with the athlete's knee extended, passively raise the leg with one hand on the posterior aspect of the lower leg while the other hand is on the anterior surface of the thigh to keep the knee extended.

Passively flex the hip until an end feel is reached.

The opposite leg remains in neutral and should not flex.

Repeat bilaterally.

This test stretches the hamstring muscles to determine if they are strained. The athlete should have at least 90° of hip flexion with knee extension.

This test also stretches the dural sleeve and can elicit pain if there is a dural problem or a lumbar nerve root impingement (see Straight-Leg Raise, Lumbar Spine Special Tests).

Active Hip Abduction (30° to 50°)

Method 1

The athlete abducts his or her leg as far as possible by sliding it along the top of the plinth. Do not allow hip flexion during the test. The pelvis should be fixed by the therapist with one arm across the athlete's iliac crests.

Method 2

This can be done in the side-lying position. The athlete abducts the leg as far as possible against gravity. Do not allow the athlete's body to roll. The therapist may need to stabilize the athlete's pelvis during abduction.

Pain, limitation of range of motion, or weakness can be caused by an injury to the hip abductor muscles or their nerve supply. The prime mover is the gluteus medius—superior gluteal N. (L4, L5, S1).

The accessory movers are:
- Gluteus minimus—superior gluteal N. (L4, L5, S1)
- Gluteus maximus (upper fibers)—inferior gluteal N. (L5, S1, S2)
- Sartorius—femoral N. (L2, L3)
- Tensor fascia lata (which only assists when the hip is flexed)

Limited hip abduction occurs in the coxa varum hip because of the impingement of the greater trochanter against the acetabulum. Limited hip abduction occurs in congenital hip dysplasia or dislocation because the affected limb is shortened with the femoral head riding out of the acetabulum.

ASSESSMENT

INTERPRETATION

Passive Hip Abduction (50°)

With the athlete lying supine, abduct the leg with one hand on the medial distal thigh while your other hand stabilizes the pelvis on the opposite side. Abduct the leg until an end feel is reached. This can also be done in a side-lying position with the upper leg passively abducted, but stabilization of the pelvis can be difficult with this method.

Pain or limitation of range of motion can come from the following:
- adductors on either leg (pectineus, adductor longus, adductor brevis, adductor magnus, gracilis)
- iliofemoral, ischiofemoral, or pubofemoral ligaments if a sprain or partial tear exists
- osteitis pubis

Resisted Hip Abduction (Supine or Side-lying Position)

The athlete's legs should be slightly abducted.

Pain or weakness can come from any of the muscles or their nerve supply (see Active Hip Abduction).

Pain and weakness can come from osteitis pubis and a clicking sensation may be present during the resisted test (Nicholas and Hershmann).

Pain can also come from iliac crest injuries (i.e., avulsion of iliac epiphysis or iliac crest periosteal contusion).

Weakness can come from a superior gluteal nerve problem or an L5 nerve root problem. If one leg is resisted, the abdominal muscles, spinal extensors, and the quadratus lumborum help to stabilize the pelvis.

Method 1

Place your hands on the lateral aspect of the malleoli bilaterally and resist toward the midline. If the athlete has a knee problem the resistance should be applied above the knee joint—this is difficult with a strong athlete and the side-lying method may be easier (see Method 2).

Method 2

This can be done with the athlete in a side-lying position. Resist abduction with one hand on the lateral thigh and the other hand stabilizing the pelvis.

Active Hip Adduction (30°) (Fig. 2-24)

The athlete in supine lying flexes one knee on the chest and holds it there with the arms. The other leg is abducted as far as possible, then adducted without moving the pelvis or flexing that hip. Stabilize the pelvis. This can be done in the side-lying position—the athlete lifts the lower leg to meet the

Pain, limitation of range of motion, or weakness can be caused be an injury to the adductor muscles or their nerve supply. The prime movers are:
- Adductor longus—obturator N. (L2, L3, L4)
- Adductor magnus—obturator N. (L2, L3, L4)
- Adductor brevis—obturator N. (L2, L3, L4)
- Pectineus—femoral N. (L2, L3, L4)
- Gracilis—obturator N. (L3, L4)

ASSESSMENT   INTERPRETATION

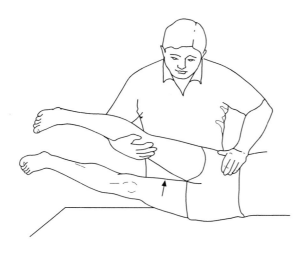

Fig. 2-24 Active hip joint adduction (side lying).

upper leg. You must stabilize the athlete's pelvis and upper leg. Stabilizing is difficult in the side-lying position.

Passive Hip Adduction (30°)

With the athlete' hip and knee on one side flexed to the chest, passively adduct the opposite leg (which is held straight) until an end feel is reached.

Pain or limitation of range of motion can come from compression of the iliopectineal bursa or from the greater trochanteric bursa as the iliotibial band tightens over it. An iliotibial band syndrome or strain may also cause discomfort.

Resisted Hip Adduction (Fig. 2-25)

With an athlete's legs slightly abducted, cross your arms between the athlete's legs and resist adduction just above the medial malleolus bilaterally, provided that no knee problems exist.

If there are medial knee joint problems, resistance can be applied above the knee.

Pain or weakness can come from the muscles or their nerve supply as above (see the section on Active Hip Adduction).

Pain may be felt in the pubic area if there is:
- instability in the symphysis pubis
- osteitis pubis
- an adductor avulsion (which is acutely painful)

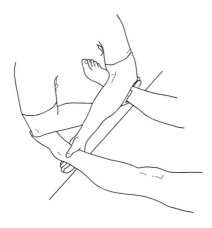

Fig. 2-25 Resisted hip joint adduction.

ASSESSMENT

INTERPRETATION

This can be done in the side-lying position as in the active test. Resist adduction at the knee joint. In the side-lying position, stabilization may be difficult.

Tests in Sitting

Resisted Hip Flexion (Knee Flexed)

The athlete sits with legs over the edge of the plinth, with hands gripping the plinth to stabilize the body.

The athlete flexes the hip and raises the thigh off the plinth.

Resist proximal to the knee with one hand while the other hand stabilizes the pelvis.

Pain or weakness can be caused by an injury to the iliopsoas muscle or its nerve supply, iliopectineal bursitis, and avulsion injuries of the anterior superior iliac spine, anterior inferior iliac spine, or the lesser trochanter. Weakness may also be part of a hip capsular pattern (flexion, abduction, medial rotation).

Active Hip Medial Rotation (35°; Internal Rotation) (Fig. 2-26)

The athlete sits as above, holding the plinth. The athlete swings the lower leg outward to rotate the hip joint medially.

Do not allow the athlete to lift the pelvis on the side that is being tested.

You can control this with one hand on the iliac crest on the side that is being tested.

Pain, limitation of range of motion, or weakness can be caused be an injury to the medial rotators or their nerve supply.

The prime movers are:
- Gluteus minimus—superior gluteal N. (L4, L5, S1)
- Gluteus medius—superior gluteal N. (L4, L5, S1)
- Tensor fascia lata—superior gluteal N. (L4, L5)

The accessory movers are:
- Adductor magnus (posterior fibers)—obturator N. (L2, L3, L4)
- Semitendinosis —tibial branch of sciatic N. (L5, S1, S2)
- Semimembranosus—tibial branch of sciatic N. (L5, S1, S2)

Passive Hip Medial Rotation (Internal Rotation)

The athlete sits as above, holding the plinth. Kneel in front of the athlete and carry the hip through medial rotation with one hand stabilizing the distal femur and the other hand on the distal tibia pushing outward until an end feel is reached. The athlete's pelvis should not rise on the side that is being tested.

Pain or limitation of range of motion may come from the ischiofemoral ligament or by tension or injury to the hip lateral rotators.

Limitation in medial rotation occurs in the athlete with a slipped capital femoral epiphysis.

A piriformis syndrome will cause pain at the end of range of motion. Osteoarthritis can limit motion in all planes, but especially limits medial hip rotation and abduction.

Resisted Hip Medial Rotation (Internal Rotation; 35°) (Fig. 2-27)

The athlete sits as above, holding the plinth. The hip should be in midrange.

Resist medial rotation of the hip with one hand stabilizing the femur and your other hand applying inward pressure to the lateral distal tibia.

Weakness or pain can be caused by an injury to the medial rotators or their nerve supply (see Active Hip Medial Rotation.) Hip arthrosis causes restriction and pain in medial rotation first and then in flexion.

Weakness may be part of a capsular pattern (flexion, abduction, medial rotation).

ASSESSMENT

INTERPRETATION

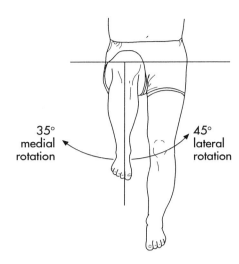

Fig. 2-26 Active hip joint medial and lateral rotation.

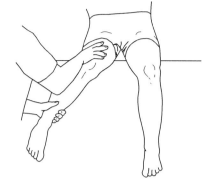

Fig. 2-27 Resisted hip joint medial rotation.

A nerve root problem of L4, L5, S1 often occurs with lower back injuries and therefore resisted medial rotation may be weak.

Active Hip Lateral Rotation (External Rotation; 45 °) (see Fig. 2-26)

With the athlete in the sitting position, holding the plinth, he or she swings the lower leg inward to rotate the hip joint laterally. Do not allow the hip or pelvis to elevate on the side being tested.

Pain, limitation of range of motion, or weakness can come from an injury to the lateral rotator muscles or to their nerve supply. The prime movers are:
- Obturator internus—sacral plexus (L5, S1, S2, S3)
- Obturator externus—obturator N. (L3, L4)
- Quadratus femoris—sacral plexus (L4, L5, S1)
- Piriformis—sacral plexus (L4, L5, S1)
- Gemellus superior—sacral plexus (L5, S1, S2, S3)
- Gemellus inferior—sacral plexus (L4, L5, S1, S2)

Passive Hip Lateral Rotation (External Rotation; 45°)

Kneel in front of the athlete and carry the tibia through hip lateral rotation with one hand stabilizing the distal end of the femur and the other hand on the distal tibia, pushing it inward until an end feel is reached.

Pain or limitation of range of motion can come from:
- injury to the medial rotators that are put on stretch
- injury to the lateral band of the iliofemoral ligament
- injury to the pubofemoral ligament

Femoral anteversion causes excessive hip medial rotation and reduces the range of lateral rotation. Femoral retroversion causes excessive hip lateral rotation and reduced medial rotation (during rapid growth at puberty, a young patient may develop a slipped capital femoral epiphysis, which results in hip joint retroversion).

Resisted Hip Lateral Rotation (External Rotation)

With the tibia in midrange, resist lateral rotation with one hand stabilizing the distal femur and the other hand on

Pain and/or weakness can be caused be an injury to the lateral rotators or to their nerve supply (see Active Hip Lateral Rotation).

ASSESSMENT

INTERPRETATION

the medial distal tibia, pushing out-ward.

Weakness can be caused be an L4, L5, S1 nerve root problem with associated low back problems (disc herniation symptomology).

A piriformis syndrome may cause pain here.

Active Knee Extension

The athlete extends the knee fully through the range of motion.

Pain, limitation of range of motion, or weakness can be caused by an injury to the knee extensor muscles or to their nerve supply. The prime movers are:
- Rectus femoris—femoral N. (L2, L3)
- Vastus medialis—femoral N. (L2, L3)
- Vastus intermedius—femoral N. (L2, L3)
- Vastus lateralis—femoral N. (L2, L3)

A quadriceps hematoma will also cause pain.

Resisted Knee Extension

Place one hand on the distal femur and the other on the lower tibia and resist knee extension. This test can also be done in the supine position.

NOTE: Active, passive, and resisted knee tests are done to rule out knee dysfunction and to test muscles that cross the hip and the knee joints.

Pain or weakness can be caused by an injury to the knee extensors or their nerve supply (see Active Knee Extension).

Weakness without pain may indicate an L3 nerve root problem (disc) and painless weakness bilaterally can indicate a localized myopathy.

Tests in the Prone Position

Active Knee flexion (120° to 130°)

The athlete flexes the knee actively through the full range of motion. The pelvis should be stabilized.

Pain, limitation of range of motion, or weakness can be caused by an injury to the knee flexors or to their nerve supply.

The prime movers are:
- Biceps femoris—sciatic N. (L5, S1, S2)
- Semitendinosus—sciatic N. (L5, S1, S2)
- Semimembranosus—sciatic N. (L5, S1, S2)

During the knee flexion, if the buttock on that side rises up, it could be because of:
- tight hip flexors
- a quadriceps hematoma
- an injury to the rectus femoris muscle

Passive Knee Flexion (130°)

Carry the knee through full flexion with one hand on the anterior distal tibia and the other hand stabilizing the pelvis and the posterior superior iliac spine. The buttocks should not rise up off the plinth during testing.

Pain of limitation or range of motion can be caused by knee-joint swelling or dysfunction, and tightness or a lesion of the rectus femoris muscle.

ASSESSMENT

INTERPRETATION

Resisted Knee Flexion

The athlete flexes the knee while you resist with one hand around the distal tibia and the other hand stabilizing the pelvis.

Medial (semimembranosus, semitendinosus) and lateral (biceps femoris) hamstrings can be tested by resisting knee flexion with the tibia rotated medially and laterally, respectively.

Pain or weakness can be caused by an injury to the knee flexors or to their nerve supply (see Active Knee Flexion). Ischial tuberosity bursitis will cause pain. Painless weakness of the hamstrings characterizes lesions of the first and second sacral nerves.

Injuries to the hamstrings have been associated mainly with lack of flexibility and training error (overstretching, overtraining, fatigue). Recently, hamstring injuries have also been associated with lumbar spine and/or sacroiliac pathologic conditions with or without neural tissue involvement (i.e., sciatic nerve, dural tube) (Cibulka, Kornberg et al.).

Active Hip Extension With Knee Extension (30°) (Fig. 2-28)

Place one arm and hand over the posterior pelvis and lower lumbar spine to stabilize them while the athlete lifts one leg (knee extended) about 30°. Lumbar extension should not occur.

Pain, limitation of range of motion, or weakness can be caused by injury to the hip extensor muscles or to their nerve supply.

The prime movers are:
- Gluteus maximus—inferior gluteal N. (L5, S1, S2)
- Hamstrings—sciatic N. (L5, S1)

Full extension of the hip and knee is needed for normal relaxed standing and gait. Full hip extension is required during the terminal part of stance phase or compensation will occur at the body segments above or below the hip. For example, the lumbar spine or knee must hyperextend if hip extension does not occur. Therefore, with time, lumbar spine and knee problems can develop because of the lack of hip extension range of motion.

Passive Hip Extension With Knee Extension (30°)

Stabilize the pelvis but the other hand goes under the athlete's anterior thigh and lifts it upward until an end feel is reached at the hip joint.

Pain or limitation of range of motion can be caused by the hip flexors putting pressure on the iliopectineal bursa or an iliofemoral or ischiofemoral ligament injury.

In the older athlete, a limitation in hip extension and some restriction in abduction and medial rotation is a sign of osteoarthritis with the resulting fibrosis of the capsule.

Resisted Hip Extension With Knee Extension

Stabilize the pelvis as above while the other hand resists the athlete's hip extension.

Pain or weakness can be caused by an injury to the hip extensors or to their nerve supply (see Active Hip Extension with Knee Extension).

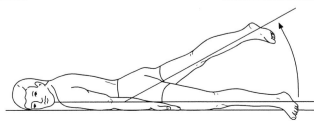

Fig. 2-28 Active hip joint extension with knee joint extension.

ASSESSMENT

INTERPRETATION

One hand resists the distal posterior thigh while the other hand stabilizes the pelvis.

Active Hip Extension With Knee Flexion

Place one arm and hand over the posterior pelvis and lower spine to stabilize them.

The athlete lifts the leg with the knee flexed to an angle of approximately 90°.

Do not allow lumbar extension.

By flexing the knee, the hamstrings relax and the gluteus maximus can be tested individually.

Pain, limitation of range of motion, or weakness of hip extension can lead to low back dysfunction because the athlete is not able to extend the hip.

Passive Hip Extension With Knee Flexion

Stand beside the plinth on the involved side.

Stabilize the pelvis with one hand while the other hand goes under the athlete's thigh.

Lift the leg while maintaining the athlete's knee flexion with your testing arm or shoulder.

The hip is gently extended until an end feel is reached.

Do not allow lumbar spine extension.

Any tightness or injury to the hip flexors will elicit pain.

Iliopectineal bursitis will also cause pain during this test.

The iliofemoral and ischiofemoral ligaments are put on stretch during this test so any injury to them will elicit pain.

This position stretches the femoral nerve, and pain experienced in the lateral hip or anterior thigh may indicate an impingement of the nerve or L2 or L3 nerve roots.

The lateral femoral or femoral cutaneous nerve may also elicit pain if impinged.

Ely's Test (Fig. 2-29)

Slowly flex the athlete's knee as far as possible so that their heel comes close to the buttocks. Observe the buttock and hip during the knee flexion. The point at which the athlete's buttock rises (pelvis lifts off the plinth) on the tested side indicates the degree of hip-flexor tightness. You can palpate the iliac crest posteriorly or the ASIS under the hip to determine when the pelvis begins to rise.

The athlete should be able to flex the knee to an angle of at least 90° before the hip and buttock rise. If this is not possible, the athlete has a tight rectus femoris muscle or even a contracture of this muscle. When the knee is flexed, the length of rectus femoris limits the motion and the ilium on that side rotates anteriorly. This rotation is then translated into lumbar extension.

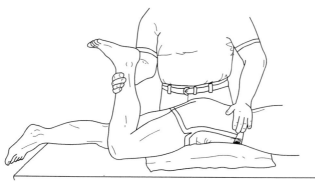

Fig. 2-29 Ely's test.

ASSESSMENT

INTERPRETATION

Resisted Hip Extension With Knee Flexion

Stabilize the pelvis with one hand and resist the athlete's hip extension with the other hand on the posterior thigh. The athlete maintains knee flexion on the leg being tested.

Weakness or pain can be caused by a gluteus maximus strain or injury to the inferior gluteal nerve or to the nerve root serving the muscle (L5, S1, S2).

SPECIAL TESTS

Thomas Test (Fig. 2-30)

The athlete lies supine on the plinth with his or her legs to midthigh hanging over the edge.

The athlete pulls one knee to the chest using the arms. The lumbar spine must be flattened to the table by having the athlete do a pelvic tilt during the test.

If the athlete's other leg rises off the plinth and/or the knee extends, the test is positive.

Palpate the hip flexors during the test. Normal flexibility of the hip flexors allows the extended hip to rest on the plinth and the knee to flex to an angle of 90°.

If the leg rises off the plinth on the extended hip and knee side, the athlete has tight hip flexors and adductors.

If the knee extends, the athlete has a tight rectus femoris. If the leg abducts, the iliotibial band is tight. If the femur rotates, the lateral rotators may also be shortened or tight.

Adaptive shortening of the iliopsoas occurs with hip bursitis, prolonged bed rest, poor posture, prolonged positions with the hips flexed (sports such as hockey and basketball) and osteoarthritic or hip degenerative joint disease.

Pain may be felt with an iliopectineal bursitis or if there is a strain lesion in either of the hip flexors.

Ober's Test (Fig. 2-31)

The athlete lies on his or her side with the involved leg uppermost. The lower leg is flexed at the hip and knee for stability.

Abduct the upper leg as far as possible and slightly extend the hip so that the tensor fascia lata and iliotibial band are over the greater trochanter. Then release the leg while maintaining stabi-

If the leg remains abducted this is a positive test. In most cases it shows that the iliotibial band has a contracture or is tight—this can be tight because of poor posture, poor flexibility, poliomyelitis, or meningomyelocele. The iliotibial band can become adhesed after severe trauma and this will also result in a positive test.

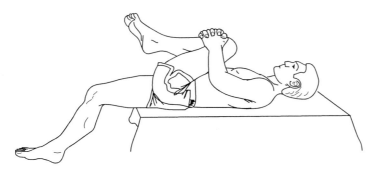

Fig. 2-30 Thomas test.

ASSESSMENT   INTERPRETATION

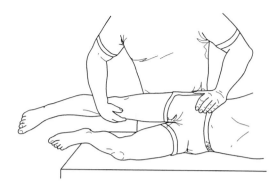

Fig. 2-31 Ober's test with knee extended.

lization of the pelvis with the opposite hand. To ensure pelvic stabilization, lean your body weight over the iliac crest. Allowing the pelvis to move or the leg to roll inward permits the iliotibial band to slide anteriorly, giving you an unreliable test.

If the iliotibial band is normal the leg will drop to the adducted position.

If the iliotibial band is tight or has a contracture, the hip will remain abducted.

The test can be repeated with the knee on the test leg flexed to 90° to test the short fibers of the tensor fascia lata.

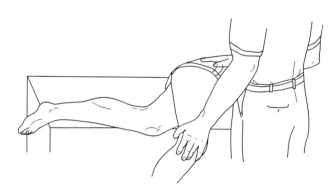

Fig. 2-32 Piriformis test.

Piriformis Test (Fig. 2-32)

With the athlete lying on his or her side the hip and the knee are flexed to 90°. Place one hand on the pelvis for stabilization and with the other hand apply pressure at the knee, pushing it toward the plinth. If tightness of the piriformis is impinging on the sciatic nerve, pain may be produced in the buttock and even down the leg.

This test tightens the external (lateral) rotators and specifically the piriformis muscle (Fig. 2-33). If the piriformis is tight or if the sciatic nerve passes through the muscle, sciatic pain can be elicited.

Trendelenburg Test

When the athlete stands on one leg with the other knee flexed, the pelvis on the opposite side should rise or stay level. If the pelvis drops on the opposite side, it is a positive sign.

This tests the stability of the hip and the ability of the hip abductors (gluteus medius primarily) to stabilize the pelvis on the femur.

ASSESSMENT   INTERPRETATION

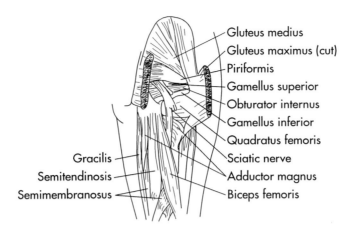

Fig. 2-33 Location of piriformis muscles.

Hip stability can be affected by the following:
- abduction weakness (see Interpretation Section on Resisted Hip Abduction)
- coxa vara, because the high position of the greater trochanter against the ilium often causes an abductor inefficiency or contracture, resulting in a positive Trendelenburg sign on the involved side.
- osteoarthritis

See the section on Trendelenburg gait under Observations.

Scouring Test (Quadrant Test) (Fig. 2-34)

The athlete's hip is in a position of flexion and adduction while his or her knee is flexed comfortably.

Encircle the knee joint with your arms and hands and apply a posterolateral force through the hip joint as the femur is rotated in the acetabulum.

The femur is passively flexed, adducted, and then medially rotated while longitudinally compressed to scour the inner aspect of the joint.

To test the outer aspect of the hip joint, the hip is abducted and laterally rotated while maintaining flexion and again longitudinally compressed.

A positive test occurs if a grating sound or sensation is experienced by the athlete or if pain is elicited.

This test stresses inner and outer aspects of the joint surface as well as the anteromedial and the posterolateral capsule for injury, and the grating sensation or sound occurs if osteoarthritis or degenerative joint changes are present in the hip joint. Any roughness or lack of smoothness can also indicate acetabulum rim or labrum tears.

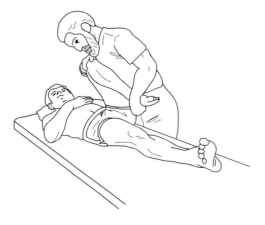

Fig. 2-34 Hip joint quadrant test (joint scouring).

ASSESSMENT   INTERPRETATION

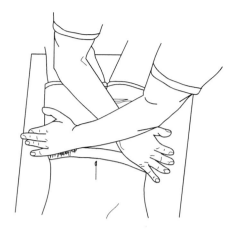

Fig. 2-35 Gapping test.

Sacroiliac Joint Tests

Pelvic Rocking Test

Place your palms on both anterior superior iliac spines, press firmly posteriorly to take up the slack and initiate a gentle rocking motion. Conduct a gentle overpressure for each innominate several times. During this you feel for symmetry of motion and the resiliency of the end feel.

The end feel should be equal, soft, pain free, and slightly springy on each side. If the sacroiliac joint is injured, this test may cause pain and the capacity for motion on the injured side is either reduced (hypomobility) or excessive (hypermobility) compared to the other side. A hard end feel indicates a restriction on that side.

Gapping Test (Fig. 2-35)

Cross your hands over the pelvis with the palms against the anterior superior iliac spines and take up the slack.

Pressure is then applied downward and outward on the ilia.

The slack is taken up and a gentle spring-like overpressure is applied to the ASIS. This compresses the sacroiliac joints posteriorly.

The test is positive if there is unilateral sacroiliac pain or posterior leg pain. It also stresses the sacroiliac ligaments.

Hip Flexion and Adduction Test

With the athlete's knee flexed, flex and adduct the hip to stress the sacroiliac joints.

In this hip position the sacroiliac joint on that side is stressed. Hip joint problems can cause pain during the test (see Scouring Test).

Gaenslen's Sign

With the athlete supine instruct the athlete to draw both legs up to the chest.

Shift the athlete to the edge of the plinth and allow one leg to drop over

When the leg is dropped over the side, the sacroiliac joint rotates forward on the same side and posteriorly on the contralateral side, causing pain if there is sacroiliac joint dysfunction.

ASSESSMENT   INTERPRETATION

the edge while the opposite leg is held to the chest by the athlete.

Sacroiliac Joint Test (Side lying Gaenslen's Test)

The athlete is in the side-lying position with the nonpainful side down.

On the injured side the hip and knee are flexed and the athlete hugs the knee to lock the pelvis and lumbar spine.

The uppermost hip is now extended to its limit, while the knee is kept extended.

Pain indicates a positive test.

As the upper hip is extended there is a rotary stress applied to the ilium against the sacrum on that side. This movement causes pain if a sacroiliac joint sprain or dysfunction exists.

Patrick's or Faber Test—(F) lexion, (Ab) duction, (E) xternal (R) otation (Fig. 2-36)

The athlete is in the supine position with one leg straight.

The other knee and hip are flexed so that the heel is placed on the knee of the straight leg. The flexed knee is then slowly lowered into abduction and the range observed.

Apply gentle pressure to the flexed knee while the opposite hand stabilizes the pelvis (the hand should be placed over the opposite anterior superior iliac spine).

The knee should lower almost parallel to the floor in the normal hip and pelvis.

Inguinal pain that is experienced when the leg is in this position suggests a hip problem.

If the athlete experiences pain in the sacroiliac joint with the overpressure, the joint is injured.

With the hip in this position the flexibility of the adductor muscles, as well as the integrity of the iliofemoral and pubofemoral ligaments, and the joint capsule are also tested.

A tight hip capsule that does not allow abduction causes excessive forces to reach the lumbopelvic joints. There are excessive forces through the ilium that is in anterior rotation on that side, leading to sacroiliac joint problems. The lumbar spine is forced to move into excessive extension during ambulation and activities to compensate for the lack of hip motion.

Pelvic Compression Test (Fig. 2-37)

The athlete is side lying. Apply pressure below the iliac crest over the iliac fossa.

This test compresses the sacroiliac joint. Dysfunction here will elicit pain.

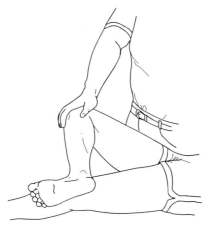

Fig. 2-36 Patrick's or Faber test (overpressure).

ASSESSMENT   INTERPRETATION

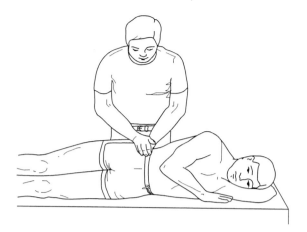

Fig. 2-37 Pelvic compression test.

You should be above the athlete and should push in a downward direction.

Sit up Test for Iliosacral Dysfunction (see Fig.1-58)

The athlete is in the supine position and the pelvis is made symmetrical through the Wilson-Barstow maneuver as follows:

The athlete flexes the knees and lifts the pelvis about 4 inches off the plinth, then drops the pelvis down to the table.

Passively extend the knees and lower the legs one at a time to the plinth.

Palpate and observe the level of the distal medial malleoli.

The athlete is instructed to sit up and the levels of the malleoli are checked again.

The sit up test can be used to determine if anterior or posterior iliac rotation exists.

As the athlete forward bends, the spinal segments lock together and the sacrum allows for the end mobility. Once the lumbar forward bending reaches the sacrum the sacroiliac joint should move 2° to 6° in a mobile joint.

If the right sacroiliac joint is blocked or hypomobile (e.g., posterior iliac rotation) the mobility on that side is missing. Therefore, during the sit up the sacrum and ilium move together. The acetabulum is thrust forward on the right side and the leg will appear to lengthen (medial malleolus migrates downward). The right malleolus goes from a shortened length in the supine position to a longer length in the sitting position.

If the right sacroiliac joint is in an anterior iliac rotation, the leg may appear longer (or the same length) in the supine position but the leg will get shorter after the athlete sits up (see Lumbar Spine, Special Tests).

Tests for Leg-length Discrepancy

See Observations section on leg-length discrepancy and pelvic posture for a more detailed discussion.

Anatomic Leg-length Discrepancy

Measurements of the athlete's leg length should be taken while the athlete is standing—measure from the ASIS to

An anatomic leg-length difference can be caused by:
- poliomyelitis of the lower limb
- fracture of the femur or tibia

ASSESSMENT

the floor and from PSIS to the floor bilaterally. If the ASIS and PSIS are lower on one side, an anatomic leg-length difference exists.

Functional Leg-length Discrepancy

If the ASIS is lower and PSIS is higher on the same side, a functional leg-length discrepancy exists.

True Leg-length (Anatomic) Measurements

When the observations indicate a leg-length discrepancy, the athlete lies in the supine position and is asked to flex the knees. Then the athlete is asked to raise the pelvis about 3 inches off the plinth and to let it drop to the plinth.

Extend the knees to the plinth and measurements are taken of each leg from the ASIS to the medial malleolus. A slight difference of up to half an inch is common. Reid recommends measurements from the ASIS to the lateral malleolus.

To determine whether there is a discrepancy in length of femur or tibia, ask the athlete to flex his or her knees 90° with the feet together and flat on the plinth. If one knee projects higher than the other, the tibia is longer. If one knee comes forward further, the femur is longer.

Measurements can be made from:
- iliac crest to greater trochanter to determine if coxa vara is present

INTERPRETATION

- bone growth problems of the lower limb (a damaged epiphyseal plate)

If coxa valgum is present on one side, the athlete will have a longer leg on the involved side with resulting pelvic obliquity and adductor weakness on that side—this condition can be confirmed by an x-ray.

If coxa varum exists, there will be a shortening of the involved leg and, as a result, the pelvis will drop on weight bearing (Trendelenburg gait and sign) and abduction will be restricted on that side.

A functional leg-length difference can be caused by:
- one pronated foot and/or one supinated foot
- muscle spasm in one hip
- hip capsule tightness
- adductor muscle spasm on one side
- more genu valgus on one side
- femoral anteversion on one side (if combined with pronated foot)

With posterior iliac rotation, the ilium and the sacrum sit posteriorly and the acetabulum is pulled backward also, making that limb appear shorter.

Either the femur or tibia is shorter or coxa vara exists.

ASSESSMENT

- greater trochanter to knee for femur length
- knee joint line to medial malleolus for tibial length.

Leg-length differences can also be caused by iliac rotation.

Apparent Shortening

If no true leg-length discrepancy is found, this measurement can be taken: measure from the umbilicus (or xiphisternal junction) to the medial malleolus; unequal distances signify an apparent leg-length discrepancy.

Tests for Dermatomes and Cutaneous Nerves

If the history includes sensory loss or hypersensitivity, test the dermatomes and cutaneous nerves.

With a pin, check the sensation of dermatomes T10 to L3 and of the cutaneous nerve regions.

Prick the pin over the dermatome and cutaneous nerve areas bilaterally (approximately 10 locations per dermatome) while the athlete looks away.

Compare the sensations bilaterally and have the athlete report his or her feelings on whether the pin prick feels sharp or dull.

If the sensations are not the same bilaterally or from one region to another on the same limb, repeat the test in those areas. Different test sensations can be done using test tubes containing hot and/or cold water or cotton balls.

Dermatomes vary and overlap in each individual so the dermatome mapping given (Gray's) is an approximation of the nerve root supply.

Dermatomes (see Fig. 1-50)

INTERPRETATION

Shortening may be caused by pelvic obliquity, adduction, or flexion deformity in the hip joint, or spasm or contracture of trunk muscles on one side.

Sensation is supplied to the hip, pelvic region, and thigh by nerves originating in the thoracic, lumbar, and sacral spines.

T10 dermatome is level with the umbilicus.

T12 dermatome is immediately above the inguinal ligament.

T11 dermatome is in the area between the dermatomes of T10 and T12.

ASSESSMENT

INTERPRETATION

L1, L2, L3, dermatomes band down the anterior thigh.
S2 dermatome is in the posterior thigh
Any problem with sensation suggests a nerve root problem.

Cutaneous Nerves (see Fig. 2-13)

Meralgia paresthetica is numbness and/or tingling of the skin that is supplied by the lateral femoral cutaneous nerve of the thigh. This condition can develop if there is friction as the nerve passes through the inguinal ligament or if the nerve has been injured by trauma—do not confuse this with an L2 nerve root lesion. Tapping at the ASIS or inguinal ligament can elicit a tinel sign.

The anterior or posterior cutaneous nerve supply to the thigh may also cause numbness if it is traumatized or damaged.

The medial (obturator) nerve on occasion can also be injured.

Circulatory Tests

Palpate the femoral artery in the femoral triangle to check for a normal pulse (Fig. 2-38)

If the hip area has sustained severe trauma, it is important to check the femoral pulse to ensure that a good blood supply is going to the lower limb. Pulses should be monitored down the limb if a fracture is suspected (popliteal artery, posterior tibial artery, and dorsal pedal artery; see Fig. 1-61).

Specific Hip Pointer Test

The athlete will experience pain when side bending away from the hip pointer side. Abduction of both legs together in the side-lying position will also cause pain and limitation of movement. The athlete may also experience pain when lying supine and lifting the pelvis on that side.

An iliac crest avulsion or contusion will cause point tenderness during this test. Pain is produced on side bending because of the pull of the quadratus lumborum or the abdominals from the crest.

The attachment of the external oblique muscle can avulse part of the iliac crest if the force is significant. In the young athlete, the avulsion can occur through the apophyseal plate. There can be significant pain and swelling and marked disability during walking if there is an avulsion.

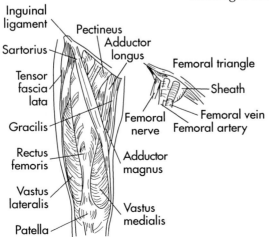

Fig. 2-38 Anterior muscles of the thigh and femoral triangle.

ASSESSMENT

INTERPRETATION

ACCESSORY MOVEMENTS

Inferior Glide (Fig. 2-39)

The athlete is in the supine position with a belt around the pelvis to fixate it.

The athlete's hip is flexed 60° to 90° and the knee is flexed 90° with the elevated lower leg over the therapist's shoulder.

Grasp the anterior aspect of the proximal femur as close to the hip joint as possible with the fingers intertwined.

An inferior glide or distraction force on the proximal femur is performed by leaning backward while simultaneously rocking the athlete's hip into more flexion.

The inferior glide of the hip joint is necessary for full hip flexion but it helps increase the overall range of motion of the hip joint also. If there is hypomobility, the joint needs to be mobilized to regain full range. If there is hypermobility, strengthening exercises are recommended for stability.

Excessive movement can lead to hip dislocation (especially in children) and degenerative changes with time.

Gentle inferior glide motions also decrease joint pain and help to increase nutrition to the articular cartilage of the hip joint.

Posterior Glide (Fig. 2-40)

The athlete is in the supine position with an inch of padding placed under the pelvis, just proximal and medial to the acetabulum.

Support the slightly flexed knee with the right hand around the medial side of the knee and under the popliteal fossa.

The mobilizing left hand contacts the anterior aspect of the proximal femur.

Rock your body weight gently over the hip joint, pushing gently posteriorly to achieve a posterior glide of the hip joint.

This posterior movement is needed for full internal rotation and flexion at the hip joint. If there is hypomobility, mobilization techniques are needed to regain the range. This glide can decrease hip joint pain and help the nutrition in the articular cartilage of the joint.

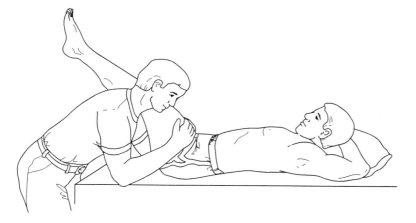

Fig. 2-39 Hip joint inferior glide.

ASSESSMENT   INTERPRETATION

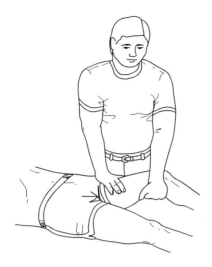

Fig. 2-40 Hip joint posterior glide.

Anterior Glide (Fig. 2-41)

The athlete is lying prone with the knee flexed to 90°, with 30° of abduction and slight external rotation.

A towel or wedge can support the anterior distal aspect of the pelvis.

Support the knee on the anterior aspect of the distal femur with the right hand.

The heel of the mobilizing hand (left) contacts the posterior aspect of the proximal femur level with the greater trochanter.

The left hand gently pushes the proximal femur anteriorly to cause an anterior glide of the hip joint.

PALPATION

Palpate for point tenderness, temperature differences, swelling, and muscle spasm. Note any adhesions, tendonitis, tenosynovitis, myofascial trigger points, or boney masses.

Anterior Structures

Boney (Fig. 2-42)
Iliac Crest

This movement is necessary for full external rotation. Any hypomobility tells you of the loss of this accessory movement and mobilization is needed.

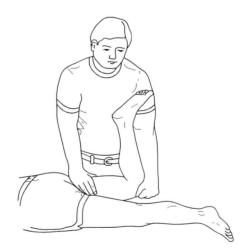

Fig. 2-41 Hip joint anterior glide.

Periosteitis, epiphyseal, or an avulsion fracture may cause exquisite point tenderness over the bone. A contusion in this area may have associated swelling with the point tenderness.

ASSESSMENT   INTERPRETATION

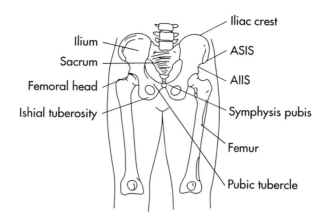

Fig. 2-42 Anterior structures (boney).

Anterior Superior Iliac Spine (ASIS)

Sartorius strain or avulsion at the ASIS may be extremely tender and an incongruity of the muscle may be palpable—this can occur in the adolescent athlete.

The heights of the ASIS should be level in lying and should be equidistance from the body's midline (xyphoid process or umbilicus).

Pelvis drop should be done first. Uneven ASIS heights can indicate an ilium rotation. A pelvic inflare or outflare can be present if the midline to ASIS measurements are not equal.

Anterior Inferior Iliac Spine (AIIS)

A rectus femoris strain or avulsion at the AIIS may be accompanied by muscle deformity and acute point tenderness in the athlete (usually adolescent). The iliofemoral ligament attaches here and may be point tender if sprained.

Symphysis Pubis

A sprain of the anterior inferior pubic, superior pubic, or arcuate pubic ligament may cause pain over the symphysis pubis.

One pubic tubercle may be higher than the other—this is caused by a displacement on that side. To evaluate their height, slide the heel of your hand down the abdomen until contact is made with the pubic bone. Locate the pubic tubercles with the fingertips and compare bilaterally (see Lumbar Spine Palpations for more detail). If the tubercles are uneven, the athlete can have sacroiliac problems and adductor problems associated with it.

Pubic Ramus

A pubic ramus stress fracture causes exquisite point tenderness over the bone on deep palpation.

ASSESSMENT   INTERPRETATION

Soft Tissue
Femoral Triangle (see Fig. 2-38)

The femoral triangle is best palpated with the athlete's hip abducted and laterally rotated. The following areas should be checked:

- lymph node
- inguinal ligament
- iliopectineal bursa or ligament

Enlarged inguinal lymph nodes in the femoral triangle area indicate a lower limb infection or a systemic infection. The lymph glands here cannot be felt unless they are inflamed.

An inguinal ligament sprain can cause tenderness over the ligament but is not to be confused with an inguinal hernia; a palpable lump may be felt to protrude when the athlete coughs.

Acute point tenderness of the inguinal area overlying the hip joint occurs with femoral neck stress fractures.

It is difficult to differentiate between iliopectineal bursitis or a ligament sprain because the bursa is too deep to be readily palpated. However, pain on passive hip flexion is often present in the case of a bursitis and not of a ligament sprain.

Anterior Muscles (see Fig. 2-38)

Sartorius; gracilis; pectineus; adductor longus, brevis, and magnus; rectus femoris; vastus lateralis; vastus medialis.

Myositis ossificans (boney mass) may be palpable in the quadriceps muscle (especially the vastus lateralis) after a severe quadriceps hematoma or repeated trauma.

Strains or tears of the sartorius; gracilis; pectineus; adductor longus, brevis, and magnus; rectus femoris; vastus lateralis; and medialis muscles are possible. Palpate from origin to insertion to determine any muscle defects or swelling. A point-tender site on the muscle, local swelling or increased temperature (inflammation) in the muscle, or lack of continuity of the muscle can help to diagnose the injury.

According to Simons and Travell, myofascial trigger points for the iliopsoas muscles are located at the lateral wall of the femoral triangle (femoral attachment), inside the edge of the iliac crest, and lateral to rectus abdominus over the psoas muscle. Iliopsoas referred pain can be into the anterior thigh or lumbar spine.

The trigger points of the adductor magnus are within the muscle belly and pain is referred to the upper medial thigh and inside the groin and pelvic area.

The trigger points for the adductor brevis and longus are in the upper medial thigh with the referred pain down the anteromedial thigh and even into the anteromedial lower leg.

Pectineus has a trigger point in the muscle and the referred pain pattern stays locally in the muscle.

The myofascial trigger point for the quadriceps femoris is over the upper portion of the muscle and pain is referred on the front of the thigh and medial knee region.

Vastus medialis has a trigger point in the muscle belly with pain referred to the patella.

Vastus lateralis has a trigger point on the lateral thigh in the lower third of the iliotibial band while the referred pain extends up the lateral thigh and can extend into the lateral buttock area.

ASSESSMENT   INTERPRETATION

Lateral Structures

Lateral structures are best palpated with the athlete in the side-lying position.

Boney (Fig. 2-43)
Greater Trochanter

This structure can appear tender because of greater trochanteric bursitis. Local warmth and localized point tenderness will determine its presence.

Iliac Crest

The iliac crest can be affected by contusions, periosteitis, epiphysitis, or avulsion fractures. All these conditions will cause severe point tenderness. Tenderness can be palpated at the origin of the external obligue or tensor fascia lata muscle (whichever muscle is involved).

Ilium

The ilium can become contused; fractures of the ilium are rare. If a contusion exists, the athlete will show signs of point tenderness, often accompanied by some local swelling and/or ecchymosis.

Soft Tissue (Fig. 2-44)
Gluteus Medius

The gluteus medius can suffer insertion strain or spasm, in which case local point tenderness and tightening of the muscle will be present. Myofascial trigger points may be present.

According to Simons and Travell, the trigger points for gluteus medius are on the posterior upper gluteal area below the

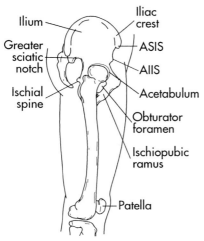

Fig. 2-43 Lateral structures (boney).

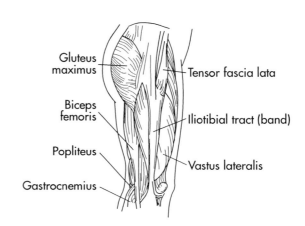

Fig. 2-44 Lateral structures (soft tissue).

ASSESSMENT

INTERPRETATION

iliac crest and opposite the sacrum. Pain is referred into the posterior gluteal region and upper posterior thigh. This referred pain is often misdiagnosed as sacroiliac dysfunction pain.

Tensor Fascia Lata and Iliotibial Band

The tensor fascia lata can become injured through a muscle strain or from repeated microtrauma as it snaps over the greater trochanter. This mechanical irritation can cause greater trochanteric bursitis—local point tenderness is usually present.

Palpate the length of the muscle and the iliotibial band for irregularities and muscle spasm.

The trigger points for the tensor fascia lata are in the muscle and its referred pain pattern is to the upper half of the lateral thigh and it may extend to the knee joint.

Posterior Structures

Boney (Fig. 2-46)
Ischial Tuberosity

Hamstring origin strain or avulsion will cause local point tenderness here and is difficult to distinguish from ischial tuberosity bursitis except by the history.

Check for the anterior and superior-inferior position of the ischial tuberosities. A change in the anteroposterior relationship may indicate an iliac rotation. One tuberosity higher or lower may indicate an upslip or downslip (rare).

Sciatic Notch

Sciatic nerve pain may be present at the sciatic notch and can spread down the length of the limb if the nerve is irritated by an intervertebral disc or if the piriformis muscle is in spasm and compressing the nerve.

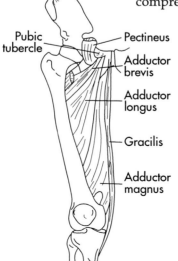

Pubic tubercle
Pectineus
Adductor brevis
Adductor longus
Gracilis
Adductor magnus

Fig. 2-45 Medial structures (muscles).

ASSESSMENT

INTERPRETATION

Lumbar Spine

Lumbar spine dysfunction and pain may be elicited by palpation. It can be the primary lesion or it can be secondary to the hip problem. L5 is just superior to the sacrum and any pressure on the lumbar spinous process can elicit pain if dysfunction exists.

Sacrum and Coccyx

Contusions, periosteitis, or fractures of these structures will elicit point tenderness.

A gentle compression force with the entire hand on the sacrum can elicit sacroiliac joint pain if there is joint dysfunction. The depth of the sacral sulci around the PSIS should be palpated with the finger tips. Palpate for sulcus depth and for local tenderness in the ligaments. If one side is deeper than the other, a sacral torsion may exist. Tenderness in the sulcus or the ligaments can also indicate sacroiliac dysfunction.

Palpate the inferior lateral angles of the sacrum (ILA) to determine if they are level. If they are not level, sacral torsion problems can exist. If they are level and one sulcus is deeper, there is a sacral rotation present.

Soft Tissue (Fig. 2-46)
Hamstrings

Contusion, strain, or avulsion of the hamstrings will elicit local point tenderness, swelling, or incongruity of the muscle. Scar tissue may be palpable as a lump or thickening in the tissue in a chronic hamstring strain.

According to Simons and Travell, the hamstring trigger points are in the muscle belly midthigh. The referred pain pattern for biceps femoris is mainly in the popliteal space with pain extending up the posterior thigh slightly and down into the upper section of the gastrocnemii. The referred pain pattern for semimembranosus and semitendinosus muscle is at the junction of the posterior thigh and buttock with it radiating down to the midleg.

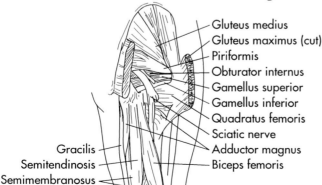

Gluteus medius
Gluteus maximus (cut)
Piriformis
Obturator internus
Gamellus superior
Gamellus inferior
Quadratus femoris
Sciatic nerve
Gracilis
Semitendinosis
Semimembranosus
Adductor magnus
Biceps femoris

Fig. 2-46 Posterior structures (soft tissue).

ASSESSMENT   INTERPRETATION

Gluteus Maximus

According to Simons and Travell, the gluteus maximus has three trigger points in the muscle. One is opposite the coccyx in the middle of the muscle belly, another is in the middle of the lower third of the muscle, and the third is just above the gluteal fold close to the center of the body. These trigger points can refer pain in practically any part of the buttock and in the coccyx.

Strains or contusions will be point tender.

Gluteus Medius

See lateral structures.

Gluteus Minimus

Gluteus minimus has a posterior trigger point midbelly that refers pain down the buttock and posterior thigh and into the gastrocnemius. This trigger point may mimic sciatica caused by nerve root irritation, but with trigger points there are no neurological deficits. There is an anterior trigger point in gluteus minimus that refers pain down the lateral thigh and lateral lower leg (as far as lateral malleolus). Gluteus minimus is deep to gluteus medius and may not be able to be palpated separately.

Piriformis

Piriformis has a trigger point midbelly and can refer pain into the sacroiliac region, buttock, down the back of the thigh and gastrocnemius, and into the sole of the foot.

Piriformis tenderness on one side or tightness may indicate a sacral torsion.

Hip Lateral Rotators

Piriformis, gemelli, obturator internus, and quadratus femoris are difficult to palpate because of their depth and also because they are covered by gluteus maximus. Muscle spasm of the lateral rotators can occur from any low back, pelvic, or hip condition.

Sciatic Nerve

Sciatic neuritis can be caused by a direct blow to the nerve or surrounding area, disc herniation, or piriformis spasm compressing the nerve.

Lumbar Musculature

Paraspinal muscle spasm can be protecting a primary lumbar problem or can be due to compensation of the lumbar musculature for hip dysfunction.

The soft tissue can be palpated from the twelfth rib to the iliac crest for protective spasm or trigger points.

ASSESSMENT	INTERPRETATION

Sacroiliac Joint Ligaments

The dorsal sacroiliac ligaments running from the sacrum to the posterior superior iliac spine and inner lip of the dorsal part of the iliac crest will be point tender if sprained or if the sacroiliac joint is in dysfunction.

Sacrotuberous Ligament

The sacrotuberous ligament running from the ischial tuberosity to the posterior iliac spine and sacrum can also be point tender with sacral or sacroiliac injury. The ligamentous tissue and the surrounding tissue may feel thicker or tighter on the side with dysfunction.

Iliolumbar Ligament

The iliolumbar ligament runs from the transverse process of the fifth lumbar vertebra to the upper lateral surface of the sacrum (blends with ventral sacroiliac ligament) and the crest of the ilium in front of the sacroiliac joint. Lumbar spine or sacroiliac dysfunction can make this ligament point tender. This ligament is important in stabilizing the L5-S1 segment, particularly during forward bending and rotation. If the lumbosacral joint is injured or hypermobile this ligament becomes acutely point tender.

*These ligaments are very deep and may not be directly palpable.

Medial Structures

Soft Tissue
Adductor Group (see Fig. 2-45)
- Gracilis
- Pectineus
- Adductor Longus
- Adductor Brevis
- Adductor Magnus

Strain, tendonitis, or spasm of any of the adductor muscles will cause point tenderness and local swelling. For the trigger points and referred pain, see Anterior Structures.

Avulsion or strain at the origin of the gracilis, adductor longus, pectineus, or adductor brevis may cause point tenderness, local swelling, or even tracking. Palpate the muscle from origin to insertion to determine if there are any muscle defects.

REFERENCES

Anderson JE: *Grant's Atlas of Anatomy*, Baltimore, 1983, Williams & Wilkins..

Bloom M and Crawford A: Slipped capital epiphysis—an assessment of treatment modalities, Orthopaedics 8:36, 1985.

Booher JM and Thibodeau GA: Athletic injury assessment, Toronto, 1985, Times Mirror/Mosby College Publishing.

Brody: Running injuries, Ciba Clinical Symposia, Ciba Pharmaceutical Co 32:4, 1980.

Cibulka MT et al: Hamstring muscle strain treated by mobilizing the sacroiliac joint, Phys Ther 66:1220-1223, 1986.

Coole G and Geick H: An analysis of hamstring strains and their rehabilitation, J Orthop Sports Phys Ther 9(2):77, 1987.

Crawford A: Current concepts review—slipped capital femoral epiphysis, Bone Joint Surg 70-A(9):1422, Oct 1988.

Cyriax J: Textbook of orthopedic medicine: diagnosis of soft tissue lesions, vol 1, London, 1978, Bailliere Tindall.

Daniels L and Worthingham C: Muscle testing techniques of manual examination, Toronto, 1980, WB Saunders Inc.

Donatelli R and Wooden M: Orthopaedic physical therapy, New York, 1989, Churchill Livingstone.

Edmund SL: Manipulation Mobilization: Extremity and spinal techniques, Toronto, 1993, Mosby-Yearbook.

Fullerton L and Snowdy H: Femoral neck stress fractures, Am J Sports Med 16(4):365, 1988.

Godshall RM and Hansen CA: Incomplete avulsion of a portion of the iliac epiphysis, J Bone Joint Surg 59A:825, 1977.

Glick JA: Muscle strains: prevention and treatment, Physician Sports Med 8(11):73, Nov 1980.

Goodman C and Snyder T: Differential diagnosis in physical therapy, Toronto, 1990, WB Saunders.

Gould JA and Davies GJ: Orthopaedic and sports physical therapy, Toronto, 1985, Mosby.

Hanson PG, Angerine M, Juhl JH: Osteitis pubis in sports activities, Physician Sports Med, Oct 1978, 111-114.

Hoppenfeld S: Physical examination of the spine and extremities, New York, 1976, Appleton-Century Crofts.

Kaltenborn F: Mobilization of the extremity joints, ed 3, Oslo, 1980, Olaf Norlis Bokhandel Universitetsgaten.

Kapandji IA: The physiology of the joints, vol 2, Lower Limb, New York, 1983, Churchill Livingstone.

Kelsey JL: Epidemiology of slipped capital epiphysis: a review of the literature, Pediatrics 51:1042, 1973.

Kendall FP and McCreary EK: Muscles testing and function, Baltimore, 1983, Williams & Wilkins.

Kessler RM and Hertling D: Management of common musculoskeletal disorders, Philadelphia, 1983, Harper and Row.

Kornberg C and Lew D: The effect of stretching neural structures on grade one hamstring injuries, JOSPT, June 1989, p 481-487.

Kulund D: The injured athlete, Toronto, 1982, JB Lippincott.

Lee D: The pelvic girdle, New York, 1989, Churchill Livingstone.

Liebert P, Lombardo J, Belhobek G: Acute posttraumatic pubic symphysis instability in an athlete—case report, The Physician and Sportsmedicine 16(4):87, April 1988.

Magee DJ: Orthopaedics conditions, assessments and treatment, vol 2, Alberta, 1979, University of Alberta Publishing.

Magee D: Orthopedic physical assessment, Toronto, 1987, WB Saunders.

Maitland GD: Peripheral manipulation, ed 2, Boston, 1977, Butterworths.

Mannheimer JS and Lampe GN: Clinical transcutaneous electrical nerve stimulation, Philadelphia, 1986, FA Davis.

Martens MA et al.: Adductor tendinitis and musculus rectus abdominis tendopathy, Am J Sports Med 15(4):353, 1987.

Metzmaker JN and Pappas AM: Avulsion fractures of the pelvis, Am Sports Med 13(5):349, 1985.

Nicholas J and Hershman E: The lower extremity and spine in sports medicine, vol 2, St Louis, 1986, Mosby.

Nitz A et al.: Nerve injury and grades II and III sprains, Am J Sports Med 13(3):177, 1985.

Noakes T et al: Pelvic stress fractures in long distance runners, Am J Sports Med 13(2):120, 1985.

Norkin C and Levangie P: Joint structure and function: A comprehensive analysis, Philadelphia, 1987, FA Davis.

O'Donaghue D: Treatment of injuries to athletes, Toronto, 1984, WB Saunders.

Pappas A: Osteochondroses: Diseases of growth centers, Physician and Sports Medicine, 17(6):51-62, June 1989.

Peterson L and Renstrom P: Sports injuries—their prevention and treatment, Chicago, 1986, Year Book Medical Publishers.

Porterfield JA and DeRosa C: Mechanical low back pain, Toronto, 1991, WB Saunders.

Puranen J and Orava S: The hamstring syndrome—a diagnosis of gluteal sciatic pain, Am J Sports Med 16(5):517, 1988.

Raether M and Lutter L: Recurrent compartment syndrome in the posterior thigh—report of a case, Am J Sports Med 10:40, 1982.

Reid D et al.: Lower extremity flexibility patterns in classical ballet dancers and their correlation to lateral hip and knee injuries, Am J Sports Med 15(4):347, 1987.

Reid DC: Functional anatomy and joint mobilization, Alberta, 1970, University of Alberta Publishing.

Reid DC: Sports injury assessment and rehabilitation, New York, 1992, Churchill Livingstone.

Roy S and Irwin R: Sports medicine prevention, evaluation, management, and rehabilitation, New Jersey, 1983, Prentice-Hall.

Rydell N: Biomechanics of the hip joint, Clin Orthop 92:6, 1973.

Schaberg J et al.: The snapping hip syndrome, Am J Sports Med 12(5):361, 1984.

Simons D and Travell J: Myofascial origins of low back pain. 1. Principles of diagnosis and treatment, Postgraduate Medicine 73:81, 1983.

Simons D: Myofascial pain syndromes, Basmajian JV and Kirby C (eds): Medical Rehabilitation, Baltimore, 1984, Williams & Wilkins.

Staton P and Purdam C: Hamstring injuries in sprinting—the role of eccentric exercise, J Sports Phys Ther 10(9):343, 1989.

Smith R, Sebastian B, and Gajdasik JR: Effect of sacroiliac joint mobilization on the standing position of the pelvis in healthy men, J Sports Phys Ther 10(3):77, 1988.

Subotnik S: Sports medicine of the lower extremity, New York, 1989, Churchill Livingstone.

Tarlow S et al.: Acute compartment syndrome in the thigh, complicating fracture of the femur, J Bone Joint Surg 9:68, 1986.

Tomberlin JP et al.: The use of standardized evaluation forms in physical therapy, J Orthop Sports Phys Ther 348-354, 1984.

Travell J and Simons D: Myofascial pain and dysfunction: The trigger point manual, vol 1, Baltimore, 1983, Williams & Wilkins.

Williams L and Warwick: *Gray's Anatomy*, New York, 1980, Churchill Livingstone.

CHAPTER 3
Knee Assessment

The knee is made up of three joints: the tibiofemoral joint, the patellofemoral joint, and the superior tibiofibular joint. All three joints are important to normal knee function. During the assessment it is important to attempt to rule out the two knee joints that you believe are not injured and then assess thoroughly the joint that is injured. On occasion, there will be more than one joint involved, i.e., tibiofemoral meniscal injury with patellofemoral dysfunction. All three joints should be assessed, and all three should be addressed in rehabilitation to return the knee to full function.

TIBIOFEMORAL JOINT

The tibiofemoral joint is reinforced by powerful muscular structures but depends primarily on ligamentous structures for joint stability. The tibiofemoral joint is very susceptible to injury because it forms the junction between two boney levers, the femur and the tibia. Valgus, varus, anterior, posterior, or rotational forces to either lever have direct effects on the joint.

Overuse conditions develop at this joint because of the repeated sagittal, frontal, horizontal, or multiplane plane actions that are required when the athlete is participating in sports. The tibiofemoral joint also must absorb or transmit the shock from the foot and ankle. This joint is a modified hinge joint with two degrees of freedom of motion; it allows flexion, extension, medial and lateral rotation, and a small amount of abduction and adduction.

There are menisci (medial and lateral) attached to the tibia that add to the joint's congruency and shock absorbency and provide protection for the articular cartilage. These menisci are susceptible to injury, particularly when there are rotational forces during weight bearing.

The ligaments that stabilize this joint are very susceptible to injury, especially during contact sports. There are no boney limitations to the tibiofemoral motion in the sagittal plane, and as a result, anterior and posterior stability is afforded by the ligaments and muscles around the joint. Each ligament and separate portions of each ligament stabilize the tibiofemoral joint in different planes and at different joint angles. These ligaments include the medial and lateral collaterals, the anterior and posterior cruciates, and the posterior oblique ligaments.

During flexion and extension, the incongruency between the femoral and tibial condyles creates a combination of accessory movements: roll, slide (glide), and spin.

In a closed kinetic chain (weight bearing) during knee flexion there is initially rolling and spinning of the femoral condyles over the fixed tibia, and the femoral condyles glide forward in an anterior direction while they continue rolling posteriorly on the tibial condyles. This anterior translation, or glide, is imperative to prevent the femoral condyles from rolling off the tibial plateaus. To initiate knee flexion from an extended position the femur must spin with lateral rotation of the femur on the tibia. This is called *unlocking* the knee.

In a closed kinetic chain during knee extension from full flexion the femoral condyles roll anteriorly over a fixed tibia while simultaneously gliding posteriorly. In the last few degrees of extension, the condyles roll and spin on the tibia. During the last few degrees of knee extension, the femur must spin with medial rotation of the femur on the tibia. This is called *locking* or the *screw home mechanism* of the knee.

The closed-packed position for this joint is knee extension and tibial lateral rotation. The resting or loose-packed position is 25° of knee flexion. The capsular pattern for this joint is flexion more limited than extension: proportions of the restriction are 90° of restricted flexion to 5° of restricted extension.

PATELLOFEMORAL JOINT

This joint consists of the largest sesamoid bone of the body, the patella, which articulates with the articular surface of the femur. The patella allows greater mechanical advantage for the quadriceps during extension of the knee.

The patella and the surrounding soft tissue are very susceptible to overuse injuries, especially if there is excessive femoral or tibial rotation during walking or running (i.e., prolonged pronation, internal tibial torsion, and internal femoral torsion). With repeated prolonged pronation and the resulting excessive internal tibial rotation, the tibial tubercle and attached patellar tendon pull medially, which can cause the patella to develop malalignment problems.

SUPERIOR TIBIOFIBULAR JOINT

The superior tibiofibular joint is a plane synovial joint between the head of the fibula and the tibia. It is not normally included in the joint capsule of the knee and mechanically it is affected by the inferior tibiofibular joint. According to *Gray's Anatomy*, 10% of the population has the synovial membrane of the joint continuous with the knee joint through the subpopliteal recess.

The superior and inferior tibiofibular joint moves with talocrural plantar flexion and dorsiflexion. These movements are small accessory movements. During plantar flexion the fibula moves laterally, anteriorly, and inferiorly, resulting in inferior movement of the superior tibiofibular joint. During dorsiflexion, the fibula moves medially, posteriorly, and superiorly, resulting in superior movement of the superior tibiofibular joint.

Superior fixation of the fibula increases the potential for foot and ankle over pronation (foot assumes calcaneal valgus, dorsiflexed, and everted position) and the resulting femoral and tibial internal rotation, therefore stressing the knee. Inferior fixation of the fibula results in a compensatory foot supination (foot assumes calcaneal varus, plantar flexed, and inverted position) with stresses then passing through the lateral side of the tibia and knee. Hypermobility of the fibula can also alter the lower limb kinetic chain by allowing extra foot and ankle mobility and resulting in lower limb overuse conditions. Damage to this joint can also cause knee flexion discomfort because of the insertion of the biceps femoris into the head of the fibula.

ASSESSMENT

INTERPRETATION

HISTORY

Mechanism of Injury

Direct Force (Fig. 3-1)
Was it a direct force?

Contusion
QUADRICEPS MUSCLE

The anterior or lateral aspects of the quadriceps muscle group are often contused by a direct blow, especially in contact sports. If poorly treated or left unprotected during the acute phase, the hematoma may increase or develop into myositis ossificans (heterotopic bone).

HAMSTRING MUSCLE, POPLITEUS

The hamstrings and popliteus can also be contused, causing a hematoma, but this is not as common as contusion of the quadriceps.

CAPSULE

A traumatic force to the capsular tissue around the joint can lead to synovitis or a hemarthrosis of the joint. Repeated blows can lead to chronic synovitis.

ASSESSMENT INTERPRETATION

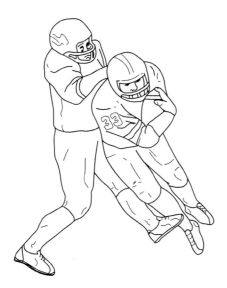

Fig. 3-1 Direct trauma to the knee.

BURSA

A direct blow to any of the bursa around the knee can cause a bursitis to develop: for example, the prepatellar bursa is often inflamed because of repeated kneeling, e.g., wrestler, baseball catcher. The suprapatellar bursa, the infrapatellar bursa (deep and superficial), and the pes anserine bursa can all develop chronic bursitis if they are subjected to repeated mild trauma.

ADDUCTOR MUSCLES

The adductor muscles are seldom contused because of the protection of the opposite leg. However, they are occasionally contused in sports when players' legs get entangled with each other, as in soccer and hockey, for example.

PATELLAR OR TIBIAL PERIOSTEUM

When the patella receives a direct blow, a periosteal contusion with an associated prepatellar bursitis often results. The tibial periosteum is often contused in sport because it lacks muscular protection.

Fractures
PATELLA

The patella can be fractured transversely, longitudinally, or in a stellate (star shaped) pattern from a direct blow or fall on the knee.

FEMUR, FIBULA, TIBIA

Femoral fractures occur most frequently in the shaft of the femur, which requires a great deal of force to break. These fractures are usually sustained in contact sports such as hockey and

ASSESSMENT   ## INTERPRETATION

high-speed sports such as skiing. Fractures around the knee joint can occur to:

- intercondylar area of the femur
- medial or lateral condyle of the femur
- fibula (neck or shaft)
- medial or lateral condyle of the tibia

OSTEOCHONDRAL (FIG. 3-2)

Osteochondral fractures are more common in the young athlete between the ages of 16 to 18. Osteochondral fractures of the medial femoral condyle are a result of compression and rotary forces on a flexed, weight-bearing knee or from direct trauma to the condyle.

Osteochondral fractures of the lateral femoral condyle are the result of compression and rotary forces on an internally rotated tibia or direct trauma to the condyle.

Osteochondral fractures of the medial aspect of the patella occur from a violent dislocation of the patella.

CHONDRAL

Central weight-bearing fractures of either condyle are most common and are often associated with anterior cruciate ligament tears, according to Wenner et al.

Anterolateral lesions of the lateral condyle following valgus or valgus plus torque injuries are usually osteochondral and are often associated with patellar dislocation.

Medial condyle fractures can occur near the notch from a valgus stress, and condyle fractures on nonweight-bearing surfaces are rare and usually the result of a direct blow to the anterior surface of the knee.

Chondral fractures are more common in the skeletally mature athlete.

EPIPHYSEAL

Epiphyseal fractures of the distal femur or tibia in the adolescent athlete can occur in football and hockey but are infrequent. The peak age for these injuries is between the ages of 12 to 15 in boys and 10 to 13 in girls—boys more commonly incur this kind of fracture.

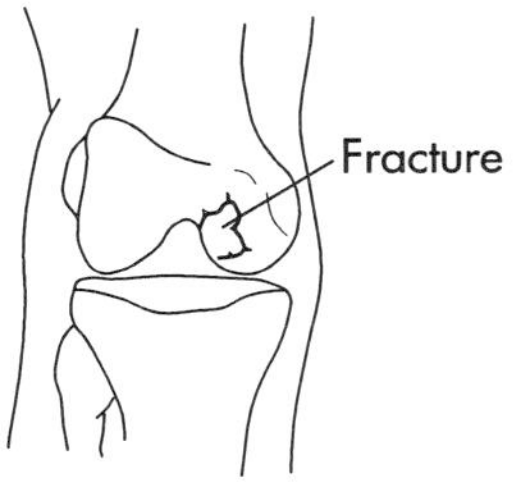

Fig. 3-2 Osteochondral fracture of the medial femoral condyle.

ASSESSMENT   INTERPRETATION

Tibial Anterior or Posterior Shift

Was it a direct force that shifted the tibia under the femur anteriorly or posteriorly (Fig. 3-3) ?

A direct blow to the tibia or a fall on a flexed knee can force the tibia backward under the femur, damaging the posterior cruciate ligament—causing it to sprain or rupture (Fig. 3-3). Repeated blows or chronic posterior instability may eventually cause the arcuate ligament complex and posterior oblique ligament to sprain or rupture.

A direct blow forcing the tibia forward under the femur, which results in hyperextension injuries, can damage the anterior cruciate ligament, causing it to sprain or rupture. The lateral and medial capsular ligaments can also sprain or tear—a severe blow to the knee can completely dislocate it with resulting popliteal artery damage or popliteus strain. According to Butler et al., the anterior cruciate provides 86% of the total resisting force to anterior displacement of the tibia on the femur. They also found that the posterior cruciate provides 95% of the total resisting force to posterior displacement of the tibia.

Force to Anteromedial Tibia

Was it a direct force to the anteromedial tibia?

A direct blow to the anteromedial tibia can cause posterolateral rotary instability with damage mainly to the arcuate-popliteus complex (arcuate ligament, lateral collateral ligament, popliteal tendon, and posterior third of the capsule; some authors include the lateral head of the gastrocnemius).

Force to Medial Knee

Was it a direct force to the medial side of the knee?

A direct blow to the medial aspect of the knee tends to straighten the valgus position and can cause:
- medial tibial condyle fracture or dislocation
- rupture of the lateral collateral ligament

Force to Lateral Knee

Was it a direct force to the lateral side of the knee?

A direct blow to the lateral aspect of the knee moves the lateral femoral condyle medially—it then contacts the lateral tibial condyle and splits the cortical bone of the lateral aspects of the tibial condyle. It usually sprains or tears the medial collateral ligament.

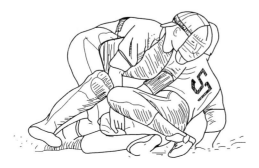

Fig. 3-3 Fall on the flexed knee, posterior cruciate injury mechanism.

ASSESSMENT

INTERPRETATION

Force to Fibula
Was it a direct force to the fibula?

A direct blow to the fibula can:
- damage the peroneal nerves as they curve around the fibular head
- sprain or rupture the superior tibiofibular joint (fibular subluxation or dislocation)
- fracture the fibula

Overstretch
Was the overstretch caused by a force?

Valgus Stress (Fig. 3-4)
Valgus stress is caused by a blow to the outside of the thigh or knee when the foot is fixed, producing a valgus overstretch on the knee joint.

Valgus stress can damage:
- medial collateral ligament
- medial capsular ligament
- medial meniscus
- anterior cruciate ligament
- lower femoral epiphysis in the teenage athlete
- posterior oblique ligament
- medial portion of the posterior capsule
- posterior cruciate (rare)

If the knee is extended during the blow, the femoral insertion of the medial collateral ligament is most commonly injured; however, both the deep and superficial fibers of the ligament are taut and can tear.

If the knee is nearly extended, the posterior deep fibers of the medial collateral ligament are taut and are more likely to tear than the superficial anterior fibers.

If the knee is flexed significantly, the injuries to the ligament occur more at the joint line, and the anterior superficial fibers of the medial collateral ligament are taut and are more likely to tear than the deep posterior fibers.

The medial collateral ligament sprain occurs most commonly at the joint line; it also occurs at the femoral origin, and occasionally at the tibial origin.

The valgus injury is very common in contact sports, especially football, but also in hockey and rugby. The cleated footwear in football, soccer, and rugby help fix the foot to the ground and therefore the ligaments are more vulnerable to injury. During sporting activities, the lateral side of the knee is vulnerable to impact when the foot is fixed and the knee is slightly flexed. The knee is forced medially when it sustains a direct lateral blow or when the medial side of the tibia is hit while the momentum of the athlete throws the knee into a valgus position. This can result in medial instability or, if the force is sufficient, anteromedial instability may result.

A

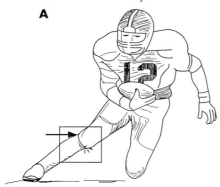

B

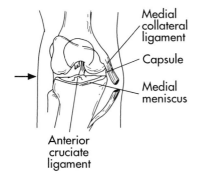

Medial collateral ligament

Capsule

Medial meniscus

Anterior cruciate ligament

Fig. 3-4 A, Lateral blow to the femur or knee joint results in a valgus stress. **B,** Structures damaged by a valgus knee injury.

ASSESSMENT   INTERPRETATION

Varus Stress (Fig. 3-5)

Varus stress is caused by a blow to the medial side of the thigh or knee, producing a varus overstretch of the knee joint.

Varus stress can damage the following:
- lateral collateral ligament—this ligament is injured less often than the medial collateral ligament because the force that damages the ligament must be applied to the medial side of the knee. This is difficult because the other leg is often in the way. The lateral collateral ligament is injured more often when the knee is extended.
- posterolateral capsule
- iliotibial band (Gurdy's tubercle attachment)—the iliotibial band is tightest at 15° to 30° of knee flexion and therefore it strains when the knee is flexed.
- arcuate-popliteus complex (arcuate ligament, popliteal tendon, lateral collateral ligament, and posterior third of the lateral capsule)
- biceps tendon at the head of the fibula
- peroneal nerve
- anterior and/or posterior cruciate ligament

Knee Flexion and Tibial Medial Rotation (Fig. 3-6)

Knee flexion with medial tibial rotation under the femur (or lateral rotation of the femur over the fixed tibia)

Knee flexion and medial rotation of the tibia under the femur (or lateral rotation of the femur over the fixed tibia) can damage the:
- posterolateral capsule
- anterior cruciate ligament (some research shows that the medial rotation of the tibia is the primary cause for an anterior cruciate tear)
- popliteal tendon
- arcuate ligament

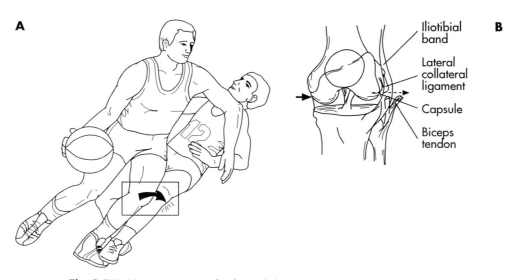

A   **B**

Iliotibial band

Lateral collateral ligament

Capsule

Biceps tendon

Fig. 3-5 A, Varus stress to the knee joint. **B,** Structures damaged by a varus knee injury.

ASSESSMENT

INTERPRETATION

- lateral collateral ligament
- iliotibial band (this is uncommon)
- biceps femoris muscle (this is uncommon)
- lateral meniscus (this is uncommon)
- lateral femoral condyle (osteochondral fracture)
- lateral coronary ligament

Knee Flexion and Tibial Lateral Rotation

Knee flexion with lateral tibial rotation under the femur (or medial rotation of the femur over the fixed tibia)

Knee flexion and lateral rotation of the tibia under the femur (or medial rotation of the femur over the fixed tibia) can damage the:

- posteromedial capsule
- medial collateral ligament (superficial and deep)
- coronary ligament (peripheral attachment of the meniscus)
- pes anserine tendons
- anterior cruciate ligament
- medial meniscus
- medial femoral condyle (osteochondral fracture)
- medial coronary ligament

This mechanism can cause a patellar subluxation or dislocation.

Lateral Rotation of the Tibia with a Valgus Force (Fig. 3-7)

Was there lateral rotation of the tibia with a valgus force?

Lateral rotation of the tibia with a valgus force is the most common traumatic knee injury; it is very common in skiing when one ski becomes trapped in the snow while momentum carries the skier forward and the tibia externally rotates with the trapped ski. It also occurs readily in contact sports. This injury can damage the:

- medial capsule
- medial meniscus
- medial collateral ligament

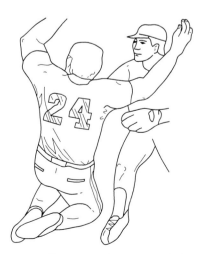

Fig. 3-6 Knee flexion and tibial medial rotation.

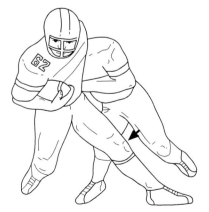

Fig. 3-7 Lateral tibial rotation and valgus stress.

ASSESSMENT

INTERPRETATION

- posterior oblique ligament
- anterior cruciate ligament

This results in anteromedial instability if damage occurs.

Deceleration with a Sudden Twist

Was there deceleration with a sudden twist?

A major mechanism causing an isolated anterior cruciate tear is a running athlete who suddenly decelerates and makes a sharp cutting motion.

This also occurs in the skier whose body quickly twists over a fixed lower extremity.

Knee Hyperextension

Was the knee hyperextended?

Knee hyperextension can damage the:
- posterior capsule and its ligaments
- anterior cruciate ligament
- posterior cruciate ligament
- lateral collateral ligament
- medial collateral ligament
- arcuate ligament
- oblique popliteal ligament
- fat pad (impingement)
- hamstring muscles
- gastrocnemius muscle

Knee Hyperflexion

Was the knee hyperflexed?

Knee hyperflexion can damage the:
- posterior cruciate ligament
- posterior horns of the menisci

Sudden Change of Direction
Patellar Dislocation (Fig. 3-8)

Was there a sudden change in direction with the quadriceps contracted?

Dislocation of the patella can result from a sudden change in direction from the weight-bearing foot and is associated with a quadriceps contraction (see Fig. 3-8). The knee is usually flexed 30° to 90°. This dislocation is often sustained by the adolescent athlete (between the age of 14 to 18 years). Female athletes with pronounced genu valgus and weak quadriceps are especially vulnerable. It can also result from a violent impact on a normal patella or a minor blow on a small, underdeveloped or unstable patella. Other predisposing factors include a shallow femoral groove, patellar hypermobility, genu recurvatum, or an underdeveloped lateral femoral condyle. The patella usually dislocates laterally and the injury can be combined with:
- medial retinaculum tear
- vastus medialis muscle avulsion
- medial joint capsule tear
- knee joint hemarthrosis
- medial ridge of the patella osteochondral fracture

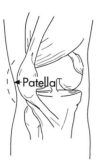

Fig. 3-8 Lateral patellar dislocation.

ASSESSMENT

INTERPRETATION

- osteochondritis dissecans of the patella—in up to 28% of cases, according to Cash and Hughston.

Forceful Contraction

Was there a forceful muscle contraction against a great resistance?

A forceful muscle contraction against a resistance that is too great can cause muscle strains, especially in muscles that cross two joints. The muscle attempts to contract when it is on stretch (eccentric contraction) and is unable to overcome the resistance, resulting in a muscle strain. These strains can occur at their origin, insertion, or midbelly.

The most common muscle strains occur to the hamstrings, the biceps femoris, and the semimembranosus in particular, especially in athletes who indulge in explosive sprinting action while having poor flexibility, e.g., sprinters, linemen.

The quadriceps are frequently strained, especially the rectus femoris muscle, which contracts when stretched over the hip and knee joint. Athletes like kickers and sprinters usually sustain this injury. The quadriceps muscles can tear at their superior patellar attachment or in the patellar tendon when the athlete is landing from a jump or hyperflexing the knee during weightlifting.

The adductor muscles are strained in sports that require a lot of quick lateral mobility, such as hockey, soccer, and squash.

The triceps surae, especially the medial gastrocnemius head, can be strained or ruptured. The achilles tendon can rupture just above the calcaneus from an overforceful plantar flexion contraction or excessive dorsiflexion beyond the tendons range.

Overuse (Fig. 3-9)

Was it an overuse, repetitive mechanism?

Overuse and repetitive conditions involve several variables.

Common overuse conditions of the knee and its related soft tissue are often sport specific.

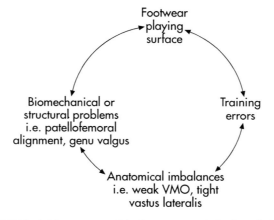

Fig. 3-9 Variables responsible for overuse injuries of the knee.

ASSESSMENT   INTERPRETATION

Running Knee Problems
Patellar Chondromalacia

Chondromalacia is the most common cause of runner's knee pain. It usually begins with patellar malalignment syndrome that progresses to chondromalacia. It consists of the softening and eventual degeneration of cartilage and even of subchondral bone on the under side of the patella. It occurs in the runner because of the repeated microtrauma and/or malalignment of the patella. A mechanical problem at the foot (pronation), the tibia (internal tibial rotation), or the hip (anteversion) can lead to patellar tracking problems and eventually patellar degeneration. Muscle tightness or weakness, asynchronous muscle firing, or connective tissue tightness can lead to chondromalacia also (e.g., tight vastus lateralis, iliotibial tract, and lateral retinaculum, and a weak vastus medialis).

Patellar Malalignment Syndrome (Patellofemoral Pain Syndrome)

Inflammation of the patellar retinaculum or synovium is usually due to patellar malalignment and overtraining. There are many predisposing factors:
- patellar flat shape (jockey-cap shaped patella)
- patella alta
- increased Q-angle
- genu valgus
- femoral anteversion
- weak VMO
- tight vastus lateralis
- L3 dysfunction
- tight rectus femoris
- anterior pelvic tilt
- overpronation (compensated subtalar varus or forefoot varus)
- internal tibial torsion
- tight lateral retinaculum
- tight iliotibial band
- asynchronous quadriceps muscle firing
- weak gluteus medias

Iliotibial Band Friction Syndrome

The iliotibial band friction syndrome usually occurs in long-distance runners. It is caused by friction between the lateral femoral epicondyle and the iliotibial band during flexion and extension of the knee. It is most common in varus knee alignment—in athletes who run 20 to 40 miles per week and have recently changed their running training habits (e.g., terrain, speed, distance, running surface, or footwear). It is often present with a rigid cavus (nonshock-absorbing) foot because stress is transferred to the lateral side of the knee. A prominent lateral femoral epicondyle and/or tight iliotibial band can lead to the problem.

ASSESSMENT   INTERPRETATION

Infrapatellar Tendonitis

The patellar tendon may develop tendonitis if patellar malalignment exists, but this is a less common running injury.

Popliteus Tendonitis

Popliteus tendonitis sometimes causes lateral knee pain, especially in athletes with deficient anterior cruciate ligament or athletes who do a great deal of downhill running. The popliteus with the anterior cruciate ligament, normally limits the femur's anterior translation over the tibia. When the cruciate is torn, the popliteus works overtime controlling the anterior glide, and therefore, the popliteus can develop tendonitis. Excessive pronation causes excessive tibial internal rotation that can lead to popliteal tendonitis also.

Pes Anserine Bursitis, Medial and Lateral Gastrocnemius Bursitis

Any of the extra-articular bursae around the knee can become inflamed through overuse.

Synovitis

Any internal derangement in the knee joint can cause an increase in synovial fluid, especially when combined with activity. Examples of internal derangement of the knee that can cause synovitis are:
- cartilage tear
- osteochondritis
- severe ligament laxity (especially of the anterior cruciate or posterior cruciate ligaments)

Jumping Knee Problems

Jumping knee problems are common in basketball, volleyball, high jump, and long jump.

Patellar Tendonitis

Patellar tendonitis is an inflammation of the patellar tendon at the attachment of the patellar tendon at the inferior pole of the patella or at the insertion of the quadriceps tendon at the base of the patella (David). In late adolescence to age 40, the most common patellar tendonitis (jumper's knee) occurs at the attachment of the patellar tendon at the inferior pole of the patella (Curwin and Stanish). After age 40, the most common location is the insertion at the base of the patella (Curwin and Stanish). The patellar tendon becomes inflamed from overuse during the take off and landing (during jumping). This tendonitis can affect any athletic group that overloads the extensor mechanism (e.g., basketball, cycling, volleyball, soccer, weight lifting). There is often patellar malalignment, patella alta (high-riding patella), or excessive foot pronation associated with this tendonitis.

ASSESSMENT

INTERPRETATION

Overtraining, and weakness in the hamstrings and abdominal muscles, predisposes the athlete to this condition. If, on landing or take off, the knees move into a valgus or adducted position, the patellar tendon is forced to contract on an angle and is more likely to develop tendonitis.

Sinding-Larsen-Johansson Disease

Sinding-Larsen-Johansson disease consists of traction apophysitis of the distal end of the patella and causes calcification in an avulsed portion of the patellar tendon. A tight rectus femoris with repeated concentric and eccentric loading of the patellar tendon during jumping can cause this to develop.

Osgood Schlatter Disease

Osgood Schlatter disease is a traction apophysitis of the tibial tubercle in the adolescent—the condition is aggravated by repetitive jumping.

Again, a tight rectus femoris or patella alta are often associated with this injury.

Swimming Knee Problems
- Medial collateral ligament
- Medial synovitis

The breaststroke whip kick, which puts the tibia into extreme external rotation with flexion and valgus force at the knee, can lead to medial synovitis, medial collateral ligament sprain, and medial patellar facet wear.

Squatting Knee Problems

Repeated hyperflexion, as practised by curlers, goalies, baseball catchers (Fig. 3-10) results in a constant progressive load on the menisci that leads to meniscal degeneration.

Chronic
Has the injury occurred before?
Is it a chronic knee problem?

Chronic knee problems and recurring soft tissue injuries include:
- repeated synovitis from meniscal lesions
- bursitis from overuse or repeated trauma
- repeated patellar subluxation/dislocations
- chondromalacia
- recurring lateral pivot shift episodes (torn anterior cruciate ligament)
- chronic hamstring strains
- chronic adductor strains
- chronic tendonitis (patellar, hamstring, popliteal) from overuse

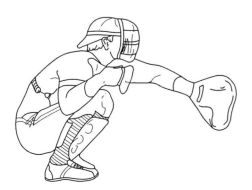

Fig. 3-10 Repeated knee joint hyperflexion.

ASSESSMENT

INTERPRETATION

Reenacting the Mechanism

Can the athlete reenact the mechanism using the opposite limb?

Determine:
- body position
- leg position
- foot position

Relevant information about the force of the blow or twist and the forces involved in the sport should be obtained.

Reenacting the mechanism using the uninjured limb helps clarify the forces and the stressed structures. It is important to know the forces involved in the sport to understand the mechanics of the problem.

Injuries involving overstretch or a direct blow over a fixed foot (i.e., one in cleated footwear or a ski boot) are usually more severe than if the foot is not fixed.

Determine if there was repeated microtrauma because of overtraining, biomechanical malalignment (such as limb-length differences, foot dysfunction, or patellar malalignment), or muscular weakness or imbalances (such as tight hamstrings, weak quadriceps, or tight iliotibial band).

Sports that involve direct contact, such as football, soccer, and rugby, have a high incidence of knee injury.

Individual sports that are carried out at high speeds, such as downhill skiing and bobsledding, can subject the knee to forces that can cause severe fractures or dislocation.

Pain

Location

Where is the pain located?

Can the athlete point to it with one finger?

Ascertaining whether the pain is local or referred depends on the depth of the involved structure more than on the type of pain. Superficial structures give rise to pain the athlete can easily localize because it is perceived at the location of the lesion, i.e., in the skin, superficial fascia, ligaments, tendon sheaths, and periosteum.

Local Pain

DeLee et al. believe that point tenderness and swelling in the posterolateral knee combined with a positive varus stress test with the knee in 30° of flexion is indicative of posterolateral rotary instability. Damage occurs to the arcuate ligament complex mainly. This consists of the arcuate ligament, the lateral collateral ligament, the popliteus muscle tendon, and the posterior third of the lateral capsule. Damage can occur to the biceps femoris tendon or occasionally to the lateral gastrocnemius head. According to DeHaven, anterior cruciate tears often cause posterolateral knee pain.

Point tenderness over the adductor tubercle and along the intermuscular septum at the insertion of the vastus medialis can suggest a patellar subluxation or dislocation if the history indicates this extensor injury.

The medial or lateral collateral ligaments are locally point tender if they are sprained or partially torn.

The bursa (pes, semimembranosus, suprapatellar, or others) is specifically point tender if bursitis exists.

Local medial joint line pain is a very positive clinical indica-

ASSESSMENT

INTERPRETATION

tion of a meniscus lesion (anterior or posterior peripheral detachment).

Referred Pain (Somatic)

Deeper structures are more difficult to localize and have a tendency to manifest referred pain. Deep somatic pain can be referred along the myotomal or sclerotomal distribution. For example, a hamstring strain can elicit pain down the back of the leg.

An osteochondral fracture can cause aching in the entire femur.

Chrondromalacia causes referred pain to the retropatellar aspect of the knee—with time, it radiates, most commonly to the medial joint line.

A slipped capital femoral epiphysis can refer pain into the knee. Legg-Calve'-Perthes disease can cause referred pain in the anteromedial thigh or knee with the usual age onset from 4 to 10 years.

Radiating Radicular Pain (Nerve Root)

Radiating pain from a nerve-root irritation goes mainly to the lower leg dermatomes (L4, L5) but occasionally can radiate to the posterior thigh (S1) or to the anterior thigh (L3, L4).

Onset of Pain
How quickly did the pain begin?

Immediate

Usually pain that begins immediately suggests a more severe injury.

6 to 12 Hours After Injury

Pain that develops after a few hours usually indicates a less severe problem (e.g., synovial swelling or lactic acid buildup).

Type of Pain
Can the athlete describe the pain?

Different musculoskeletal structures give rise to different kinds of pain.

Sharp

Sharp pain is experienced with damage to the following structures:
- skin, fascia (e.g., laceration)
- muscle—superficial (e.g., rectus femoris)
- muscle tendon—superficial (e.g., biceps femoris at insertion)
- ligament—superficial (e.g., medial collateral ligament)
- bursa—subcutaneous (e.g., prepatellar bursa)
- periosteum (e.g., patellar contusion)

ASSESSMENT

INTERPRETATION

Dull, Aching

Dull, aching pain is experienced with damage to the following structures:
- bone—subchondral (e.g., chondromalacia pain is often dull, aching, throbbing)
- tendon sheath (e.g., patellar tendonitis)
- muscle—deep (e.g., semimembranosus midbelly)
- ligament—deep (e.g., anterior cruciate ligament)
- bursa—deep (e.g., infrapatellar bursa)
- fibrous capsule (e.g., around knee joint—synovitis)
- joint (e.g., osteochondral lesion of femur)

Tingling

Tingling pain may be experienced in the following structures:
- peripheral nerve (e.g., the common peroneal nerve)
- nerve root problem (e.g., the L3 nerve root can cause tingling on the anterior thigh)
- circulation problem (e.g., popliteal artery)

Twinges with Movement

Twinges of pain with movement can occur in superficial ligaments or muscles (e.g., the medial collateral ligament or adductor muscle), which hurt when stretched.

Stiffness

Stiffness is usually muscular or capsular in origin—stiffness of the knee is a common complaint with chondromalacia but it usually diminishes with activity. Any joint effusion will cause stiffness in the joint regardless of the cause. Rheumatoid arthritis, osteochondritis, and osteoarthritis can cause recurring joint effusion and stiffness.

Severity of Pain
How severe is the pain?
- Mild
- Moderate
- Severe

Whether the athlete expresses the pain as mild, moderate, or severe is *not* a good indicator of the severity of the problem.

The amount of pain felt is often influenced by the athlete's emotional state, cultural background, and previous experiences with pain rather than the degree of tissue damage.

In some cases a mild sprain is more painful than a complete ligamentous tear because in the complete tear there are no intact afferent fibers to carry the pain message. This painless tear sometimes occurs with a complete anterior cruciate ligament tear.

Timing of Pain
What makes it better?
- Rest
- Heat or cold
- Elevation of the limb

Usually, acute injuries feel better when rested and chronic conditions improve once they are moved. Overuse conditions improve when the action that causes the irritation is stopped.

Chronic lesions or arthritic conditions usually feel better

ASSESSMENT

INTERPRETATION

when heat is applied, whereas acute lesions respond better to ice pack applications.

If the pain decreases when the limb is elevated, it is usually a sign that active inflammation is still occuring.

What makes it worse?
- •Walking
- •Squatting
- •Climbing Stairs
- •Jumping

Flexed-knee positions with prolonged sitting (also called the movie sign) and walking aggravate patellofemoral injuries (i.e., chondromalacia). Squatting and climbing stairs also aggravate chondromalacia. Deep squats with rotation will aggravate meniscal tears.

In patellofemoral disorders, more pain is felt on descending stairs because of the greater tension developed with the eccentric contraction of the quadriceps.

Jumping can cause the following:
- patellar tendonitis
- Sinding-Larsen-Johannson disease
- Osgood-Schlatter disease
- quadriceps strains
- hamstring strains
- meniscal lesions

Pain on Movement

Acute muscle strains and tendonitis become worse when the muscle is required to move and ligaments become painful when they are stretched.

The bursae are painful if the structures over or under them are moved or if they are pinched by joint movement.

Any internal derangement of the knee joint is aggravated by activity (i.e., meniscal lesions, synovitis, osteochondritis dessicans, osteochondral fractures, hemarthroses, and anterior cruciate tears).

Periosteal pain or bone injuries (stress fractures) are aggravated by vibration of the bone.

Synovial plica* problems and iliotibial band syndrome are aggravated by repeated flexion and extension of the knee; the prepatellar bursa is aggravated by kneeling.

Synovial plica is a fold in the synovium that is present in 20% to 60% of the population. It is a remnant of the embryological septum that can persist into adult life. It can be irritated after a knee injury or from friction during knee flexion and extension movements (Kegerreis et al., Blackburn et al., and Nottage et al.).

Morning Pain

Pain in the morning that subsides with joint movement and increases as the day progresses is typical of degenerative joint disease (i.e., osteoarthritis).

ASSESSMENT   INTERPRETATION

Swelling

Location

Where is the swelling located?

Local (Fig. 3-11)

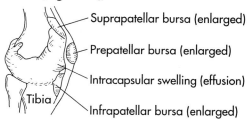

Suprapatellar bursa (enlarged)

Prepatellar bursa (enlarged)

Intracapsular swelling (effusion)

Tibia

Infrapatellar bursa (enlarged)

Fig. 3-11 Local knee joint swelling.

Local swelling is often present in the bursae around the knee. These include the:
- infrapatellar bursa
- suprapatellar bursa
- prepatellar bursa
- pes anserine bursa

Local swelling can occur inside the joint (intracapsular). This can be synovial swelling or a hemarthrosis (bleeding inside the joint).

Diffuse

Swelling outside the joint in the soft tissue is called extracapsular swelling. This is more diffuse. Intramuscular (within the muscle) or intermuscular (between the muscles) swelling is usually palpable (especially in the quadriceps muscle).

Time of Swelling

How quickly did the knee swell in the adult and adolescent athlete?

Immediate—Within 30 Minutes to 2 Hours

Swelling that develops quickly—immediately to within 2 hours usually is a hemarthrosis. The joint becomes tense with the swelling. Such swelling is usually indicative of severe injury. The swelling is usually warm, which indicates injury to a structure with a rich blood supply.

Gross swelling that develops immediately in the adult athlete can be the result of:
- isolated partial or complete rupture of the anterior cruciate ligament (this is the most common)
- lateral subluxation/dislocation of the patella
- intra-articular fracture (chondral or osteochondral)
- isolated partial or complete tear of the posterior cruciate ligament
- traumatic effusion from a direct blow
- epiphyseal fracture
- fracture of the patella
- major meniscal tear from its vascular-enriched periphery

In the adolescent athlete the most common causes of hemarthrosis (according to Nisonson) in order of frequency are:
- patellar dislocation/subluxation
- epiphyseal injury (especially the distal femoral epiphysis)
- anterior cruciate ligament disruption

ASSESSMENT   INTERPRETATION

• chondral/osteochondral fracture

Immediate swelling into the soft tissue of the thigh can indicate a severe muscle injury from a quadriceps hematoma or tear.

After 6 to 24 Hours

Joint swelling that develops 6 to 24 hours after injury is usually of synovial origin, caused by traumatic synovitis. Common irritants of the synovium are:

• meniscal tear
• bone chips (osteochondritis dissecans)
• capsular sprain
• medial collateral ligament damage
• patellar subluxation/dislocation

Occasionally a hemarthrosis takes longer to develop, especially if it is an anterior cruciate partial tear when the swelling remains in the synovial sheath around the ligament (Reid). A meniscal tear may also slowly bleed, forming a hemarthrosis.

Amount of Swelling

What is the amount of swelling?

The amount of swelling does not always indicate the severity of the injury. Gross ligamentous injuries with a torn capsule will allow the hemorrhaging to move outside the joint and into the surrounding soft tissue; as a result, severe injuries may not have much visible swelling. On occasion, minor injuries may cause a gross synovial effusion. Swelling caused by an anterior cruciate tear starts immediately and is extensive within 4 to 6 hours.

When the Knee Swells

When does the knee swell with activity?

• Rotation
• Jumping
• Kneeling

Does the knee swell at the end of the day?

Rotational activities aggravate ligamentous and meniscal problems. Jumping activities aggravate the patellar tendon and infrapatellar bursa. Prolonged kneeling aggravates chondromalacia and the prepatellar and infrapatellar bursae.

Swelling at the end of the day suggests that daily activities or prolonged weight bearing is aggravating the joint. If swelling occurs only after activity and subsides with rest, it may indicate a reactive synovitis due to some pathologic process that is aggravated by overuse.

Function

Degree of Disability

Return to Play

Could the athlete continue playing?

The degree of immediate incapacity can be misleading and is not always related to the severity of the injury. A player with a total rupture of the medial collateral ligament, posteromedial capsule, and anterior and posterior cruciate can (by bracing his or her quadriceps) stand or even walk after injury. (According to Hughston, Cross, and Crichton, 75% of the players who sus-

ASSESSMENT

INTERPRETATION

tained this injury were able to walk to a clinic or hospital.) Total ligamentous and capsule ruptures tend to be painless because the pain in these structures is usually generated when they are still partially intact.

Knee injuries severe enough that the player does not want to return to play are?
- patellar dislocation (first time)
- second-degree medial and lateral ligament sprains
- meniscal tears (medial or lateral)
- anterior cruciate sprains and tears
- hamstring strains and tears
- posterior cruciate sprains and tears
- quadriceps strains and tears

Weight Bearing

Could the athlete weight-bear immediately?
- Walking and running
- Cutting
- Jumping

Significant problems within the knee joint that cause effusion to develop quickly will limit weight bearing immediately and later.

Feelings of insecurity and unwillingness to weight-bear immediately suggests a severe injury has occurred, and therefore the knee should be assessed fully before allowing any weight on the limb.

Being able to walk and run immediately suggests a less severe knee problem.

Instability when cutting and changing direction can suggest gross ligamentous and surrounding soft-tissue tears.

The ability to jump after injury tests the quadriceps mechanism and the integrity of the hamstrings, as well as patellofemoral joint function.

Range of Motion

How much range of motion did the knee have immediately after the injury?

How much range of motion is there 6 to 12 hours after the injury?

The amount of range of motion available immediately is an indication of the function of the knee but also of the athlete's willingness to move the joint. Limitations to movement or a reluctance to move the joint immediately can be an indication of a substantial injury such as:
- second-degree muscle strain
- second-degree ligament sprain
- second-degree quadriceps muscle contusion

If the range of motion is not affected until 6 to 12 hours after the injury was sustained, the injury is less severe and could be:
- traumatic synovitis
- gradual hemorrhaging with first-degree muscle strain or first-degree ligament sprain
- muscle spasm

Weakness

Was there any weakness in the joint immediately after or at the time of the injury?

Immediate weakness can be a clue from the body that the limb should not be pushed to weight-bear or to return to func-

ASSESSMENT

INTERPRETATION

tion too quickly. The weakness may be from muscle-guarding or neural trauma to the area.

If the weakness at the injury site persists, there may be:

Did the weakness persist to the following day (after 12 hours)?

- significant damage to the muscles involved
- neural damage to the nerves supplying the muscle
- significant injury that is causing reflex inhibition of the local muscles

Locking

Was there locking in flexion or extension?

Meniscal Tear (Fig. 3-12)

The athlete should demonstrate the position in which the knee was fixed and recall the feelings at the time—true locking, in the acute case, from a meniscal tear limits the knee from full extension and usually occurs with a rotary component during injury. A history that the knee locked and that extension gradually returned in the course of a few hours or days is indicative of a meniscal tear. True-locking takes place at a range between 10° to 40° short of full extension. Once a meniscal tear causes locking, it has a tendency to recur.

Loose Body

Locking in the knee from a loose body (i.e., osteochondral fragment, piece of cartilage) is usually momentary and occurs quite unexpectedly during weight bearing.

Isolated Tear of Anterior Cruciate Ligament

An anterior cruciate ligament tear can cause momentary locking when its superior or midportion ruptures and a flap of the ligament catches between the femur and tibia during weight bearing.

Peripheral Hemorrhage

A hematoma in the infrapatellar fat pad or in the anterior peripheral attachment of the meniscus may limit or block flexion and extension and may simulate locking.

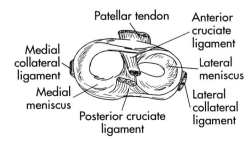

Fig. 3-12 Superior view of the right knee joint.

ASSESSMENT

INTERPRETATION

Posterior Hemorrhage

A hematoma in the popliteal space also can limit full extension and simulate locking.

Daily Function

How limiting is the injury to daily function?
- Stairs
- Deceleration, twisting
- Knee flexion and rotation

Daily function reports usually indicate degree of severity and degree of incapacitation. Hughston and Jacobson found that patients with posterolateral instability were unable to fully extend the knee and therefore had trouble ascending and descending stairs or slopes.

Anterolateral instability with a complete anterior cruciate tear can cause episodes of the knee giving way or of the tibia shifting, especially when the knee is decelerating or twisting.

Cartilage tears can also cause a slipping, or shift, between the femur and tibia when the knee is flexed and either bone is rotated.

Instability

Is there a feeling of instability?

Medial Instability

The athlete expresses an apprehension that the knee will buckle inward—this is a sign of a severely torn medial collateral ligament that is often associated with damage to the capsule, medial meniscus, and anterior cruciate. This is a common injury of contact sports like football (Fig. 3-13, *A*), soccer, and rugby.

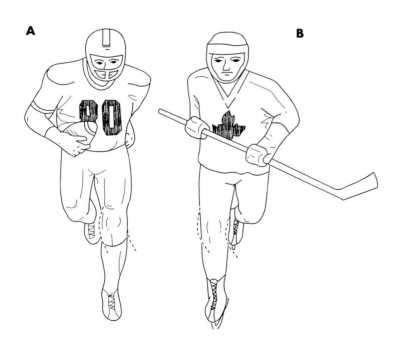

A   **B**

Fig. 3-13 A, Football is often a cause of medial knee joint instability. **B**, Hockey is often a cause of lateral knee joint instability.

ASSESSMENT

INTERPRETATION

Lateral Instability

The lateral opening of the joint is a sign of a severe lateral ligament injury that can include the iliotibial band, the lateral capsule, and the arcuate complex. Single-plane laxity rarely causes functional instability—if the athlete describes functional instability and rotary instability, a combined ligamentous or capsular injury is present. Lateral instability is more common in hockey (Fig. 3-13, *B*).

Giving Way

Is there a feeling that the knee is likely to give way?
- Meniscus tear
- Cruciate tear
- Chondromalacia
- Patellar subluxation
- Osteochondritis dissecans

When this is caused by a torn meniscus, the giving way occurs suddenly with such movements as turning around, walking on uneven ground, or stepping on a small stone.

Giving way that is due to a rupture of the cruciate ligament, quadriceps insufficiency, or loss of full extension occurs on descending stairs or jumping from a height.

Giving way or buckling during weight bearing can also occur with chondromalacia and is commonly associated with climbing stairs or walking down an incline.

The patella momentarily slipping over the edge of the condyle (patellar subluxation) gives a feeling of giving way, especially when the athlete turns over a flexed knee. Recurrent patellar subluxations occur when the athlete is turning with a sudden change of direction away from the affected side.

Osteochondritis dissecans of the tibia, femur, or patella can cause giving way if a loose body gets between the articular surfaces during weight bearing.

Weakness of the quadriceps can also cause giving way episodes.

Sensations

Describe the sensations felt at the time of injury and now.

Clicking

Clicking is usually indicative of a meniscus tear. However, clicks can come from the patella rubbing over the femoral condyles or in the joint with hypermobile menisci with loose attachments.

Snapping

Snapping is usually a sign of a synovial plica or a tendon snapping over bone; for example, the biceps tendon snapping over the fibula. Snapping deep in the joint can be caused by a congenital discoid, lateral meniscus, or an osteochondral fracture.

ASSESSMENT

INTERPRETATION

Grating

Grating can be caused by chondromalacia, osteochondritis, or osteoarthritis. It is necessary to determine if the patellofemoral joint or the tibiofemoral joint is making the noise.

Tearing

Tearing is usually felt by the athlete at the time of injury when the muscle or ligament involved is torn.

Catching

Catching can indicate a meniscal tear or subluxing patella. Often, in patellar subluxations, the catching is produced as the patella slips into the patellofemoral groove during walking or running when the weight-bearing leg begins to extend from the flexed position.

Tingling

Tingling can be caused by a neural or circulatory problem.

Hypesthesia/Hyperesthesia

Hypesthesia/hyperesthesia indicate a local nerve or nerve root problem (see the section on dermatomes and cutaneous nerve supplies in Functional Assessment).

Warmth

Warmth is usually caused by local inflammation but an infection or gout can also cause a joint to flare up.

Popping

If the athlete heard or felt a pop, especially after a hyperextension or internal tibial rotation injury, it is usually indicative of an anterior cruciate tear.

In a few cases, it may be a subluxed patella, though a tearing sensation is more common in this injury.

In a small number of cases the pop will be a meniscal tear, although a crackling sound is more common in this case.

A complete hamstring, rectus femoris, gastrocnemius, or adductor tear may also pop on rupturing.

Particulars

Has this happened before?

If so, has the athlete seen a physician, orthopedic surgeon, physiotherapist, physical therapist, chiropractor, osteopath, or any other medical personnel?

- Diagnosis
- X-ray results
- Recommendations

If the athlete has seen a physician, record the physician's name, address, diagnosis, recommendations, and name of any medications prescribed. Also record whether x-rays were taken where they were taken, and the results. Record the name of the previous therapist, his or her address, and what treatment and rehabilitation exercises were done. What part of the treatment was successful and/or unsuccessful?

ASSESSMENT

INTERPRETATION

• Prescriptions

At the time of injury, what was the method of transportation: car or ambulance?

What is the position of most comfort, then and now?

Do the athlete's occupation or daily habits aggravate the injury?

Is the athlete still able to participate in his or her sport?

The description of the method of transportation may indicate the severity of the injury at the time it occurred.

The position of comfort is usually a position that puts the damaged structures at rest. Attempt to put the athlete in this position as much as possible during the remainder of the assessment (e.g., pillow under the knee, leg elevated).

If the athlete's occupation or activities aggravate the problem, advise the athlete on ways to alleviate.

Sport participation helps determine the degree of injury and the willingness or ability to return to participation.

OBSERVATIONS

Observe the entire lower limb in weight bearing and in nonweight-bearing positions. The entire lower limb should be exposed as much as possible—the athlete should wear shorts or a bathing suit. Compare the lower limbs bilaterally. Note the degree of pain and whether there is any instability. Is the athlete capable of full weight bearing, partial weight bearing, or is he or she unable to weight-bear.

Standing

Anterior View
Alignment
PELVIS

The pelvis should be level bilaterally. If one anterior superior iliac spine and the iliac crest is higher, a leg-length problem may exist. According to Klein, the shorter leg has more injuries to the knee than the longer leg.

The pelvis may drop on one side due to gluteus medius weakness on the opposite side. This can lead to many mechanical problems during gait and in sporting events. At the knee, the pelvis dropping causes the knee on that side to go into valgus, which can lead to patellofemoral dysfunction.

ANTERIOR SUPERIOR ILIAC SPINE

If the anterior superior iliac spines are not level, observe (in the posterior view) the level of the posterior superior iliac spine and determine if there is a leg-length difference.

FEMORAL ANTEVERSION (SEE FIG. 3-15)

Femoral anteversion causes an internal rotation of the femur. This type of hip is associated with patellar malalignment syndromes, patellar subluxations, and chondromalacia.

| **ASSESSMENT** | **INTERPRETATION** |

FEMORAL RETROVERSION

Femoral retroversion causes an external rotation of the femur, which can cause some patellar malalignment problems also.

GENU VARUM (COXA VALGUM) (FIG. 3-14, *A*)

Genu varum puts an extra load through the lateral collateral ligament of the knee and causes a crossover running style—this can lead to overuse problems.

GENU VALGUM (COXA VARUM) (FIG. 3-14, *B*)

Genu valgum (more common in women because of the wider pelvis) is susceptible to medial collateral ligament problems. This can also cause calcaneal valgus and the resulting pronation, which can cause patellar malalignment and internal rotation of the tibia at the knee joint. A genu valgum deformity causes an increased Q-angle and this is associated with patellofemoral malalignment problems.

Patella
Q-ANGLE

An increased Q-angle can lead to patellofemoral malalignment conditions (chondromalacia, patellar tendonitis, patellar retinaculum problem, retropatellar irritations) and may predispose the patella to dislocations or subluxations. An inward facing patella (squinting patella) is more typical in the athlete who has chondromalacia or patellar malalignment problems.

SQUINTING PATELLAE (FIG. 3-15)

Squinting patellae are suggestive of femoral anteversion or increased femoral rotation and are usually accompanied by an apparent genu valgum.

FISHEYE PATELLA

An outward facing patella is more susceptible to subluxation and dislocation. The usual cause is femoral retroversion. Tightness in the lateral retinaculum and/or iliotibial band can pull the patella laterally or pull the lateral border of the patella posteriorly.

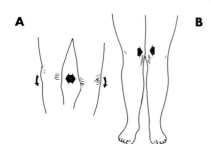

Fig. 3-14 A, Genu varum. **B**, Genu valgum.

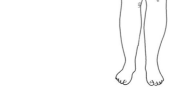

Fig. 3-15 Femoral anteversion "squinting patellae."

ASSESSMENT

INTERPRETATION

PATELLA ALTA

Patella alta (high-riding patella) is frequently associated with malalignment problems, chondromalacia, and patellar instability. The rectus femoris muscle is too tight and often the athlete has just had a growth spurt.

PATELLAR SIZE

A small patella is often unstable in the femoral groove and is more susceptible to subluxation and dislocation.

Tibial Torsion

Internal or external tibial torsion can affect the patellar tendon alignment, which increases susceptibility to malalignment syndromes, chondromalacia, or patellar tendonitis.

Tibial Varum

Tibial varum usually causes a compensatory calcaneal eversion and resulting pronation when the heel contacts the ground.

Pronated Foot or Feet

A foot that remains in pronation too long in midstance of gait will cause excessive internal tibial rotation. This excessive internal rotation puts added stress on the patellofemoral joint, the patellar tendon, lateral joint structures, and the medial meniscus.

Muscle Wasting
  Quadriceps (especially VMO)

Vastus medialis atrophy can be caused by pain inhibition, inactivity, or restriction of joint movement (lacking full extension). There will be decreased knee protection and stability when the quadriceps muscle strength is decreased. The weakness of the vastus medialis leads to poor patellar tracking, which can lead to malalignment conditions such as patellar tendonitis and chondromalacia. The patella will pull laterally because vastus lateralis will overpower medialis during a quadriceps contraction. Susceptibility to patellar subluxation and dislocation is also very common if there is deficiency in the vastus medialis muscle strength.

Swelling (see Fig. 3-11)
SUPRAPATELLAR BURSA

Swelling in the suprapatellar pouch may be intra-articular or extra-articular. Swelling that is intra-articular will lift the patella off the femoral condyles but swelling that develops just in the bursa or is extra-articular will not affect the patella.

Significant intra-articular joint effusion collects in the suprapatellar bursa and the prepatellar recesses when the knee is extended.

ASSESSMENT

INTERPRETATION

INFRAPATELLAR BURSA

Swelling in the infrapatellar bursa is located between the patellar tendon and proximal tibia and appears as a small local inflammation.

PREPATELLAR BURSA

Swelling in the prepatellar bursa appears as a lump between the front of the patella and the skin.

PES ANSERINE BURSA

Swelling in the pes anserine bursa is local swelling under the tendinous insertion of the gracilis, semitendinosus, and sartorius muscles.

Posterior View
Alignment
LUMBAR SPINOUS PROCESSES
- Scoliosis
- Prominent L5 spinous process

An alignment problem may indicate that scoliosis exists. The scoliosis may be a functional or a structural problem. A structural scoliosis can be caused by leg-length difference, which in turn can affect the mechanics of the entire lower quadrant.

A prominent L5 spinous process can be indicative of spondylolithesis, which can lead to referred pain down the leg. A lumbar spine assessment should be done if this is the case.

PARASPINAL MUSCLE SPASM

Lumbar paraspinal muscle spasm can indicate lumbar facet joint dysfunction or intervertebral disc pathology that can radiate pain into the lower limb. If this is suspected, a full lumbar spine assessment should be done.

A facilitated segment at L3 is often associated with patellofemoral malalignment problems.

ILIAC CRESTS

The iliac crests should be level. If one is higher and the PSIS on that side also is higher, a leg-length discrepancy may exist. A leg-length difference will upset the lower quadrant kinetics. Also the short leg is more susceptible to injury (Klein).

POSTERIOR SUPERIOR ILIAC SPINE

The posterior superior iliac spines should be level unless a leg-length discrepancy or pelvic rotation exists. Any frontal or horizontal plane asymmetry will upset the lower leg mechanics.

POPLITEAL CREASE

Popliteal creases should be level—if they are not, the cause can be a functional or structural leg-length discrepancy with its related problems.

ASSESSMENT

INTERPRETATION

CALCANEAL INVERSION

Calcaneal inversion during weight bearing may be compensated for by excessive pronation in midstance (compensated subtalar varus foot type); therefore the inverted calcaneus should be viewed during gait. Prolonged pronation can cause patellofemoral problems. If the calcaneus remains inverted during weight bearing and gait (uncompensated subtalar varus foot type), limited pronation occurs and the lateral aspect of the lower limb and knee are subjected to excessive force.

CALCANEAL EVERSION

Calcaneal eversion (subtalar valgus) during weight bearing causes excessive pronation during gait. This keeps the tibia internally rotated too long and can cause patellar malalignment conditions.

Muscle Wasting (Atrophy)
- Hamstrings
- Gastrocnemius

Atrophy of the buttock and hamstrings can occur from hip arthritis. Atrophy of just the hamstrings occur from:
- previous muscle strain or contusion
- previous knee surgery
- muscle imbalance

Atrophy of both the hamstrings and gastrocnemius can indicate an S1-S2 nerve root irritation.

Atrophy of the gastrocnemius can indicate:
- previous muscle strain, Achilles tendon tear, or tendonitis
- previous ankle joint injury
- previous knee surgery

A decreased strength in the hamstring or gastrocnemius muscle groups means that the posterior aspect of the joint is not as well protected or supported, since both these groups cross the back of the knee joint.

Muscle Hypertrophy
- Hamstrings
- Gastrocnemius

Hamstring hypertrophy is common in athletes in sports where sprinting is predominant.

Gastrocnemius hypertrophy often develops in athletes in jumping events.

Hamstring and gastrocnemius tightness should be noted, since muscle imbalances or lack of flexibility leads to knee joint and patellofemoral dysfunction.

Swelling
- Baker's cyst
- Popliteus bursitis

NOTE: A knee that is kept at 15° to 20° of flexion can indicate gross joint effusion because this angle of knee flexion

A Baker's cyst (synovial effusion in the gastrocnemius or semimembranosus bursa) is caused by:
- lesion of the posterior segment of the medial meniscus—this is probably the most common cause of a popliteal cyst in middle age

ASSESSMENT	INTERPRETATION

provides the synovial cavity with the maximum capacity for holding swelling (joint's resting position).

- inflammation from trauma
- asymptomatic hernia of a tendon sheath
- defect or degeneration of the posterior joint capsule

Swelling in the popliteal bursa between the popliteus tendon and the fibular collateral ligament may be seen in this position.

Lateral View
Alignment
EXCESSIVE LUMBAR LORDOSIS

An excessive lordotic curve can be associated with lumbar spine dysfunction. If a lumbar problem is suspected, a full lumbar assessment should be done. Lumbar spine dysfunction can refer pain anywhere in the lower quadrant but particularly into the hip and knee area.

ANTERIOR PELVIC TILT

An anterior pelvic tilt can lead to or be caused by:
- tight low back muscles or hip flexors
- weak and stretched abdominals, hamstrings, and glutei muscles

This tilt leads to excessive lumbar lordosis and can lead to lower quadrant dysfunction.

GENU RECURVATUM

Genu recurvatum is often associated with a hypermobile patella with its attendant subluxation and dislocation problems. Genu recurvatum is often associated with generalized ligament laxity.

FLEXED KNEE

A flexed knee can be caused by:
- acute spinal derangement (i.e. intervertebral disc protrusion, facet dysfunction)
- knee joint effusion
- acute medial collateral ligament sprain
- meniscal tear (that has locked the joint)
- quadriceps insufficiency or reflex inhibition
- acute chondromalacia

Lesion Site
Bruising, Tracking, Ecchymosis

Local bruising, tracking, or ecchymosis can be caused by a contusion in the soft tissue or from a severe ligamentous injury.

Bruising that tracks down the thigh or calf can indicate an intermuscular strain, tear, or severe contusion (e.g., of the hamstring muscles).

ASSESSMENT	INTERPRETATION

Scars

Previous surgery (e.g., anterior cruciate repair, menisectomy, lateral release) can affect your assessment and your interpretation of the findings.

Skin Color

An inflamed area may be redder in color over or around the lesion site. Cyanosis over the lower leg can be caused by a reflex sympathetic dystrophy (post-trauma or post-surgical) or a circulatory occlusion. In either case this should be referred to a physician for further evaluation immediately.

Deformity

Any boney or soft tissue deformities should be observed and noted. If the boney deformities are significant, immobilize the area and refer the athlete to a physician for further evaluation as soon as possible.

Gait (if the athlete is able to weight-bear) (Fig. 3-16)

What to look for during walking:
- watch the movement of the entire lower quadrant (lumbar spine, pelvis, hip, knee, ankle, and foot).

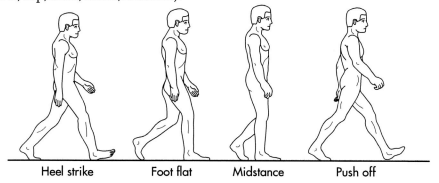

Heel strike   Foot flat   Midstance   Push off

STANCE PHASES

Fig. 3-16 Gait.

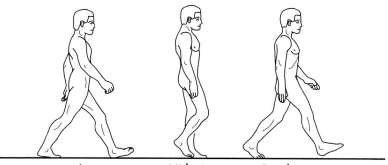

Acceleration   Midswing   Deceleration

SWING PHASES

ASSESSMENT

INTERPRETATION

Stride Length

Stride length is determined by measuring the distance from heel strike of one limb until the heel strike of the same limb.

The average stride length should be the same bilaterally. Stride length varies according to the athlete's leg length, height, age, and sex. Stride length may decrease if the athlete suffers from low back pain, limb pain, or fatigue.

Step Length

Step length is the linear distance between two successive points of contact of opposite limbs. It is usually measured from heel strike of one foot to the heel strike of the opposite foot.

The step length measurement is used to analyze gait symmetry—the more equal the step length, the more symmetry and, usually, the less the lower limb dysfunction.

Degree of Toe Out

The degree of toe out is determined by the angle of foot placement—this angle can be measured by drawing a line from the center of the heel to the second toe.

The angle of foot placement is normally 7° from the sagittal plane. An angle of toe out that is greater than 7° can cause:
- excessive pronation problems
- longitudinal arch collapse
- decreased stride length
- rotational torsion through the entire lower limb

Stride Width

Stride width is the distance from the midpoint of one heel to the midpoint of the opposite heel.

The width of the stride is usually 2 to 4 inches—the base is widened if the athlete has heavy thighs, balance problems, or decreased sensation in the heel or sole of the foot.

Rhythm

Rhythm is indicative of the coordination between the limbs and of the weight distribution on each limb.
- Weight distribution
- Antalgic gait (limp)
- Ability to lock knee in midstance

Rhythm indicates the coordination between the limbs and the weight distribution on each limb.

An antalgic gait occurs when the time spent on the injured limb is shortened; it can result from an injury to any segment or joint in the lower quadrant.

The knee should go into full extension and lock in midstance. If the knee cannot extend fully it can indicate:
- joint effusion
- meniscal blocking
- quadriceps inhibition
- significant ligamentous injury (i.e. medial collateral ligament)
- significant patellofemoral dysfunction

Walking Cycle (see Fig. 3-16)

Carefully examine the knee during each phase of the walking cycle.

Heel Strike

When the athlete is unable to extend the knee fully, he or she will put the entire foot down carefully.

ASSESSMENT

INTERPRETATION

Foot Flat and Midstance

The knee needs to reach full extension in this phase of walking. If the knee has posterolateral rotary instability, the athlete will walk with marked genu varus and will hyperextend during midstance.

Any problem that limits full extension such as a meniscus tear or joint effusion will affect this part of the gait.

During foot flat, the tibia internally rotates while the foot pronates and the midtarsal joints unlock, enabling the foot to adapt to the terrain.

During the midstance phase, the tibia externally rotates while the foot supinates and the midtarsal joint locks—the foot can become rigid for a strong push-off. If prolonged pronation occurs in late midstance and the foot does not get resupinated, the tibia will stay internally rotated and, as a result, the patellar tendon and indirectly, the patella, will have undue stress. This prolonged pronation can cause patellar malalignment problems—these are very difficult to observe. What the therapist will see is a pronated foot that does not get resupinated before push-off.

A foot that is turned out (usually on the short leg side or because of a retroverted hip) can develop compensatory pronation problems. This can lead to superior fibular fixation. The resulting overpronation can lead to excessive tibial internal rotation and the resulting patellofemoral problems.

A foot that is turned in can develop an inferior fibular fixation and compensatory supination. This leads to excessive lateral forces through the knee.

Push-off and Acceleration

A weak push-off is evident with most knee joint injuries.

Instability here and in midstance comes with a significant injury to the collateral ligaments.

An injury to the hip flexors and, sometimes, to the adductors will cause pain during the acceleration phase.

Midswing and Deceleration

During the swing phase, there are no weight-bearing forces through the joint so usually there are fewer symptoms during this part of the gait. The length of the swing phase for deceleration may be shortened if there is a hamstring strain or tightness.

Alignment
Anterior View
PELVIC CONTROL

During gait there must be good concentric and eccentric control of the muscles that stabilize the pelvis. Weakness in the gluteals (especially gluteus medius) or quadratus lumborum can cause dropping of the pelvis on one side. If the pelvis drops on

ASSESSMENT	INTERPRETATION
	one side, uneven forces move up to the lumbar spine, as well as down through the lower quadrant. If the knee musculature is also weak (especially vastus medialis) the knee will move into a valgus position and the patellofemoral joint may go into dysfunction.
PATELLAR TRACKING	In the anterior view, the quadriceps should contract smoothly, pulling the patella straight upward. If the patella deviates, patellar malalignment problems may exist. Weakness or atrophy of the quadriceps, especially of the vastus medialis obliquus, should be looked for. Weakness in the vastus medialis obliquus allows the patella to track laterally during a quadriceps contraction, which not only causes malalignment conditions but also makes the patella susceptible to subluxation or dislocation.
Posterior View KNEE RANGE	In the posterior view, look for full knee extension during heel strike and midstance.
ACHILLES ALIGNMENT	Look for a good alignment of the Achilles tendon.
PROLONGED PRONATION See prolonged pronation in Foot and Ankle Assessment.	A sign of prolonged pronation is a calcaneus that everts and an Achilles that bows. This prolonged pronation with the longitudinal arch collapse causes the tibia to remain in internal rotation—this subjects the patellar tendon and patella to unwanted rotational forces.
NO PRONATION (STAYS SUPINATED) See fixed supination in Foot and Ankle Assessment.	If the foot does not pronate at all and the calcaneus stays inverted (uncompensated subtalar varus type foot) the foot does not act as a shock absorber or conform to the terrain. As a result, shock is transmitted up the limb and can result in stress fractures or microtrauma up the lateral aspect of the lower extremity.

Muscle Wasting
    Anterior View
        Quadriceps
	Look for quadriceps wasting when the muscles are actually contracting. If there is wasting of vastus medialis in particular, the patella may track laterally (malalignment).

Posterior View Gastrocnemius, hamstrings	Look for hamstring and gastrocnemius wasting when the muscles are actually contracting.

ASSESSMENT	INTERPRETATION

Sitting

Long Sitting

Observe both knees while the athlete is long sitting.

In the resting position (position of comfort) is the knee flexed or extended?

Observe for:
- swelling
- bruising
- quadriceps atrophy
- scars
- patellar position

If the position of comfort for the athlete while long sitting is with the knee in slight flexion this can suggest that joint effusion is inhibiting full extension (15° to 20° flexion allows maximum capacity for knee joint swelling) or may be indicative of a collateral ligament sprain (usually medial-superficial fibers) because they are on stretch and are painful in the extended position.

This is a good position to observe if there is swelling because any joint effusion moves under the patella or to the suprapatellar bursa and is readily visible.

Bruising, quadriceps atrophy, and scars are easy to note when the athlete is in this position.

The patella, its positions, and characteristics can be observed and a small, high-riding or bipartite patella can be noted.

According to Jenny McConnell's work, the patella may sit laterally (see Fig. 3-36, *A*) or may tilt downward on the lateral edge (see Fig. 3-37, *A*) if the lateral retinaculum or iliotibial band is tight (static lateral glide and static lateral tilt respectively). The patella may be rotated so that the inferior pole of the patella is either lateral or medial (see Fig. 3-38, *A* and *B*) to the midline of the femur. The superior or inferior (see Fig. 3-39, *A* and *B*) pole of the patella may also be more posterior than the opposite pole. Any of these patellar positions can cause patellofemoral dysfunction and should be tested further in the functional tests for the dynamic changes that occur. These positions should be analyzed, since McConnell tape jobs and techniques can be done to help rehabilitate the knee.

High Sitting

Observe both knees in the high-sitting position.

Patellar position (Fig. 3-17)

Alignment of the patellar tendon

In the high-sitting position, if the patellae sit laterally, this is an indication of vastus medialis weakness, vastus lateralis tightness, or an underdeveloped lateral femoral condyle. Lateral tilting of the patella is also considered to be a diagnostic sign for patellar subluxation problems.

The normal patella should sit deeply in the patellofemoral sulcus and the patellar tendon should be in a straight vertical alignment. If the tibia is excessively rotated the tibial tubercle will be rotated and the patellar tendon with be malaligned.

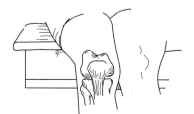

Fig. 3-17 Patellar alignment in sitting.

ASSESSMENT

INTERPRETATION

Tendon malalignment is associated with peripatellar pain, tendonitis, and chondromalacia. A high-riding patella is indicative of a tight rectus femoris muscle.

FUNCTIONAL TESTING

Establish a testing order that does not require the athlete to change positions too often, especially if the knee is acutely painful.

Most of the tests are done in the supine position. Make sure that the athlete is comfortable. Support the knee as often as possible during and between tests, for example, with a rolled-up towel or pillow under the knee and with hand support during testing.

SUMMARY OF TESTS

Rule Out
    Inflammatory disorders
    Lumbar spine
    Hip joint
    Superior tibiofibular joint
    Foot and ankle
    Fracture
Tests in Supine Position
    Joint effusion tests
        Wipe test
        Fluctuation test
        Patellar tap test
Functional Tests
    Active knee flexion
    Passive knee flexion
    Active knee extension
    Passive knee extension
    Bounce home sign
    Active medial and lateral rotation of the tibia on the femur
    Passive medial and lateral rotation of the tibia on the femur
    Resisted medial and lateral rotation of the tibia on the femur
    Resisted knee extension
    Resisted knee flexion
Special Tests – Tibiofemoral joint
    Valgus test (medial collateral ligament)
        In full extension
        In 30° flexion
    Varus test
        In full extension

ASSESSMENT   INTERPRETATION

      In 30° flexion
   McMurray's meniscus test
   Drawer sign or test
      Anterior
      Posterior
   Modified drawer test for rotary instability
   Anteromedial rotary instability (Slocum and Larsons test)
   Anterolateral rotary instability
   Posterolateral rotary instability
   Lachman test (anterior cruciate)
   Pivot shift tests for anterolateral instability
      Jerk test method 1 (Hughston)
      Method 2
      MacIntosh test
      Losee test
      Slocum's test
      Bach et al. test
   Posterior sag sign (posterior cruciate)
   External rotation recurvatum test
   Quadriceps active test
Special Tests – Patellofemoral joint
   Patellar orientation
   Patellar mobility
   Patellar apprehension sign
   Critical test (McConnell)
   Patellofemoral compression test
   Patellar retinaculm test
   Clarke's sign
   Plica test
   Q-Angle
   Lower extremity girth
   Patellar reflex
   Dermatomes
   Cutaneous nerve supply
   Circulatory tests
Tests in Prone Position
   Apley's compression and distraction test
Tests in Standing
   Functional tests to observe
      Step tests
      Full squat
      Return from squat
      Knee-circling
      Duck walk
      Jumps
      Crossover test
      Proprioception test

ASSESSMENT   INTERPRETATION

Accessory Movement Tests
    Tibiofibular joint
        Superior tibiofibular joint anterior and posterior glide
        Superior tibiofibular joint inferior and superior glide
    Tibiofemoral joint
        Posterior glide of the tibia on the femur
        Anterior glide of the tibia on the femur
        Internal rotation
        External rotation
    Patellofemoral joint
        Superior and inferior glide
        Medial and lateral glide

Rule Out

Rule out inflammatory disorders and involvement of the lumbar spine, hip joint, superior tibiofibular joint, and the foot and ankle joints because knee pain can be referred from these areas.

Inflammatory Disorders

Arthritic joint changes should always be considered and ruled out during your history-taking and observations.

Rule out arthritis, gout, and osteoarthritis when any of the following occur:
- there is an insidious onset of pain
- both knees or other joints are also painful
- the athlete feels unhealthy when the joints are also painful
- the athlete experiences repeated joint discomfort without a predisposing cause

If any of the above occur, test the joints as usual but also refer the athlete to his or her family physician for a complete checkup.

Lumbar Spine

Rule out involvement of the lumbar spine through the history-taking and observations.

Active tests of forward bending, back bending, side bending, and rotation can be done.

Radiating pain to the anterior knee area can come from an L3 nerve root irritation. If there is L3 disc herniation, pain usually begins in the groin and later moves to the anterior knee area. Pain can be referred to the posterior knee area from an S1 nerve root irritation as a result of an L5-S1 disc herniation. A lumbar spine nerve root irritation can also cause motor weakness of the muscles around the knee:
- knee extension (quadriceps) weakness can come from an L3 nerve root irritation
- knee flexion (hamstrings, gastrocnemius) weakness can come from an S1and/or S2 nerve root irritation

If the lumbar spine cannot be ruled out, a full lumbar spine assessment is necessary.

ASSESSMENT

INTERPRETATION

Hip Joint

Rule out involvement of the hip joint throughout the history-taking and observations.

Active hip flexion and medial rotation with an overpressure will rule out hip joint involvement.

Referred pain to the anterior knee area can come from the hip joint. This pain is more diffuse than a nerve root irritation.

The knee may even give way with hip conditions (i.e., slipped capital femoral epiphysis), but other hip signs and symptoms should come up in the history.

If the hip is involved, active hip movements or overpressures will elicit pain. If the hip joint cannot be ruled out, a full hip joint assessment is necessary.

Superior Tibiofibular Joint

Rule out the superior tibiofibular joint through the history-taking and observations.

Passive anterior/posterior and superior/inferior joint play movements can be done.

The superior tibiofibular joint can cause lateral leg and knee pain. Its joint play movements should be pain free and equal bilaterally.

The superior tibiofibular joint should be ruled out because limitations or dysfunctions in this joint can also alter foot and ankle mechanics that in turn will influence the knee joint.

This joint can also affect the function of the biceps femoris muscle that has a direct influence on the knee joint. With recurrent or chronic subluxations or dislocations of the superior tibiofibular joint, the knee can pseudolock when the athlete deep knee bends and rotates.

Foot and Ankle

Rule out foot and ankle pathology throughout the history-taking and observations.

Active plantar flexion, dorsiflexion, inversion, and eversion can be done, as can an overpressure in each of these ranges to ensure that the foot and ankle joints are not involved.

Injuries of the foot and ankle can refer pain into the knee, especially if the tibia is involved.

Dysfunction in foot mechanics can also lead to overuse conditions at the knee, particularly in the patellofemoral joint.

If foot and ankle pathology cannot be ruled out, a full foot and ankle assessment is necessary (see Chapter 4).

Fracture

If a fracture is suspected or your observations show deformity, complete the following fracture tests and do *not* carry out any further functional tests.

Tap the involved bone along its length (not over the potential fracture site). Gently palpate the fracture site to check for specific boney tenderness or deformity.

If a fracture is suspected the athlete should be immobilized and transported for treatment immediately. Treat the athlete for shock and monitor his or her pulses (femoral, popliteal, posterior tibial, and dorsal pedis).

Suspect a fracture if:
- the mechanism indicated sufficient force
- athlete felt or indicated a fracture
- athlete is reluctant to move the neighboring joints
- tapping the bone above or below the site elicits pain at the injury site
- there is deformity in the boney or soft-tissue contours
- athlete shows signs of sympathetic nervous system involvement or shock

ASSESSMENT

INTERPRETATION

Femur

The mechanism of injury of a femoral shaft fracture usually involves a violent torsional force.

Condyle fractures can occur in the adolescent through the epiphyseal growth plates, especially if there is a valgus or varus force.

Condyle chondral fractures can also occur after a patellar dislocation.

A medial femoral condylar avulsion fracture can occur with a posterior cruciate injury.

Patella

Patellae can be fractured by direct trauma, quadriceps strain, or patellar dislocation. The avulsion fracture occurs most often on the medial side when the patella is forced laterally or when the quadriceps contract and the patella is hit inferiorly or superiorly.

Direct trauma can fracture the medial or lateral margin or the upper or lower pole of the patella. Chondral fractures are common, especially with a patellar dislocation or a shearing force to the patella.

Palpating the patella may indicate the location of the fracture. Gross swelling may be present at the site of the fracture.

Tibia

Tibial condyle fractures can occur, especially chondral fractures of the tibial plateau. Chondral fractures occur with a compression force through the femur or up the tibia.

The upper tibia can be avulsed with an anterior cruciate tear.

An avulsion fracture of the tibial tuberosity can also occur, especially in the adolescent with previous or present Osgood-Schlatter disease—this fracture is usually caused by a vigorous quadriceps contraction in a flexed knee.

Fibula

Direct trauma can fracture the fibular head or neck—this can result in peroneal nerve, peroneal muscle, biceps tendon, and/or lateral collateral ligament damage.

The fibular head can also be dislocated—this injury must not be confused with a fracture.

Tests in the Supine Position

Joint Effusion Tests

These tests are done to determine if joint effusion exists.

All these tests are done with the ath-

Attempt these swelling tests before testing the knee joint because effusion will alter the active and passive ranges of flexion and extension. It is helpful in your interpretation of your

ASSESSMENT   INTERPRETATION

lete's knee fully extended and resting on the plinth.

testing results to determine if joint effusion is present and the amount of swelling present. With joint effusion, the ranges will be limited in flexion and extension and the knee will sit in approximately 15° of flexion.

Wipe Test (Fig. 3-18)

Begin medial to the patella below the joint line and stroke two or three times upward around the patella and over the suprapatellar pouch. This moves the swelling proximally.

The opposite hand strokes down on the lateral side of the patella.

Look on the medial side of the joint for fluid movement.

This test is used to determine slight-to-moderate intracapsular swelling. A wave of fluid will bulge on the medial side of the joint (as little as 4 to 8 ml will show).

Fluctuation Test (Fig. 3-19)

Place the palm of one hand over the suprapatellar pouch. The other hand is placed over the front of the joint just below the patella. By pressing one hand and then the other you may be able to feel the fluid.

This test is used to determine slight-to-moderate intracapsular swelling—blood fluctuates in a block (like jelly moving), whereas clear effusion runs down smoothly.

Patellar Tap Test

With one hand, press down gently on top of the patella while the athlete's knee is extended.

A floating sensation of the patella over fluid is felt or a tap occurs as the patellar goes through the swelling before hitting the condyles. (This test is only effective when moderate swelling exists, it is not effective with minimal or gross swelling.)

Moderate intracapsular swelling can be determined with this test—swelling that is intracapsular lifts the patella off the condyles. When pressing on the patella, if there is a fluid sensation under the patella or a delay before the patella hits the condyles, it is a sign of joint effusion. In the normal knee, the cartilaginous surfaces of the patella and femur are already in contact, thus no tap can be elicited.

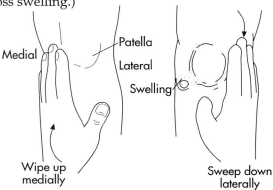

Fig. 3-18 Joint effusion "wipe test."

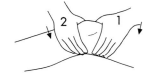

Fig. 3-19 Fluctuating test.

ASSESSMENT

INTERPRETATION

Active Knee Flexion (135°)

The athlete actively flexes one knee and then the other as far as possible.

Compare range of motion bilaterally.

Put one hand over the patella to feel for crepitus during the knee flexion.

If the athlete complains of tightness (swelling) or pain, ask its location and nature.

Pain, weakness, or limitation of range or motion in knee flexion can be caused by an injury to the muscles or to their nerve supply.

The prime movers of knee flexion are the hamstrings, which include:

- Semimembranosus—the sciatic N. (tibial branch; L4, L5, S1)
- Semitendinosus—sciatic N. (tibial branch; L4, L5, S1)
- Biceps femoris—Sciatic N. (tibial branch; L5, S1, S2)

The patella should descend into the femoral condylar groove with slight lateral tilting at the extreme range of flexion.

Patellar crepitus can be caused by chondromalacia.

Patellar clicking can occur because of a synovial plica or the patellar tendon clicking over the patella. Clicking that is lateral to the knee joint can be the iliotibial band over a prominent lateral epicondyle, which in a runner can lead to iliotibial band syndrome.

Semimembranosus tendonitis in the endurance athlete can cause pain below the joint line on the posteromedial aspect of the knee.

Limitation to the full knee flexion range of movement can be caused by joint effusion. The capsular pattern on the knee joint causes flexion to be very restricted, while extension is somewhat restricted.

Passive Knee Flexion (135°) (Fig. 3-20)

The athlete is hook-lying with the knee flexed to midrange.

Passively move the knee into as much flexion as possible until an end feel is reached.

The end feel should be tissue approximation. Pain and/or limitation of range of motion can come from:

- anterior capsule with intracapsular joint swelling
- quadriceps muscle due to a muscle strain, tear, or hematoma

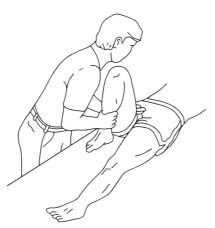

Fig. 3-20 Passive knee flexion.

ASSESSMENT

INTERPRETATION

- posterior capsule with an intracapsular swelling or a Baker's cyst
- patellar tendonitis
- patellar tendon strain or tear
- infrapatellar bursitis
- prepatellar bursitis
- suprapatellar bursitis
- medial or lateral collateral ligament sprain

Active Knee Extension (0° to - 15°)

Put your arm under the athlete's knee at an angle of 90° of flexion. Ask the athlete to extend the knee over your arm. Be aware of hyperextending knees. Look for a strong quadriceps contraction and a full range of motion bilaterally.

This can also be done with the athlete high-sitting with the knee flexed over the end of the plinth.

Pain, weakness, or limitation of range of motion during knee extension can be caused by an injury to the muscles or to their nerve supply.

The prime movers of knee extension are the quadriceps femoral N. (L2, L3, L4), which include rectus femoris, vastus lateralis, vastus intermedius, and vastus medialis.

The patella should glide proximally and slightly laterally during extension. According to Ficat and Hungerford, there are three abnormal patellar tracking trajectories. These are (1) a bayonet movement, which causes an abrupt lateral translation of the patella just before full extension, then further extension in a straight line; (2) an abrupt lateral translation at the end of knee extension; and (3) a semicircular route as if the patella is pivoting around the lateral patellar facet. Abnormalities in patellar tracking can be caused by:

- boney abnormalities of the patella or patellar sulcus
- support structure abnormalities (e.g., retinaculum, plicas)
- muscle imbalances in the quadriceps
- asynchronous muscle firing of the quadriceps

Patellar crepitus and pain that begins beyond 30° of flexion can indicate chondromalacia.

Jerky patellar tracking during extension can be caused by a weak vastus medialis obliquus or a subluxing patellar tendency.

Snapping near full extension or between 40° to 60° of flexion suggests a suprapatellar plica problem (shelf syndrome).

The patella may "stutter" during the course of knee extension rather than moving smoothly—this can also suggest a suprapatellar plica problem (shelf syndrome).

Limitation of full extension can be caused by:

- meniscus displacement
- intra-articular loose body
- joint effusion
- tear of the anterior cruciate ligament (part of the ligament gets trapped in the joint)
- acute medial collateral ligament sprain

ASSESSMENT   INTERPRETATION

Passive Knee Extension (0° to - 15°) (Fig. 3-21)

With the athlete hook-lying, extend the knee passively until an end feel is reached

The knee may hyperextend, especially in women.

If the knee hyperextends, lower the leg to the plinth and measure the amount of hyperextension.

Fix the femur with one hand just above the patella while the other hand lifts the lower leg (under the malleoli) up as far as possible. With the femur fixed on the plinth, the tibia and fibula may be lifted up so the joint goes past 0° into hyperextension. There may be as much as 15° of hyperextension.

Compare the amount bilaterally.

The end feel should be a tissue stretch.

Pain and/or limitation of range of motion can be caused by:
- medial collateral ligament sprain of the anterior superficial fibers
- hamstring strain or tear
- medial or lateral collateral ligament sprain

Pain on the anterior joint line at the end of passive extension suggests a fat pad lesion (Hoffa disease).

Pain in the popliteal fossa indicates a popliteal muscle strain or tear or Baker's cyst.

Increased extension or hyperextension accompanied by pain suggests a posterior capsule tear.

Knee hyperextension can indicate inherent joint hypermobility or severe joint laxity from severe or repeated trauma.

Bounce Home Sign

The athlete is relaxed and the knee supported by you with your hand in the popliteal space at 15° of flexion.

Let go of the posterior knee, allowing it to bounce gently into full extension.

During the bounce home test, there is usually full extension of the knee and then slight flexion. A lack of full extension suggests a torn meniscus, loose body, or significant intracapsular joint swelling.

Pain on the medial or lateral joint line at the end of range is a sign of a medial or lateral collateral ligament sprain.

A springy block as the end feel suggests a torn meniscus that is caught between the bone ends.

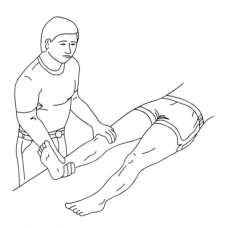

Fig. 3-21 Passive knee extension.

ASSESSMENT

INTERPRETATION

Active Medial (30°) and Lateral (40°) Rotation of the Tibia on the Femur

The athletes knee is flexed to an angle of 90° and he or she is asked to turn both feet inward (tibia rotates medially) as far as possible.

Compare the tibial movement. The athlete repeats the procedure turning the feet outward (tibial rotates laterally) as far as possible.

Stabilize the femur with a hand on the condyles. You should compare the tibial movement but must not be influenced by the ankle and foot rotation.

This can also be done in the high-sitting position.

Pain, weakness, or limitation of range of motion can be caused by an injury to the muscles or to their nerve supply.

The prime movers of medial rotation are:
- Semimembranosus—sciatic N. (tibial branch; L4, L5, S1)
- Semitendinosus—sciatic N. (tibial branch; L4, L5, S1)
- Popliteus—tibial N. (L5, S1, S2)

The prime mover of lateral rotation is the biceps femoris—sciatic N. (tibial branch; L5, S1, S2)

Pain or limitation of range of motion can also be elicited with these rotations if any of the following exist:
- meniscal tear
- joint effusion
- tibiofemoral joint injury

Passive Medial (Fig. 3-22) and Lateral Rotation of the Tibia on the Femur

With the athlete hook-lying, rotate the lower tibia without allowing any femoral movement.

This can also be done in the high-sitting position.

Medial rotation increases the tension in the posterolateral structures. Lateral rotation of the tibia increases tension in the posteromedial structures.

Pain and/or limitation of range of motion during passive medial rotation can come from:
- posterolateral capsule sprain or tear
- arcuate ligament sprain or tear
- popliteal tendon strain or tear, or tendonitis
- iliotibial band strain or tear
- lateral collateral ligament sprain

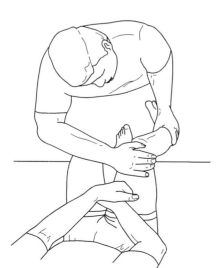

Fig. 3-22 Passive medial rotation of the tibia on the femur.

ASSESSMENT

INTERPRETATION

Pain and/or limitation of range of motion during passive lateral rotation can suggest:
- posteromedial capsule sprain or tear
- medial collateral ligament sprain or tear
- coronary ligament sprain
- pes anserine bursitis
- semimembranosus strain or tear
- semitendinosus strain or tear
- gracilis strain or tear

Resisted Medial and Lateral Rotation of the Tibia on the Femur

The athlete is hook-lying with the knees flexed to an angle of 90°.

Stabilize the femur with one hand over the femoral condyles while resisting tibial rotation with the other hand around the malleoli and under the foot.

This can also be done in the high-sitting position.

Pain and/or weakness can be caused by an injury to the muscles or to their nerve supply (see Active Medial and Lateral Rotation of the Tibia on the Femur).

According to Gollehon et al., tearing of the posterolateral structures (lateral collateral ligament, arcuate complex, and posterior cruciate ligament) will cause increases in lateral rotation of the tibia. It will also cause increased posterior drawer (translation) and varus joint opening.

Resisted Knee Flexion (Midrange)

The athlete flexes his or her knee to midrange and attempts further knee flexion against your resistance.

Resist behind the tibia just above the malleoli with one hand while the other hand stabilizes the pelvis.

Turn the tibia medially to test the medial hamstrings.

Turn the tibia laterally to test the lateral hamstrings.

This can also be done with the athlete's knees flexed and with his or her lower leg over the end of the plinth (a high-sitting athlete stabilizes the pelvis with his or her body weight).

Pain and/or weakness can occur from an injury to the muscle or to its nerve supply (see Active Knee Flexion). The accessory movers are:
- Sartorius
- Gastrocnemius
- Gracilis
- Popliteus

Resisted Knee Extension (Midrange) (Fig. 3-23)

The athlete flexes his or her knee to an angle of 90° with the feet resting on the plinth.

Place your hand on top of the flexed knee further away from you. The athlate drapes the other leg over your arm, allowing the leg to flex to midrange.

Resist extension of the draped leg by

Pain and/or weakness can occur from an injury to the muscle or to its nerve supply (see Active Knee Extension).

ASSESSMENT

INTERPRETATION

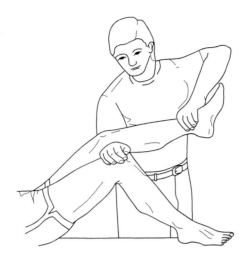

Fig. 3-23 Resisted knee extension.

applying resistance on the tibia just above the ankle.

If the athlete can easily overcome your resistance in this position, repeat the test with the athlete's legs hanging over the end of the plinth with you resisting at the ankle.

Your other hand stabilizes the athlete's pelvis.

SPECIAL TESTS—TIBIOFEMORAL JOINT

Valgus Test (Medial Collateral Ligament) (Fig. 3-24)
Full Extension (see Fig. 3-24)
Method 1

Hold the athlete's knee securely around the joint with both hands.

The athlete's right lower leg is resting on your right hip and is kept trapped there by your right elbow.

Palpate the medial joint line with the right hand while the other hand applies a valgus force to the femur.

The valgus force is accentuated gently at the knee as you lever the tibia next to your body with the right elbow in an attempt to open the joint on the medial side.

Test gently with the knee in full extension at first, and then at an angle of 30° of flexion.

ASSESSMENT

INTERPRETATION

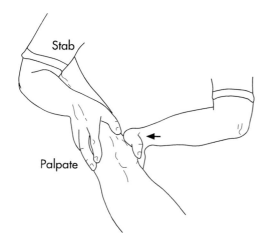

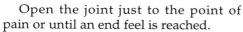

Fig. 3-24 Valgus test.

Open the joint just to the point of pain or until an end feel is reached.

The amount of joint opening is compared bilaterally.

Method 2

If the athlete has heavy thighs or is very apprehensive, this test can be done with the extremity resting on the examination table.

The hip is abducted slightly with the thigh resting on the table.

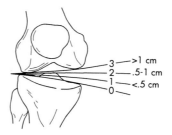

Fig. 3-25 Grades of medial instability.

Medial instability rating scale

Grade 0 = no joint opening
Grade 1+ = less than 0.5 cm joint opening
Grade 2+ = 0.5 to 1 cm joint opening
Grade 3+ = more than 1 cm joint opening

If the knee joint opens medially in full extension, it indicates the following:
- sprain or tear that involves the ligaments and structures with posteromedial attachment
- serious knee injury because the posterior capsule and the posterior cruciate ligament must be involved, since they add to the knee's stability in extension
- one-plane medial instability
- major knee joint instability problem

Grade 1 to Grade 2 instability can indicate:
- posteromedial capsular sprain
- medial collateral ligament sprain or tear (the entire medial collateral ligament is taut with full knee extension)
- posterior oblique ligament sprain or tear
- anterior cruciate ligament may be sprained

Grade 3 instability can indicate tearing of the structures above plus the following:
- anterior cruciate (posterolateral and intermediate bundles)
- medial portion of the posterior capsule
- posterior cruciate ligament may also be torn (see below)

Tears of the anterior and posterior cruciate ligaments cause gross instability.

ASSESSMENT

INTERPRETATION

30° Flexion

Place one hand on the medial malleolus and the other hand on the lateral aspect of the thigh, just above the knee.

Apply a gentle valgus force with the knee at an angle of 30° of flexion and in full extension.

This method does not allow the joint opening to be palpated as easily as in Method 1.

If the knee opens medially at an angle of 30° of knee flexion, it indicates the following:

- sprain or tear of the anteromedial structures
- one-plane medial instability—there is no rotary element involved (see Hughston et al.)

Grade 1 to Grade 2 instability can indicate:

- medial capsular ligament sprain
- posterior oblique ligament sprain
- medial collateral ligament sprain (the anterior superficial fibers of the medial collateral ligament are most taut at 30° of flexion and are most likely to sprain first)

Grade 3 instability can indicate damage to all of the above structures plus a tear of the medial bundle of the anterior cruciate ligament. Hughston et al. differ in their classification of knee instabilities. They believe that instabilities revolve around the integrity of the posterior cruciate ligament. They also believe that to get straight one-plane instability the posterior cruciate must be torn. According to them the posterior cruciate must be intact for there to be rotary instability; therefore their tests classify the results as follows: A Grade 3 valgus instability at full extension indicates a posterior cruciate ligament tear. Because it is torn there is no rotary instability and it is classified as a straight medial instability. A Grade 3 valgus instability at 30° of knee flexion with no instability at full extension has an intact posterior cruciate ligament and is classified as an anteromedial rotary instability (AMRI).

It is important to realize that this is controversial and there are shades of grey in the diagnosis of rotary and straight instabilities. It is also important to realize that there can be multiple rotary instabilities. It is fairly common to have anteromedial and anterolateral instabilities at the same time. It is important to be aware of these combinations, and it is imperative to record the test results.

Most children or adolescents who have Grade 3 opening on the valgus test (this is rare) will have failure and therefore opening at the joint epiphysis, since the ligamentous structures are stronger than their growth plates.

If the ligament does fail, it tears at the midportion or distal insertion, according to Clanton et al. The anterior cruciate ligament tear can avulse the anterior tibial spine, although this is fairly uncommon.

Varus Test

As on the medial side, tears that are more posterolateral occur in extension and structures injured in flexion are anterolateral.

ASSESSMENT

Full Extension (Fig. 3-26)
Method 1
This is the same as for the valgus test (Method 1) but apply a varus stress at the knee with the knee in full extension and at 30° of flexion.

It is important to palpate carefully for lateral joint opening because it may be hard to detect.

Ensure that the patient is relaxed and try to open the joint to the point of pain or when an end feel is reached.

You can move to the medial side of the limb if this position is more comfortable.

Method 2
If the athlete has a long or heavy thigh or is apprehensive, this test can be done with the extremity resting on the table.

The hip is abducted slightly with the thigh resting on the table—have one hand on the medial side of the thigh just above the knee with the other hand on the lateral malleolus.

A gentle varus stress is applied to open the knee joint.

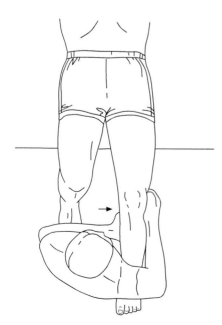

INTERPRETATION

If the joint opens laterally in full extension it represents a one-plane lateral instability (straight instability).

Grade 1 to Grade 2 instability occurs with damage that can include:
- posterolateral capsular tear
- lateral collateral ligament sprain or tear
- biceps tendon strain or tear
- arcuate complex sprain or tear

Grade 3 instability represents a major instability with problems approaching the proportions of a dislocation. The structures damaged can include tearing of the structures mentioned above plus the following:
- anterior cruciate ligament is torn
- posterior cruciate ligament is torn
- biceps femoris tendon can develop a complete tear

Fig. 3-26 Varus test.

ASSESSMENT

INTERPRETATION

30° Knee Flexion

If the joint opens laterally when the knee is in 30° of flexion, this represents a one-plane lateral instability.

Again, Hughston et al. differ in that they classify a Grade 3 varus instability in full extension as a straight lateral instability; there is no rotary component because the posterior cruciate is torn. These authors also classify a Grade 3 varus instability at 30° of knee flexion as anterolateral rotary instability (ALRI).

A Grade 1 lateral instability may be present without any injury. A Grade 1 to Grade 2 instability with an injury can cause damage (strain or tear) to:
- lateral capsule
- lateral collateral ligament
- iliotibial band
- arcuate-popliteus complex
- biceps femoris tendon

A Grade 3 instability represents significant damage to all the structures above.

McMurray's Meniscus Test (Fig. 3-27)

With the athlete in the supine position, fully flex the athlete's knee and hip (heel to buttock).

The tibia is rotated internally and externally with one hand on the distal end of the tibia (O'Donoghue Test).

The other hand palpates the joint line medially and laterally for signs of crepitus or tenderness.

Put your ear close to the joint line to listen for clicking or snapping.

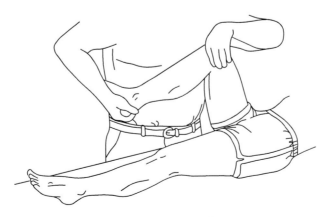

Fig. 3-27 McMurray's meniscus test.

ASSESSMENT   INTERPRETATION

Flexion

When the knee is placed in full flexion and rotated, in many cases a posterior meniscus tear will give a definite cartilage click. In fact, this procedure can actually cause the meniscus to slip forward and the knee to become locked.

With the tibia in external rotation (with a valgus force) the lateral meniscus is pulled anteriorly while the medial meniscus is drawn posteriorly where it can be caught between the femoral and tibial condyles.

With the tibia in internal rotation (with a varus force) the medial meniscus moves forward while the lateral meniscus recedes to where it can be trapped between the femoral and tibial condyles.

During knee flexion, the medial meniscus is drawn posteriorly by the semimembranosus expansion, while the anterior horn is pulled anteriorly by the fibers of the anterior cruciate ligament.

Extension

The knee is then taken into extension with a slight varus force while the tibia is internally rotated—this tests the lateral meniscus.

Repeat this with the tibia externally rotated while applying a slight valgus stress and extending the knee—this tests the medial meniscus.

Clicking, locking, or a springy block at the end of range of motion indicates a positive test.

During extension, the menisci are pulled forward by meniscopatellar fibers and the posterior horn of the lateral meniscus is pulled anteriorly by the tension in the meniscofemoral ligament. The lateral meniscus is held posteriorly by the politeus expansion.

An audible click during the McMurray test suggests a meniscal tear that catches in between the femoral and tibial condyles when the meniscus moves posteriorly in the knee joint. Joint line pain during the maneuver and on palpation is also a very positive sign of a meniscal tear. The most common lesion involves the medial meniscus with a bucket-handle tear and the mechanism is knee flexion with tibial lateral rotation in relation to the femur.

Feeling a snapping inside the joint that is level with the joint line also can indicate a tear.

Meniscal tears are frequently found in conjunction with isolated anterior cruciate ligament injuries or combination injuries of the anterior cruciate and collateral ligaments. This tear may occur at the time of injury or can develop with time.

The anterior cruciate deficient knee has progressive joint degeneration with time (Feagin and Curl, Fetto and Marshall). The pivot shift phenomenon as a result of the ACL tear causes a sudden directional change in both femoral condyles that may be responsible for the meniscal degeneration (Reuben). One or both menisci can tear and eventually augment the instability even further.

According to Cerbona et al., the most frequent meniscal tear with an isolated anterior cruciate ligament rupture is a peripheral posterior longitudinal tear of the medial meniscus. The lateral

ASSESSMENT   # INTERPRETATION

meniscus tears occasionally occur with these ruptures and are radial lesions.

The most frequent meniscal tear with the anterior cruciate ligament and collateral ligament (combination injury) is a peripheral posteromedial longitudinal tear. Once again, the lateral meniscus can tear and is of the radial type.

Drawer Sign or Test (Fig. 3-28)

According to Katz and Fingeroth, the anterior drawer test is not as accurate as the Lachman and pivot shift tests for determining anterior cruciate instability. There may be a normal anterior drawer in spite of the anterior cruciate tear in more than 25% of the cases. The drawer sign may be negative in an anterior cruciate tear because the posterior horn or the medial meniscus may act as a blocking wedge, capsular restrains may be strong and intact, or hamstring spasm may limit the drawer.

This test may be difficult to perform 12 hours after an injury because of joint effusion, hamstring spasm, and the inability to flex the knee to an angle of 90°.

Anterior

The athlete is in the supine position and should be comfortable and relaxed.

The athlete's knee is flexed to an angle of 90° and the hip is flexed to 45°—the foot is flat on the table.

Sit on the athlete's forefoot with the athlete's foot and tibia in neutral.

Place your hands firmly around the upper tibia with thumbs on the medial and lateral joint lines.

The anterior instability rating scale for a positive drawer sign is presented in the following list (Fig. 3-29).

If the tibia moves forward more than .5 cm, there is damage to the anterior cruciate ligament. If there is greater than 1 cm of anterior displacement, an anterior cruciate and medial collateral ligament rupture should be suspected.

Often the joint capsule is also stretched or torn if the anterior cruciate is injured.

The anterior cruciate is 3.8 cm long and 1.1 cm in diameter. According to Butler, it provides 86% of the total stabilizing force

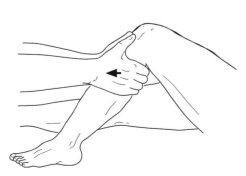

Fig. 3-28 Anterior drawer sign. Anterior glide of the tibia on the femur.

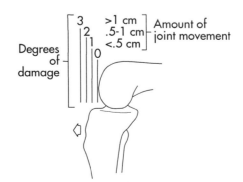

Fig. 3-29 Anterior glide of the tibia on the femur. Grades of anterior instability.

ASSESSMENT

Your fingers are around the tibia and touching the hamstring tendons in the popliteal space (the tendons must be lax to do this test).

Gently pull the tibia forward.

A slow, steady pull is more effective than a jerk, which can cause discomfort. The hamstrings must be relaxed (not in spasm) and this test must be carefully compared bilaterally.

Posterior (Fig. 3-30)

The posterior drawer sign test uses the same position as the anterior drawer sign or test. But this time, gently push the tibia straight backward.

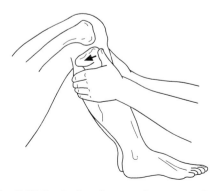

Fig. 3-30 Posterior drawer sign. Posterior glide of the tibia on the femur.

INTERPRETATION

against anterior displacement of the tibia. It is made up of three distinct bundles: anteromedial, intermediate, and posterolateral. These bundles restrict anterior tibial displacement during different knee joint positions. When the knee is flexed and during flexion, the anteromedial bundle remains taut. When the knee is fully extended, the intermediate and posteromedial bundles becomes taut.

During sports activities the knee usually assumes a flexed position so the anteromedial bundle is most often damaged. The anterior drawer sign with the knee flexed position tests this anteromedial bundle of the anterior cruciate ligament. The anteromedial band of the anterior cruciate is the only portion that is tight in knee flexion and is what prevents forward displacement. The remainder of the ligament (posterolateral and intermediate bundles) is a secondary check. The medial collateral (deep fibers) is the tertiary check.

On occasion the posterior oblique ligament, iliotibial band, and arcuate-popliteal complex may be injured to some degree.

If the anterior drawer test is positive, it must be differentiated from a false-positive test that can occur with a ruptured posterior cruciate ligament. With a posterior cruciate tear the tibia subluxes backward when the knee is flexed to an angle of 90° and therefore may appear to move forward excessively during the anterior drawer test.

Occasionally, an athlete with hypermobility and genu recurvatum may have a positive anterior drawer up to Grade 2+ without any knee pathology.

If the tibia moves posteriorly excessively, the structure most commonly injured is the posterior cruciate ligament. The arcuate ligament complex and the posterior oblique ligament may also be partially or completely torn if the displacement is great.

If posterior instability exists, the tibia may be sitting backward already and the neutral starting position for the test is difficult to determine. You may mistakenly find that the tibia moves forward excessively and suspect an anterior cruciate ligament tear. If the drawer test is positive, look at the lateral view of the knee and determine if the tibia is under the femur or if the tibia has a posterior sag (which suggests a torn posterior cruciate).

A posterior cruciate tear is an uncommon injury. According to Fowler and Messieh, the mechanism of injury is usually one of the following:
- hyperextension of the knee
- hyperflexion of the knee
- posterior displacement of the tibia on the femur

This lesion may result in progressive posterior instability with accompanying degenerative changes in the knee joint.

ASSESSMENT   INTERPRETATION

Modified Drawer Test for Rotary Instability (Slocum's Test) (Fig. 3-31)

The athlete's knee is flexed to an angle of 90°, the hip is flexed to an angle of 45°, and the foot rests on the examination table.

The hamstrings must be relaxed.

Anteromedial Rotary Instability (Slocum and Larson's Test)

The tibia is put in 15° of external rotation.

The tibia is pulled forward gently.

If the tibia comes forward, there is anteromedial instability.

If the tibia in this position of external rotation subluxes forward when an anterior force is applied, it indicates anteromedial rotary instability. This instability is caused by:

- medial collateral ligament tear
- posterior oblique ligament tear (posteromedial one third)
- anterior cruciate ligament sprain or tear (anteromedial bundle)
- medial capsule tear (posteromedial)

The medial tibial plateau rotates and displaces anteriorly from beneath the medial femoral condyle. In external knee rotation, the medial and posterior structures are placed on stretch while the cruciates are lax (unwound).

Hughston and Barrett believe that the posterior oblique ligament, semimembranosus, and medial meniscus complex are the primary deterrents to anteromedial stability.

Anterolateral Rotary Instability

The tibia is rotated internally 30°. Sit on the forefoot to stabilize it and pull the tibia forward gently with your hand around the upper end of the tibia.

Motion will occur if anterolateral instability exists.

If the tibia in this position of internal rotation subluxes forward when an anterior stress is applied, it indicates anterolateral rotary instability. This instability is caused by:

- lateral capsule tear (posterolateral aspect)
- arcuate complex partial or complete tear (especially of the lateral collateral ligament)
- partial or complete tear of the anterior cruciate ligament

On occasion, the lateral collateral ligament or posterior cruciate can also be sprained.

The cruciates tighten as the tibia is internally rotated and stress is placed on the anterolateral structures. Anterolateral instability allows the lateral tibial plateau to rotate and displace

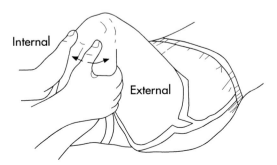

Internal

External

Fig. 3-31 Internal and external rotation of the tibiofemoral joint for rotary instability testing.

ASSESSMENT

INTERPRETATION

anteriorly from beneath the lateral femoral condyle. This is the most common instability and leads to lateral pivot shift episodes in the athlete, especially if the anterior cruciate is completely torn.

Terry et al. believe that anterolateral knee instability is a result of the combined injury of the following:
- anterior cruciate ligament
- midthird capsular ligament
- lateral meniscus and its capsular attachments
- capsulo-osseus and deep layers of the iliotibial tract

Posterolateral Rotary Instability

The tibia is rotated externally 15°. Gently push the tibia posteriorly.

If the tibia moves backward, there is posterolateral instability.

This should be differentiated from the posterior drawer test because, during this test, the posterolateral corner of the tibia drops backward with varus opening rather than the entire tibia moving backward.

The lateral tibial plateau rotates posteriorly in relation to the femur with varus knee joint opening.

This is the result of a serious injury with damage to the:
- arcuate complex
- biceps femoris tendon
- anterior cruciate ligament (posterolateral band)
- lateral capsule

At times, the posterior cruciate may be sprained. (Hughston et al. do not believe that it tears because they believe a torn posterior cruciate will not result in rotary instability.)

According to Grood et al., the posterior cruciate is an important secondary restraint to external rotation at 90° of flexion.

This athlete may walk with a marked knee varus due to posterior lateral subluxation and there is often marked hyperextension laxity as well.

The arcuate complex consists of the arcuate ligament, the popliteal tendon, the lateral collateral ligament, and the posterior third of the lateral capsule. (Hughston et al. also include the lateral head of gastrocnemius.)

Lachman Test (Anterior Cruciate) (Fig. 3-32)

The Lachman test should always be done before the pivot shift tests because of its accuracy and simplicity.

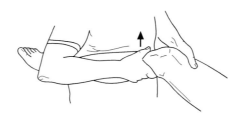

Fig. 3-32 Lachman test. Anterior cruciate ligament test.

ASSESSMENT

Method 1

The athlete lies supine with the tibia in slight external rotation and the knee flexed to an angle between 5° to 20°.

Stand on the lateral side of the knee being tested, facing the athlete's head.

Hold the injured leg with the arm closest to it so that the athlete's ankle is supported between your chest and arm.

Place one hand on the posteromedial aspect of the proximal tibia with the thumb along the anteromedial joint line.

Your other hand stabilizes the anterior aspect of the distal femur to prevent femoral movement.

Your hand on the tibia lifts upward and anteriorly while the femur is held steady.

The test is virtually an anterior drawer test performed at 5° to 20° of knee flexion.

A positive sign is indicated by a mushy, or soft, end feel when the tibia moves forward on the femur.

Palpate with your thumb for any movement of the tibia.

Method 2

An athlete with a large, heavy thigh and leg may require this alternative method of testing.

Stabilize the leg by placing a rolled towel beneath the femur to hold the knee in slight flexion.

Have an assistant hold the femur down while you grasp the tibia and move it anteriorly and posteriorly.

The athlete's heel can rest on the plinth during the test if the weight of the limb presents a problem.

Anterior tibial movement with a soft end feel indicates a positive test.

INTERPRETATION

A positive sign is indicated by a soft end feel when the tibia moves forward on the femur; you will see and feel the anterior translation of the tibia.

A positive Lachman test indicates that the anterior cruciate ligament (posterolateral bundle) has been injured.

It is generally agreed in the literature that this test is the most reliable for determining the presence of an anterior cruciate ligament rupture, especially of the posterolateral bundle (Jonsson T et al.; King S et al.).

It is often the only anterior cruciate test that can be done for the acute knee, although it is also very accurate in the detection of chronic instability.

The Lachman test is more reliable than the anterior drawer sign for determining an anterior cruciate tear. It is particularly useful when the hamstrings or iliotibial band are in spasm or difficult to relax. It is a test that is superior to the drawer sign test, according to Torg, because:

- there is less pain because the knee does not need to be flexed to an angle of 90°, which is not possible if a hemarthrosis exists
- there is less meniscus impingement
- hamstrings are less likely to spasm

The Lachman test can also be superior to the pivot shift tests when testing for an anterior cruciate tear because the knee does not have to be fully extended for the test. Therefore it can be done if joint effusion exists. This test can also be done if there is medial collateral ligament involvement because it does not stress the ligament like the pivot shift test does.

ASSESSMENT   INTERPRETATION

Pivot Shift Tests (Anterolateral Instability Tests)

For completeness, several pivot shift tests are outlined. Do not attempt every test on the athlete. Find which pivot shift test is best suited to your assessment style and most comfortable for you and the athlete. Use your favorite test to confirm previous findings from the history-taking and the Lachman test.

These pivot shift tests are most suitable for the athlete who has chronic anterolateral rotary instability (ALRI). If anterolateral displacement of the tibia under the femur causes a jerk, click, subluxation, and/or reduction, the test is positive.

A positive test indicates a torn anterior cruciate ligament (specifically the anteromedial band) and middle third lateral capsule tear or laxity. With further damage the arcuate complex may also be injured.

Meniscal tears, usually lateral, are very common with anterior cruciate tears. These menisci may be injured at the same time as the cruciate or may go onto meniscal degeneration following an anterior cruciate tear.

Injuries that can commonly accompany the anterior cruciate tears are:
- meniscal tears
- femoral osteochondral fractures
- posterior cruciate tears

Method 1 (Jerk Test; Hughston)

The athlete is in the supine position with the hip flexed to an angle of 45° and the knee flexed to an angle of 90°.

Place one hand on the lower tibia at the ankle with the tibia internally rotated.

Your other hand is placed behind the head of the fibula to apply a valgus force (use the heel of the hand).

The athlete's knee is extended while the valgus force is applied.

As the knee extends, the femur will fall back and the tibia will move forward.

There is a jerk when the tibial condyle subluxes at 30° of flexion and another pop as reduction occurs when the knee is extended.

As the knee reaches full extension the tibia will shift backward, reducing the subluxation.

The jerk test reproduces what happens during a knee pivot shift episode or "giving way." The athlete will be aware of the shift as he or she is tested.

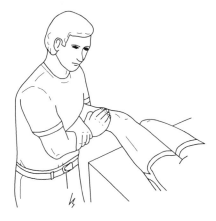

Fig. 3-33 Pivot shift test method 2.

ASSESSMENT

Method 2 (Fig. 3-33)

Put the athlete's leg under your armpit.

Your elbow locks the leg over your hip.

With the opposite hand, apply a valgus stress while the hand on the locking arm grasps your other wrist.

The knee is taken into flexion and extension.

The tibia can be seen to sublux and reduce as above.

Method 3 (MacIntosh)

The athlete is in the supine position and must be relaxed.

Lift the heel of the foot to an angle of 20° of hip flexion with the knee fully extended and with the other hand behind the upper lateral aspect of the tibia and the fibular head.

In this position, in the presence of instability, the lateral tibial plateau begins to sublux forward on the femur.

Apply internal rotation to the tibia and fibula at the knee and ankle and apply a lifting force to the back of the tibia and fibula.

The knee is allowed to flex about 2° to 5°, then apply a medial push with the proximal hand and a lateral push with the distal hand to produce a valgus force at the knee.

As the internal rotation, valgus force, and forward displacement are maintained, the knee is slowly passively flexed.

If anterior subluxation of the tibia is present, a sudden, visible, audible, and palpable reduction occurs at 20° to 40° of knee flexion.

INTERPRETATION

This method allows you to apply a valgus force while flexing and extending the knee. It is particularly effective in the athlete with a heavy or large leg that is difficult to lift and test.

This test is very similar to Method 2 but allows more tibial rotation force and leverage.

ASSESSMENT

INTERPRETATION

Method 4 (Losee Test—Flexion, Extension, Valgus FEV Test)

The athlete is relaxed in the supine position.

The athlete's right ankle is placed between your right arm and chest (above the iliac crest) while the tibia is maintained in a position of lateral rotation.

Put both hands along the joint line on each side of the knee.

Apply a valgus and superior axial force with the knee extended. Maintaining the force, slowly flex the knee, allowing the tibia to medially rotate.

At 15° to 20° of flexion, the lateral tibial plateau becomes visible or palpable, having shifted under the femoral condyle. During this shift a "clunk" may be felt.

The tibia will then move back into place with knee extension.

The Losee test may not reveal mild laxity but it will pick up chronic or gross laxity. It is an easier and less stressful test.

This test allows the therapist to palpate the joint line and determine the degree of shift.

Method 5 (Slocum's Test; Fig. 3-34)

Slocum's anterolateral rotatory instability test is often most useful in the chronic problem.

The athlete is side lying with the affected side up and the normal hip and knee flexed out of the way.

Roll the athlete's pelvis posteriorly about 30° from the supine position, with the medial side of the foot resting on the plinth and the knee flexed to an angle of 10°.

This position allows the knee to fall into a valgus position (and internal tibial rotation). Palpate the posterolateral joint and the femoral and tibial condyles. The tibia will be subluxed anteriorly and internally on the femur.

Apply a valgus force while flexing the knee.

When a positive instability is present, a reduction is felt as the knee flexes to an angle of 25° to 45°.

Slocum's test is valuable especially to test chronic anterolateral instability and in the heavier or tense athlete. If the posterior horn of the menisci and the capsular ligaments are damaged with the anterior cruciate, chronic gross instability can result.

Method 6 (Bach et al.)

The athlete is in the supine position,

Recent research by Bach et al. indicates that the hip and tibial

ASSESSMENT   INTERPRETATION

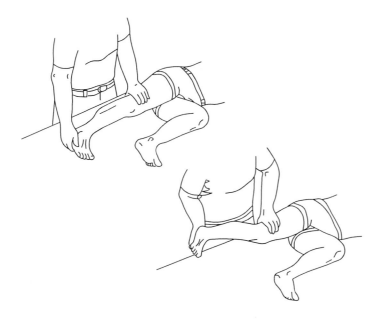

Fig. 3-34 Pivot shift test method 5.

with hip abducted to an angle of 30°, knee in extension, and tibia externally rotated approximately 20°.

Have one hand on the medial malleolus and the tibia, holding the leg in abduction and the tibia in external rotation.

Your other hand is on the lateral aspect of the knee joint.

Apply a constant axial compressive force while flexing the knee.

The best position for you is at the foot of the table, to ensure pure hip abduction without hip rotation.

positions are important in the results of the therapist's testing.

Hip abduction and tibial external rotation during the pivot test gave the highest degree of accuracy during testing, while hip adduction/tibial external rotation and hip adduction/tibial internal rotation resulted in lower scores. Bach et al. suggest that the iliotibial band, hip adduction, and internal tibial rotation may all dampen the pivot shift test.

Posterior "Sag" Sign (Posterior Cruciate) (Fig. 3-35)

The athlete lies supine and flexes both hips to angles of 45° and both knees to angles of 90°. Observe and compare the femoral tibial relationship from a lateral view.

In this position, the tibia will drop backward or sag back on the femur if the posterior cruciate is torn.

A posterior position (sag) of the tibia under the femur indicates a torn posterior cruciate ligament and capsule. Secondarily, the arcuate complex and the posterior oblique and the anterior cruciate ligaments may also be injured.

External Rotation Recurvatum Test

Hold the athlete's feet by the heels

This test indicates posterolateral rotary instability, which

ASSESSMENT

INTERPRETATION

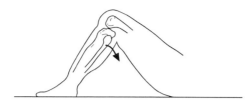

Fig. 3-35 Posterior sag sign.

with the knees extended, lift them off the plinth to an angle of 45° of hip flexion.

The athlete's quadriceps must be relaxed.

The test is positive if the tibia shows excessive hyperextension and external rotation.

allows the tibia to displace backward in relation to the lateral femoral condyle. There is damage to the arcuate complex mainly.

Quadriceps Active Test (Daniel et al.)

The athlete is in the supine position with the knee flexed to an angle of 90° in the drawer test position.

The thigh is supported so that the thigh muscles are relaxed.

The athlete gently contracts the quadriceps muscle to shift the tibia without extending the knee.

In the normal knee there is no anterior tibial shift.

The test indicates a posterior cruciate rupture if the tibia shifts anteriorly more than 2 cm.

If the posterior cruciate is ruptured, the tibia sags posteriorly, and therefore on contraction of the quadriceps the patellar tendon pulls the tibia anteriorly.

SPECIAL TESTS—PATELLOFEMORAL JOINT

Patellar Orientation Tests (McConnell)

With the athlete supine lying and the quadriceps relaxed, determine the patellar orientation in relation to the femur.

To examine the static glide component, the therapist should palpate the femoral condyles and patella and determine if the patella is sitting in the midline between the condyles, or in a medial or lateral position (Fig. 3-36, *A* and *B*). Then ask the athlete to contract the quadriceps and determine if the patella

For the **static glide component**, the patella should sit centrally, but often it sits laterally, since the lateral structures are usually tight (Fig. 3-36, *A*). The lateral structures that can contribute to the tightness include:
- lateral retinaculum
- iliotibial tract
- iliopatellar band (fascial band from the iliotibial band to lateral inferior edge of the patella)
- long head of biceps femoris
- short head of biceps femoris

The patella can sit medially but this is rare (Fig. 3-36, *B*).

The patella may sit centrally during the static glide examina-

ASSESSMENT

moves laterally or medially—**dynamic glide component.**

To examine the **tilt component**, the height of the medial patellar border is compared with the height of the lateral border (Fig. 3-37, *A* and *B*). Is it tilted medially or laterally? A severe tilt will not allow your fingers to get under the lateral patellar border. Determine what happens to the tilt when the patella is glided medially—**dynamic tilt component.**

To examine the **rotational component,** the inferior and superior poles are observed and palpated. The poles should be in line with the longitudinal axis of the femur. Determine if the inferior pole is medial or lateral to the superior pole (Fig. 3-38, *A* and *B*).

To examine the **anteroposterior component,** the **inferior** and **superior poles** of the patella are examined to see if either pole is posterior to the other pole (Fig. 3-39, *A* and *B*).

INTERPRETATION

tion, but when the quadriceps contract the patella may then track laterally—**dynamic lateral glide**. If this occurs, there is usually an asynchronous quadriceps contraction with vastus lateralis contracting first and more powerfully than vastus medialis. This creates a patellar glide problem that may respond to treatment with strengthening and a McConnell tape job.

When examining the **static tilt component**, the patellar lateral border is often held down lower than the medial border, creating a lateral tilt (Fig. 3-37, *A*). The patella may just be held at the inferior surface or at the entire lateral border. In a severe case, the lateral border and superior surface of the lateral border may also be held. Tight, deep retinacular structures can tether the lateral edge down, creating this tilt. Occasionally an athlete may have a medial tilt (Fig. 3-37, *B*).

During the **dynamic tilt component**, if the medial border of the patella rises with a manual medial glide, this is another sign of patellar malalignment and the necessity for correction through taping and exercise. It further shows that the lateral retinaculum, deep and superficial, or other lateral structures are limiting patellar motions.

The **rotational component** can indicate inferior pole restriction in a medial (internal) rotation or lateral (external) rotation (Fig. 3-38, *A* and *B*). Rotational components lead to patellar malalignment problems (patellar tendonitis, synovitis, chondromalacia, etc.).

The anteroposterior patellar position often shows a posterior inferior pole position that can lead to fat pad impingement and patellar pain, especially when it is associated with genu recurvatum (Fig. 3-39, *A*). The fat pad can become swollen and painful if this position is present. The patellar superior pole can be posterior, this is rare. McConnell recommends a taping correction for this.

For more details on McConnell assessment and treatment see the bibliography for reference materials.

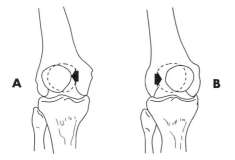

Fig. 3-36 Patillar glide component. **A**, Static lateral glide. **B**, Static medial glide.

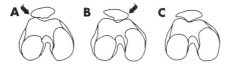

Fig. 3-37 Patellar tilt component. **A**, static lateral tilt. **B**, Static medial tilt. C, Normal.

ASSESSMENT   INTERPRETATION

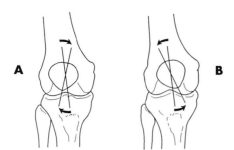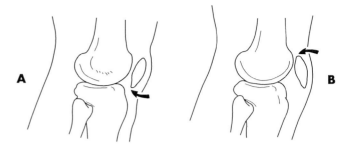

Fig. 3-38 Patellar rotational component. **A,** Lateral (external) rotation. **B,** medial (internal) rotation.

Fig. 3-39 Anteroposterior component. **A,** Inferior tilt. **B,** Superior tilt.

Patellar Mobility (Patellar Instability) (Fig. 3-40)

The athlete's knee is extended with the quadriceps relaxed.

Displace the patella medially, laterally, inferiorly, and superiorly. The patella should move freely.

If laxity is suspected, repeat the test at an angle of 30° of knee flexion. Any tightness with medial glide due to tight lateral structures should be recorded.

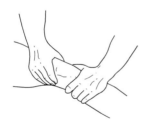

Fig. 3-40 Patellar mobility.

The patella should move smoothly over the trochlear groove of the femur. Any roughness on the articular surfaces causes crepitus and sometimes pain when the patella is moved.

Chondromalacia is the usual cause of discomfort and roughening, but osteochondral defects of degenerative changes within the trochlear groove or patella itself can precipitate these symptoms.

With the knee in full extension, the patella can displace laterally, up to one half its width. If it displaces more, there is patellar hypermobility.

At 30° of knee flexion, the patella should be secure in the sulcus with little or no lateral displacement possible. A grossly unstable patella can be subluxed over the lateral femoral condyle, both in extension and at an angle of 30° of knee flexion. Hypermobility of the patella is often associated with patella alta or recurvatum—this hypermobility makes the patella susceptible to subluxations and dislocations. Patellar hypermobility can be caused by abnormalities in the patellofemoral configuration. These abnormalities are:

- small patella
- patella alta (high riding)
- jockey cap–shaped patella
- shallow trochlear groove
- low lateral femoral condyle

Patellar alignment problems can be caused by:

- weak quadriceps, especially the vastus medialis obliquus
- weakness of the medial retinaculum
- increased Q-angle
- lax or tight lateral retinacular extensions of vastus lateralis
- abnormal tibial or foot mechanics

Patellar Apprehension Sign

With the athlete in the supine posi-

When lateral displacement is attempted, if the athlete shows

ASSESSMENT

INTERPRETATION

tion with the knee flexed to an angle of 30°, gently push the patella laterally.

If the athlete has previously dislocated the patella, he or she will contract the quadriceps, which is indicative of a positive test.

The athlete will feel apprehensive at this time.

signs of apprehension by contracting the quadriceps or grabbing your hand, this is a positive indication of a subluxing or dislocating patella.

Pain often accompanies this sign.

Critical Test (McConnell)

With the athlete high sitting, resist an isometric quadriceps contraction at 0°, 30°, 60°, and 90°; each is held for 10 seconds. Determine if pain is elicited or the athlete's symptoms are reproduced. Repeat the painful test while pushing the patella medially to determine if the symptoms decrease or disappear.

If the patellar symptoms decrease or disappear with patellar medial glide, McConnell taping and medial musculature strengthening along the lateral patellar structure and stretching will usually help the athlete recover from malalignment dysfunction.

Patellofemoral Compression Test

The athlete's knee is in full extension.

Push the patella downward against the femoral condyles.

If there is pain, the test is positive.

The patella can be gently tapped to see if pain results.

If compression did not cause pain, this test can be repeated at angles of 30°, 60°, and 90° of knee flexion.

Pain experienced under the patella during this procedure can indicate chondromalacia or a chondral fracture.

Osteochondritis dissecans of the patella will elicit a positive compression test (Schwarz et al.).

Prepatellar or suprapatellar bursitis may also cause pain during this test. Prepatellar bursitis will give rise to pain *over* the patella, not under it.

If pain is present during this test, the articular wear of the patella of the femoral condyle may be a result of recurrent patellar subluxations.

Patellar Retinaculum Test

With the athlete's knee in full extension, displace the patella medially and palpate the medial retinaculum fibers, now taut, to see if there is any localized tenderness.

Then the patella is displaced laterally and the lateral retinaculum fibers are palpated.

Retinacular inflammation due to abnormal patella tracking is fairly common.

This retinaculum test allows you to determine if the patellar problems are primarily extra-articular or intra-articular; chondromalacia and synovial involvements need to be ruled out. If the lateral retinaculum is tight and painful, a patellar malalignment problem should be investigated.

Clarke's Sign (Chondromalacia)

With the athlete in the supine position with the knee extended, trap the upper pole of the patella with the web

You may hear or feel crepitus during the Clarke's sign test if chondromalacia exists—the pain will be retropatellar. Most athletes will find this test uncomfortable, so do it gently, or you

ASSESSMENT

INTERPRETATION

between the thumb and index finger.

The athlete is asked to contract the quadriceps while the patella is pushed downward.

If the athlete expresses retropatellar pain or cannot contract the quadriceps, the test is positive.

A variation of this is to move the patella distally, then have the athlete contract the quadriceps.

If the test is performed at 0° of extension, the patella sometimes pinches the synovium, giving pain and a false positive. This can be avoided by flexing the knee to an angle of 20°.

If chondromalacia is suspected, this test should be done at the end of the assessment because it is a painful procedure.

may omit it if chondromalacia is not suspected. If chondromalacia is suspected, do this test last to confirm the results.

Plica Test (Hughston et al.)

With the athlete in the supine position, passively flex and extend the knee with the tibia in medial rotation. One of your hands is holding the lower tibia while the other hand presses the patella medially (with the heel of the hand) and palpates the medial femoral condyle with the fingers.

Feel for popping of the plica with the fingers—popping indicates a positive test.

The patella plica is the remnant of an embryonic septum that made up the knee joint capsule. The incidence of patella plica varies, according to different authors, from 18% to 60% of the population (Blackburn et al.; Nottage et al.; Kegerreis et al.). It can become inflamed as a result of the following:

- trauma
- repeated microtrauma
- repeated knee extension exercises (isokinetic or isometric exercise)
- repeated knee-bending activities (weight lifting, skiing, or while performing the swimmer's whip kick)

Q-Angle (Patellar Alignment Problems) (Fig. 3-41)

With the athlete in the supine position with the knees extended, measure the Q-angle with a goniometer.

One arm of the goniometer lines up with the ASIS. The center of the goniometer is on the center of the patella. The other arm of the goniometer is lined up with the tibial tubercl (in some texts, the inferior pole of the patella is used as the middle point).

The quadriceps should be relaxed.

The normal angle should be between 13° to 18°.

The normal Q-angle is 13° for males and 18° for females—the female Q-angle is greater due to wider hips and pelvis. A Q-angle that is greater than 18° may increase the likelihood of patellar subluxations and can also be associated with chondromalacia.

An increased Q-angle from lateral placement of the tibial tubercle or an excessive amount of external tibial rotation predisposes the patella to lateral displacement when the quadriceps contract strongly. Because of the abnormal patellar tracking, the articular cartilage of the medial, the odd, or the lateral patellar facet begins to degenerate as a result of too little or too much compression through the articular cartilage.

Habitual lateral tracking may also produce adaptive changes

ASSESSMENT   INTERPRETATION

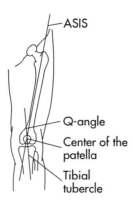

Fig. 3-41 Q-angle measurement.

According to Hughston this Q-angle can be measured with the quadriceps contracted on an extended knee. The angle should be approximately 10° in a contracted quadriceps—Q-angle that is greater than 10° is considered abnormal.

so that, with time, the vastus lateralis becomes shortened, the vastus medialis becomes stretched, and the lateral patellar retinaculum shortens.

Erosion of the articular cartilage on the condyles can also occur from a faulty Q-angle.

Lower Extremity Girth (Swelling/Atrophy)

Locate the joint line bilaterally.

Measurements of girth are made bilaterally at the joint line—3, 6, and 9 inches (7, 15, and 22 cms) above the joint line, and 2, 4, and 6 inches (5, 10, and 15 cms) below the joint line.

Increased measurements at the joint line indicate joint effusion; increased measurements 3 inches (7 cm) above the joint line can indicate gross effusion in the suprapatellar bursa.

Decreased measurements 3 inches (7 cm) above the joint line can indicate vastus medialis atrophy.

Decreased measurements 6 inches (15 cm) and 9 inches (22 cm) above the joint line indicate general upper leg strength loss.

Decreased measurements below the joint line can indicate atrophy in the gastrocnemius.

Increased measurements below the joint line can indicate swelling that has tracked down the leg due to gravity.

It is important to measure the joint and its surrounding musculature to determine the progression of the joint effusion and any girth changes.

Reflexes, Dermatomes, and Cutaneous Nerve Supply Tests

Patellar Reflex—L2, L3, L4

To test the patellar reflex, the athlete sits on the end of the plinth with legs hanging freely. It is also permissible to seat the athlete with one knee crossed over the other.

The patellar tendon is on stretch.

The patellar reflex is a deep-tendon reflex, mediated through nerves emanating from L2, L3, and L4 neurological levels (predominantly L4).

Even if the L4 nerve root is pathologically involved, the reflex may still be present, since it is innervated at more than one level. The patellar reflex may be diminished but is rarely absent.

ASSESSMENT

Hit the patellar tendon with a percussion hammer at the level of the knee joint.

Compare bilaterally.

The reflex may be increased, diminished, or absent.

Dermatomes (Fig. 3-42)

L2, L3, L4, L5, S1, and S2 sensory dermatomes should be pricked with a pin while the athlete closes his or her eyes or looks away.

The athlete will report whether the prick feels sharp or dull.

Several areas (8 to 10 points) within each dermatome should be stimulated.

The test is done bilaterally.

If the test is positive, other cutaneous tests can be used (e.g., cotton balls, test tubes, hot/cold).

INTERPRETATION

If the athlete does not feel the pinprick or describes the sensation as dull in a specific dermatome, a nerve-root problem can be suspected in the lumbar or sacral area, depending on the location of decreased sensation. Dermatomes around the knee (according to *Gray's Anatomy*) are:

- L2—anterior portion of the middle thigh
- L3—anterior thigh at and above the knee joint
- L4—anterior portion of the knee and down the medial side of the leg
- L5—lateral knee and anterolateral calf
- S2—midline of the posterior thigh and the popliteal fossa

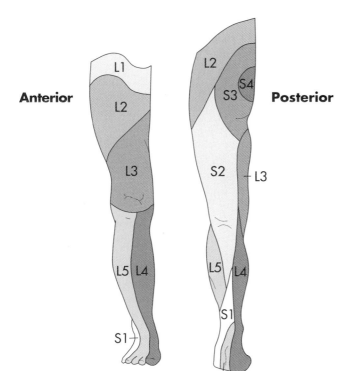

Anterior   **Posterior**

Fig. 3-42 Dermatomes of the lower limb.

ASSESSMENT

INTERPRETATION

Cutaneous Nerve Supply (Fig. 3-43)

Test the skin as above, but trace the cutaneous nerve supply areas to see if sensation is affected.

Areas of decreased sensation can be caused by damage to the cutaneous nerve that serves that area.

The cutaneous nerves that supply the knee area are:
- medial and intermediate cutaneous nerve of the thigh
- lateral cutaneous nerve of the thigh
- saphenous cutaneous nerve
- lateral cutaneous nerve of the calf
- posterior cutaneous nerve of the thigh

Circulatory Tests

If circulatory involvement is suspected, palpate the femoral, popliteal, posterior tibial, and dorsal pedis pulses (Fig. 3-44).

A reddish color or cyanosis can indicate circulatory problems.

Observe if the limb blanches when the limb is elevated or if it remains the same.

Weak pulses indicate problems of circulation through the injured site and rapid evaluation by a specialist is indicated to check for the presence of diabetes, heart disease, or other circulatory problems.

The pulses should especially be evaluated when a fracture or arterial occlusion is suspected.

Tests in the Prone Position

Apley's Compression and Distraction Test (Meniscus; Fig. 3-45)
Compression

The athlete is in the prone position with the knee flexed at an angle of 90°.

Apley's test puts force through the posterior horns of the menisci—a pain response indicates a posterior horn meniscal

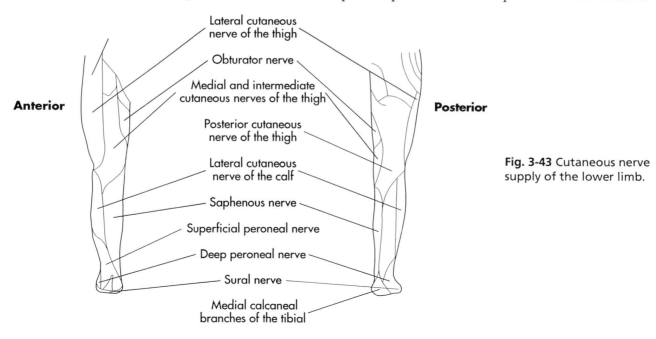

Fig. 3-43 Cutaneous nerve supply of the lower limb.

ASSESSMENT   **INTERPRETATION**

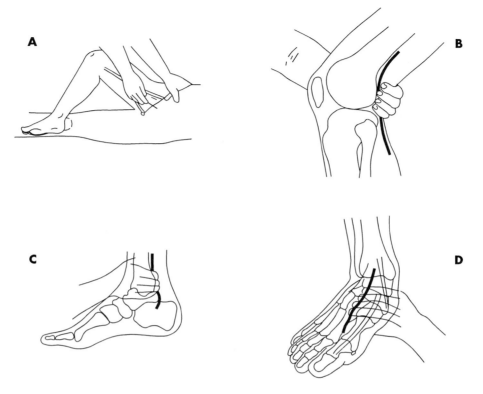

Fig. 3-44 Circulatory tests. **A**, Femoral atery. **B**, Popliteal artery. **C**, Posterior tibial artery. **D**, Dorsal pedis artery.

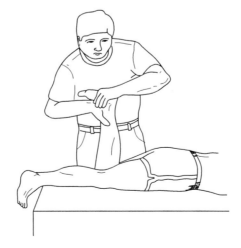

Fig. 3-45 Apley's compression test.

ASSESSMENT

INTERPRETATION

Stabilize the femur by carefully putting your knee over the athlete's thigh.

Lean on the athlete's heel to compress the medial and lateral menisci between the tibial and femur.

The tibia is rotated medially and laterally while the compression is maintained.

A positive sign is pain, clicking, or catching on the knee joint during the test.

Determine if this pain is medial or lateral (possible meniscal tear).

If the athlete has patellar discomfort, a towel can be placed above the patella.

This test can be modified slightly by compressing the joint in different ranges.

tear on the side opposite to that toward which the rotation is directed. There may be "catching" or "clicking" of the meniscus—this is also indicative of a positive test. The athlete will indicate whether the pain is on the medial or the lateral joint surface.

Distraction

Distraction is performed as above, but lift up on the athlete's tibia by pulling up on the foot.

Internal and external rotation of the tibia are repeated.

A positive sign is pain over the ligament during distraction (possible ligament damage).

The traction takes the pressure off the menisci and puts strain on the collateral ligaments. The athlete will indicate which collateral ligament hurts during your rotations of the tibia.

Tests in Standing

Functional Tests to Observe

If the athlete has a chronic injury and is able to weight-bear, have him or her attempt these progressive functional tests. If the athlete experiences pain or is reluctant to perform a test, no further tests in the progression should be done.

These tests are for the detection of chronic knee problems and not for the inflamed knee.

Ask the athlete to attempt these tests but to stop if he or she experiences any discomfort or apprehension.

Some knee conditions are only painful when stressed with the athlete's full body weight. These tests are designed for such vague or long-term chronic knee injuries.

These movements are done to determine the athlete's ability and willingness to move the joint functionally.

Weakness, proprioception, and muscle contraction synchronization can be observed. Joint mechanics of the entire lower quadrant in a closed kinetic chain activity is important to analyze in the active athlete.

If discomfort or reluctance stops the tests, determine the location of pain or the reason for the athlete's inability to perform the movement. Any malalignment (e.g., patellofemoral joint) or instability (e.g., pelvic drop) should be recorded.

Step Tests

Have the athlete step up on a stair and determine the hip and knee

If the quadriceps are weak or inhibited the athlete will have difficulty stepping up. Pain can be caused by joint dysfunction

ASSESSMENT

strength. Note if there is weakness or any symptoms produced.

Have the athlete step down and observe the knee alignment to determine if the knee goes into valgus. Also note if the pelvis remains stable and there is adequate hip and knee strength.

Full Squat

Return From Squat

Knee-circling

Duck Walk

INTERPRETATION

in the knee joint (e.g., articular cartilage degeneration, osteochondritis dissecans, meniscal tear, joint effusion).

During the step down from the stair, there is a strong eccentric contraction of the quadriceps. Any weakness or quadriceps inhibition will cause pain and problems. If the gluteus medius or quadratus lumborum is weak, the pelvis will drop and the opposite knee may move into a valgus position. This can lead to patellar malalignment pain and problems. If this occurs in the jumping athlete (basketball, volleyball), this valgus position will occur on landing and can lead to patellofemoral problems (e.g., patellar tendonitis, chondromalacia, patellofemoral malalignment syndrome).

Pain when reaching end of range of motion during knee flexion can indicate:
- patellar tendon strain (first degree)
- quadriceps strain or hematoma (first degree)
- infrapatellar bursitis
- suprapatellar bursitis
- prepatellar bursitis
- slight joint effusion (pain behind the knee)

Pain during the descent to the squat can indicate patellar malalignment problems or chondromalacia because of the compression of the patella into the condyles; a quadriceps strain or contusion may also cause pain because these structures are contracting eccentrically. Record the range(s) that cause discomfort.

Pain or difficulty returning from the squat can indicate:
- quadriceps weakness or inhibition
- chondromalacia
- joint effusion
- any of the conditions previously mentioned

According to Hughston and Jacobson, patients with posterolateral instability are unable to lock the knee in full extension and therefore experience difficulties ascending and descending stairs or slopes.

Pain or apprehension during knee-circling can indicate:
- cartilage tear if pain or clicking occurs
- instability of ligaments
- chondromalacia, patellofemoral malalignment syndrome

Pain on performing this or a reluctance to perform the duck walk can indicate:
- cartilage tear because the joint is compressed with the entire body weight

ASSESSMENT

INTERPRETATION

- medial collateral ligament sprain because of the valgus stress that is placed on the knee during the walk
- patellofemoral malalignment where the flexion hurts behind or around the patella

Jumps

Watch for quadriceps eccentric weakness or the knee moving into valgus due to weak gluteus medius on opposite side.

Pain on performing jumps or an inability to do a jump can indicate:

- extensor mechanism problems (quadriceps)
- patellofemoral problems (e.g., jumper's knee, chondromalacia patella, Osgood Schlatter disease, Sinding-Larsen-Johannson disease)
- pain on landing
- any of the conditions listed previously for jumping

Crossover Test (Fig. 3-46)

The athlete stands with his or her legs crossed, with the uninvolved leg in front.

Stabilize the foot on the injured side by gently standing on it.

The athlete rotates his or her body 90° away from the injured leg over his or her fixed feet.

During trunk flexion, stabilize the athlete's body by holding the shoulders.

The crossover test indicates a positive anterior cruciate tear if the tibia shifts anterolaterally.

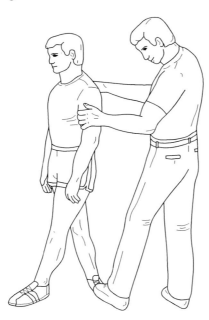

Fig. 3-46 Crossover test.

ASSESSMENT

INTERPRETATION

The athlete then contracts the quadriceps and holds the contraction while flexing the knees slightly.

Proprioception Test

Ask the athlete to stand and balance on each leg for 30 seconds with eyes open and then repeat with eyes closed.

Wavering or putting a foot down to regain balance is a positive proprioception test.

Body shift, pelvic drop, or hip wavering should be recorded.

A partial or complete ligament or capsular tear can decrease the kinesthetic awareness from the joint, and balance can be affected.

This is important to test and record because the joint is susceptible to reinjury or further injury if proprioception and kinesthetic awareness is decreased.

If the pelvis is unstable and drops (usually gluteus medius weakness) the knee often goes into a valgus position. This valgus position can lead to patellofemoral malalignment problems. Weakness in any of the pelvis or hip musculature can cause extra compensations through the knee and ankle joints that can result in injury or overuse problems.

ACCESSORY MOVEMENT TESTS

Joint Play Movements

Superior Tibiofibular Joint Anterior and Posterior Glide (see Fig. 4-53)

The athlete is in the supine position with the knees flexed 90°, the hip flexed 45°, and the foot resting on the plinth. The hamstrings must be relaxed.

Put your thumb and index finger around the head of the fibula.

Your other hand grasps and stabilizes the upper surface of the tibia.

Gently move the fibula anteriorly and posteriorly.

Anterior/posterior movements of this joint are needed because the head of the fibula must move anterior on knee flexion and posterior on knee extension. The head of the fibula must also move superiorly, laterally, and anteriorly with talocrural dorsiflexion and inferiorly, medially, and posteriorly on plantar flexion.

If plantar flexion or dorsiflexion were limited during the earlier functional testing, the accessory movements of the superior and inferior tibiofibular joints should be tested. For inferior tibiofibular accessory movements see Foot and Ankle Chapter.

Any hypomobility or hypermobility of this joint can cause pain into the knee. Normal joint play is needed in this joint to attain a full range of motion at the knee and ankle.

Superior Tibiofibular Joint Inferior and Superior Glide

The athlete is lying supine with the hip and knee flexed 90°. Support the knee with one hand posteriorly. That hand is also palpating the head of the fibula. The other hand grasps the ankle with the index finger hooked over the lower end of the fibula.

Invert the ankle and foot while pulling the lower end of the fibula inferiorly to achieve an inferior glide of the

This inferior and superior glide of the fibula is very important to the mechanics of the foot and ankle. If the fibula becomes displaced superiorly, it increases the potential for foot and ankle over pronation. This can then result in rotational forces through the tibia, therefore stressing the knee.

If the fibula is fixed inferiorly there is a compensatory foot and ankle supination, which then causes excessive lateral forces through the tibia and knee.

ASSESSMENT

INTERPRETATION

entire fibula. Then, evert the ankle and foot and push the fibula upward for a superior fibular glide.

Tibiofemoral Joint

Posterior Glide of the Tibia on the Femur (see Fig. 3-30)

The athlete is in the supine position with the knee flexed 90° and the hip flexed 45° (as for the drawer sign test). Sit on the athlete's forefoot while both hands hold the proximal end of the tibia with the thumbs over the tibial tubercle. Push the athlete's tibia backward gently.

Any hypomobility or hypermobility should be noted. Full posterior glide is needed for full knee flexion to be possible. Hypermobility can be caused by a posterior cruciate laxity or tear or by an anterior cruciate laxity in which the tibia then rests too far forward.

Anterior Glide of the Tibia on the Femur (i.e., Anterior Drawer Test) (Fig. 3-28)

Perform in the same position as for the posterior glide of the tibia on the femur. Pull the tibia forward gently as in the Anterior Drawer Sign.

This accessory movement is necessary for full knee extension.

Hypermobility can be caused by an anterior cruciate laxity or tear or by a posterior cruciate tear when the tibia then rests too far backward and for this reason appears to glide forward excessively.

Excessive mobility occurs with an anterior cruciate and medial collateral tear.

Internal Rotation

Perform internal rotation in the same position as above. Turn the tibia medially (internally).

Full internal rotation is needed for full knee flexion. Hypermobility can come from posterolateral instability.

External Rotation (Fig. 3-31)

Perform external rotation in the same position as above. Turn the tibia laterally (externally).

Full external rotation is necessary for full knee extension.

Hypermobility can come from posteromedial instability in which the damage is usually to the medial collateral ligament.

Patellofemoral Joint

Superior and Inferior Glide

The athlete is in the supine position with a pillow under the knee to slightly flex the knee. Your thumbs push caudally (inferiorly) on the top of the patella and then cephalically (superiorly) on the bottom of the patella.

The patella must glide superiorly for full knee extension and inferiorly for full knee flexion.

Medial and Lateral Glide (Fig. 3-47)

With the athlete in the supine position and with the knee over a pillow,

Patellofemoral movement is necessary for normal patellar articular cartilage nutrition.

ASSESSMENT	INTERPRETATION

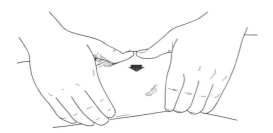

Fig. 3-47 Medial patellar glide.

gently push the patella medially with your thumbs and laterally with the index fingers.

Hypomobility will cause patellar articular degeneration and then can progress to chondromalacia.

Hypermobility or movement of the patella laterally for more than one half of its width can cause patellar subluxations or dislocations. This hypermobility can also add to patellar tendonitis, especially if there is malalignments of the lower limb or an increased "Q" angle.

Medial glide is very important to regain if there are tight lateral structures holding the patella down or pulling it laterally.

PALPATION

Palpate for point tenderness, temperature differences, swelling, muscle spasm, muscle tone, trigger points, boney and muscle congruency, adhesions, crepitus, and calcium deposits.

Anterior Structures (Fig. 3-48)

Boney
Patella

There can be the following:
- tenderness from a periosteal contusion from a direct blow
- fracture from a direct blow or after a patellar dislocation
- tenderness at the inferior pole of the patella, suggesting Sinding-Larsen-Johannson disease, which is an overuse condition that is aggravated by repetitive jumping
- bipartite patella (congenital)

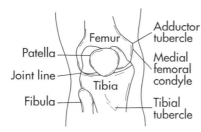

Fig. 3-48 Anterior boney structures of the knee.

ASSESSMENT

INTERPRETATION

Condyles

Tenderness on the medial and lateral condyle suggests a contusion, articular wear, or a chondral fracture. An adductor tubercle that is point tender can be caused by a medial collateral ligament sprain or an adductor magnus strain.

Joint Line

Tenderness on the joint line suggests a meniscal tear or injury to the coronary ligament.

Tibial Tubercle

Enlargement and point tenderness right on the tubercle can be Osgood-Schlatter disease in the adolescent.

Tenderness on the tendon-periosteal junction can suggest a tendon strain of the patellar tendon at its insertion.

The proximal tibia may be tender if the pes anserine group is inflamed with a bursitis or strain. The medial collateral insertion can be tender here also.

The lateral tibial tubercle area can be tender if the iliotibial band is strained or if tendonitis is present.

Soft Tissue (Fig. 3-49)
Quadriceps

Point tenderness or a lump in a quadriceps muscle can suggest a muscle strain or hematoma. A hard mass in the quadriceps from a previous blow (3 to 6 weeks old) can indicate a myositis ossificans. The quadriceps muscle can be avulsed from the anterior inferior iliac spine in the adolescent athlete, so the muscle should be palpated over its entire length. This muscle is susceptible to injury because it crosses and functions over two joints.

The vastus medialis obliquus muscle should be palpated for atrophy or hypoplasia—this muscle loses tone very quickly if

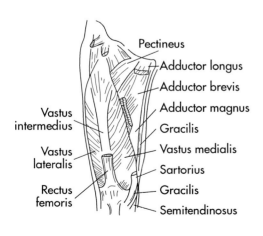
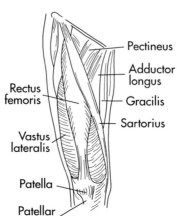

Fig. 3-49 Anterior musculature of the upper thigh and knee.

ASSESSMENT

INTERPRETATION

there is any knee dysfunction. According to Outerbridge, the lower the point of the vastus medialis obliquus insertion, the greater its effectiveness in stabilizing the patella.

According to Simons and Travell, the trigger point for the quadriceps femoris muscle is in the upper part of the muscle. The referred pain from this point centers mainly over the patella and lower anterior thigh.

Vastus medialis has a trigger point in the muscle belly and also has referred pain mainly over the patellar region.

Vastus lateralis has a trigger point on the lateral central thigh area and pain can be referred over the lateral thigh and even into the lateral buttock.

Vastus intermedius has a trigger point on the proximal central thigh with referred pain into the anterior upper thigh.

Sartorius

The sartorius muscle can be strained anywhere along its length. It can be avulsed from its origin on the anterior superior iliac spine (ASIS) in the adolescent. The injury mechanism usually involves a kicking maneuver. It is susceptible to injury because it functions over two joints.

Prepatellar Bursa

Prepatellar bursitis, an inflammation caused by a direct blow or prolonged kneeling, may be present.

Infrapatellar Bursa, Superficial and Deep

Infrapatellar bursitis, superficial or deep, can be aggravated through a direct blow or overuse. The superficial bursa is over the patellar tendon, just under the skin. The deep bursa is between the tibia and the patellar tendon.

Patellar Tendon

Patellar tendonitis from repetitive jumping or a patellar tendon strain at the insertion can cause pain here.

Pes Anserine Bursa

The pes anserine bursa can become inflamed from a direct blow or from a sprain of the medial collateral ligament.

The insertion of the sartorius, gracilis, and semitendinosus can also be strained or overused and cause tenderness in the pes anserine insertion area.

Peripatellar Tenderness

Tenderness of the soft tissue around the patella, especially on the medial side, is common after a patellar subluxation or dislocation. The medial and lateral retinculum can be strained or torn. The patella should be pushed medially and laterally to assess the retinacular structures— a tight retinaculum may

ASSESSMENT   INTERPRETATION

cause decreased mobility when the patella is pushed medially.

On pressing the medial side of the patella downward, the lateral edge of the patella should elevate; the therapist can then palpate the lateral retinaculum for tightness or tenderness, and palpate the lateral patellar facet.

On pressing the lateral edge of the patella downward, the medial edge of the patella rises, and the medial retinaculum and medial patellar facet can be palpated for pain or problems.

Medial Structures

Boney (Fig. 3-50, A)
Medial Femoral Condyle

Point tenderness on the medial epicondyle or adductor tubercle can suggest an avulsion of the medial collateral ligament. Point tenderness high on the medial condyle may also suggest Pellegrini-Steida disease (a calcification of the medial collateral ligament).

Fractures through the growth plate of the femur or tibia in the adolescent can cause tenderness along the epiphyseal plate of either of these bones.

Medial Tibial Plateau

Tenderness suggests a sprain or tear of the medial meniscus or coronary ligament.

Soft Tissue (Fig. 3-50, B)
Adductor Muscle Group

Gracilis is the most superficial and because of its many functions can easily be strained. If injured at its insertion, it will affect knee function.

Pectineus is located in the femoral triangle and functions mainly on the hip joint and pelvis.

The adductors mainly function at the hip and pelvis but are synergists during gait and posture. They are important to the

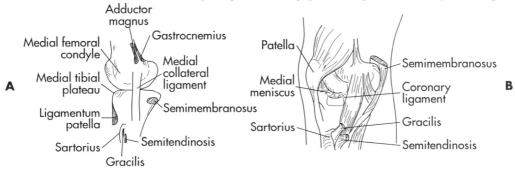

Fig. 3-50 Medial aspect of the knee joint. **A,** Boney, showing muscle insertions. **B,** Soft tissue, pes anserine group.

ASSESSMENT

INTERPRETATION

balance involved in the entire lower limb and if injured can affect knee function.

For the myofascial trigger points of the adductors, see palpations, Hip and Pelvis Chapter.

Medial Collateral Ligament

The medial collateral ligament is also part of the medial joint capsule and any defects or point tenderness along its length suggests a sprain or tear that can also result in capsular damage. Common sites for medial collateral problems are at the ligament's midpoint, at the joint line, at the adductor tubercle insertion, and at tibial insertion—avulsion fractures can occur at either of the attachments.

Pes Anserine Group (Fig. 3-50, B)
- Sartorius
- Gracilis
- Semitendinosus muscle tendons

The sartorius, gracilis, or semitendinosus muscle tendons are also along the medial side of the knee and any strain to these muscles will cause point tenderness at the lesion site.

Lateral Structures

Boney
Lateral Femoral Condyle and Epicondyle

If the lateral femoral epicondyle is prominent, often the runner will develop iliotibial band syndrome.

Lateral femoral condyle or tibial condyle point tenderness can suggest a fracture, especially in the adolescent in whom the epiphyseal plate is not closed.

Head of Fibula

The head of the fibula can be damaged from a direct blow. The superior tibiofibular joint can also be tender after a subluxation of this joint or a spontaneously reduced dislocation.

Soft Tissue (Fig. 3-51)
Lateral Collateral Ligament

The lateral collateral ligament becomes point tender with a sprain, tear, or avulsion.

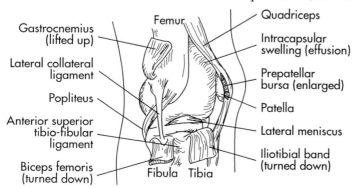

Gastrocnemius (lifted up)
Lateral collateral ligament
Popliteus
Anterior superior tibio-fibular ligament
Biceps femoris (turned down)
Femur
Fibula   Tibia
Quadriceps
Intracapsular swelling (effusion)
Prepatellar bursa (enlarged)
Patella
Lateral meniscus
Iliotibial band (turned down)

Fig. 3-51 Lateral aspect of the knee joint, soft tissue.

ASSESSMENT   INTERPRETATION

Lateral Meniscus

A lateral meniscus tear will cause point tenderness along the lateral joint line.

Coronary Ligament

A coronary ligament injury can also cause lateral joint line pain.

Anterior Superior Tibiofibular Ligaments

The anterior superior tibiofibular ligaments can be sprained if the superior tibiofibular joint has been subluxed or dislocated.

Iliotibial Band

The iliotibial band can become inflamed in the runner who has a prominent lateral epicondyle or can be strained or torn along with lateral knee injuries. It is very important to the lateral stability of the knee.

Peroneal Nerve

The peroneal nerve can be injured, since it wraps around the neck of the fibula, by a direct blow, compression, or a fibular fracture.

Biceps Femoris Tendon

The biceps femoris tendon can be strained or can develop tendonitis.

Because it functions at both the hip and knee, it is more susceptible to injury or overuse—on rare occasions it can be avulsed from the head of the fibula.

Posterior Structures

With the athlete in the prone position, the posterior part of the knee can be palpated, but deep pressure is necessary to palpate the boney structures.

Boney
Joint Line

Point tenderness along the joint line can suggest a posterior horn meniscal tear. This is most common on the medial side.

Soft Tissue
Popliteal Fossa

Point tenderness and a lump in the popliteal fossa can suggest a Baker's cyst.

Popliteus tendonitis can occur especially in downhill runners.

There is a trigger point in the midbelly of the muscle that can refer pain into the lower medial part of the popliteal space.

ASSESSMENT   INTERPRETATION

Hamstrings

Strains or hematomas in the hamstring muscles or tendons cause point tenderness, and warmth may be felt in the acute phase. Often the lesion occurs at the musculotendinous junction.

Hamstring strains are the most common soft tissue injuries of the thigh (Nicholas and Hershman) for several reasons:
- They function over two joints (hip and knee).
- They often function eccentrically during running to decelerate knee extension and hip flexion, which requires strength while the muscles are on stretch.
- Activities that require a hurdle position force the hamstring to contract while the trunk and hip is flexed fully and the knee is extended. This puts the muscle on maximal stretch.

Chronic strains lead to scar tissue that can be felt as a knot or lump in the muscle belly.

According to Simons and Travell, the trigger point for the biceps femoris is midbelly and the referred pain spreads mainly in the popliteal fossa and into the posterior upper gastrocnemius. The trigger points for semimembranosus and semitendinosus are in the muscle belly and pain can radiate down the posterior thigh and buttock and extend to midleg.

Gastrocnemii

Gastrocnemius muscle strains or contusions can be felt and will be point tender.

The medial head of gastrocnemius can be severely strained or even avulsed (sometimes termed *tennis leg*). This strain or tear can occur with the gastrocnemius on maximal stretch with the ankle dorsiflexed and knee extended and then quickly contracting in this stretched position. This mechanism occurs most frequently in racquet sports (i.e., squash, tennis).

According to Simons and Travell, the trigger point is in the upper part of the medial head of the gastrocnemius. It can refer pain from the popliteal space down to the posterior calf. There is often strong referred pain into the arch of the foot.

REFERENCES

Anderson JE: *Grant's Atlas of anatomy*, Baltimore, 1983, Williams and Wilkins.

Anno S: The A angle: A quantative measurement of patellar alignment and realignment, JOSPT 12(6):237, Dec 1990.

Antich TJ et al: Evaluation of knee extension mechanism disorders: clinical presentation of 112 patients, J Orthop Sports Phys Ther 248-254, Nov, 1986.

APTA orthopaedic section: Review for advanced orthopaedic competencies, The Knee, Terry Malone. Chicago: Aug. 10, 1989.

Arno S: The A angle: a quantative measurement of patellar alignment and malalignment, JOSPT 12(6):257, Dec 1990.

Ashcroft: Prevention and treatment in distance runners, Physiotherapy 30(1):15, 1978.

Bach B, Warren R, Wickienwicz T: The pivot shift phenomenon: results and description of a modified clinical test for anterior cruciate ligament insufficiency, Am J Sports Med 16(6):571, 1988.

Beazell J: Entrapment neuropathy of the lateral femoral cutaneous nerve: cause of lateral knee pain, J Orthop Sports Phys Ther, Vol 10(3):85, 1988.

Bechtel S, Ellman B, Jordan J: Skier's knee: the cruciate connection, Phys Sports Med 12(11):51, 1984.

Benton J: Epiphyseal fracture in sports, Phys Sports Med Nov 10(11):63, 1982.

Blackburn T, Eiland W, Brandy W: An Introduction to the Plica, JOSPT 3(4): 171-177, 1982.

Bloom MH: Differentiating between menisceal and patellar pain, The Physician and Sport Med 17(8):95, 1989.

Booher JM and Thibodeau GA: Athletic injury assessment, Toronto, 1985, Times Mirror/Mosby College Publishing.

Brody: Running injuries, Ciba Clinical Symposia, Ciba Pharmaceutical Co, 32:4, 1980.

Butler DL et al: Ligamentous restraints to anterior-posterior drawer in the human knee, J Bone Joint Surg 62(A):259, 1980.

Calliet R: Knee pain and disability, Philadelphia, 1983, FA Davis Co.

Cash J and Hughston J: Treatment of acute patellar dislocation (abstract of the annual meeting of the American Orthopaedic Society for Sports Medicine), Sports Med 15(6):621, 1987.

Cerabona F et al: Patterns of meniscal injury with acute anterior cruciate tears, Am J Sports Med 16(6):603, 1988.

Chick R and Jackson D: Tears of the anterior cruciate in young athletes, J Bone Joint Surg 7(A):60, 1978.

Clancy W: Knee ligamentous injury in sports: the past, present, and future, Med Sci Sports Exercise 15(1):9, 1983.

Coughlin L, Oliver J, Berretta G: Knee bracing and anterolateral rotary instability, Am J Sports Med 15(2):161, 1987.

Clanton T et al: Knee ligament injuries in children, J Bone Joint Surg, 61A:1195, 1979.

Cross MJ and Crichton KJ: Clinical examination of the injured knee, Baltimore, 1987, Williams & Wilkins.

Curwin S and Stanish WD: Tendonitis: Its etiology and treatment, Lexington, Mass, 1984, DC Health & Co.

Cyriax J: Textbook of orthopedic medicine: diagnosis of soft tissue lesions, vol 1, London, 1978, Bailliere Tindall.

Daniel D et al: Use of the quadriceps active test to diagnose posterior cruciate ligament disruption and measure posterior laxity of the knee, J Bone Joint Surg 70A(3):386, 1988.

Daniels L and Worthingham C: Muscle testing techniques of manual examination, Toronto, 1980, WB Saunders.

David D: Jumpers knee, J Sports Phys Ther 11(4):137, 1989.

Davies G and Larson R: Examining the knee; Physician Sports Med 4:49, 1978.

DeHaven KE: Diagnosis of acute knee injuries with hemarthrosis, Am J Sports Med 8:9, 1980.

DeHaven K et al: Chondromalacia patellae in athletes, Am J Sports Med 7(1):5, 1979.

DeLee JC, Riley M, Rockwood C: Acute posterolateral rotary instability of the knee, Am J Sports Med 11(4):199, 1983.

Depodesta Mike: Physical examination of the knee, Unpublished paper, 1980.

DiStefano VJ: The enigmatic anterior cruciate ligament, Athletic Training pp. 244-246, 1981.

Dommelen B and Fowler P: Anatomy of the posterior cruciate ligament—a review, Am J Sports Med 17(1):24, 1989.

Donatelli R and Wooden M: Orthopaedic physical therapy, New York, 1989, Churchill Livingstone.

Draper DO: A comparison of stress tests used to evaluate the anterior cruciate ligament, Phys and Sports Med 18(1):89, 1990.

Feagin JA and Curl WW: Isolated tear of the anterior cruciate: 5 year follow-up study, Am J Sports Med 4:95, 1976.

Fetto JF and Marshall JL: The natural history and diagnosis of anterior cruciate insufficiency, Clin Orthop, 14(7):29, 1980.

Ficat P and Hungerford DS: Disorders of the patellofemoral joint, Baltimore, 1977, Williams & Wilkins.

Fischer R et al: The functional relationship of the posterior oblique ligament to the medial collateral ligament of the human knee, Am J Sports Med 13(6):390, 1985.

Fowler P: The classification and early diagnosis of knee joint instability, Clin Orthop 147:15, 1980.

Fowler P and Messieh S: Isolated posterior cruciate ligament injuries in athletes, Am J Sports Med 15(6):553, 1987.

Fowler P and Regan W: The patient with symptomatic chronic anterior cruciate insufficiency, Am J Sports Med 15(4):321, 1987.

Fulkerson J: Awareness of the retinaculum in evaluating patellofemoral pain, Am J Sports Med 10(3):147, 1982.

Girgis FG et al: The cruciate ligaments of the knee joint—anatomical, functional, and experimental analysis, Clin Orthop 106:216, 1975.

Glick JA: Muscle strains: prevention and treatment, Physician Sportsmed 8(11):73, 1980.

Gollehon D, Torzill P, Warren R: The role of the posterolateral and cruciate ligaments in the stability of the human knee, J Bone Joint Surg, 69A(2):233, 1987.

Gould JA and Davies GJ: Orthopaedic and sports physical therapy, Toronto, 1985, Mosby.

Grood E, Stowers S, Noyes F: Limits of movement in the human knee, J Bone Joint Surg 70A(1):88, 1988.

Hanks G et al: Anterolateral rotary instability of the knee, Am J Sports Med 9:4, 225, 1981.

Hoppenfeld S: Physical examination of the spine and extremities, New York, 1976, Appleton-Century Crofts.

Hughston JC et al: Patellar subluxation and dislocation, Philadelphia, 1984, WB Saunders.

Hughston JC and Barrett GR: Acute anteromedial rotary instability—long-term results of surgical repair, J Bone Joint Surg 65A:145, 1983.

Hughston JC and Jacobson KE: Chronic posterolateral rotary instability of the knee, J Bone Joint Surg 67A(3):351, 1985.

Injury to the anterior cruciate ligament—a round table, Physician Sports Med 10(11):47, 1982.

Insall J: Current concepts review patellar pain, J Bone Joint Surg 64A(1):147, 1982.

Johnson B and Cullen M: The anterior cruciate ligament injuries and functions in anterolateral rotary instability, Athletic Training 4:79, 1982.

Jonsson T et al: Clinical diagnosis of ruptures of the anterior cruciate ligament, a comparison of the Lachman test and anterior drawer sign, 10(2):100, 1982.

Jonsson H, Karrholm J, Elmqvist L: Kinematics of active knee extension after tear of the anterior cruciate ligament, Am J Sports Med 17(6):796, 1989.

Kannus Pekka: Nonoperative treatment of grade II and III sprains of the lateral compartment of the knee, Am J Sports Med 17(1):83, 1989.

Kannus P and Javinen M: Conservatively treated tears of the anterior cruciate ligament, J Bone Joint Surg 69(A):1007, 1987.

Katz J and Fingeroth J: The diagnostic accuracy of ruptures of the anterior cruciate ligament comparing the Lachman test, the anterior drawer sign, and the pivot shift test in acute and chronic knee injuries, Am J Sports Med 14(1):88, 1986.

Kapandji IA: The physiology of the joints, vol II, Lower limb, New York, 1983, Churchill Livingstone.

Kegerreis Sam, Malone T, Johnson F: The diagonal medial plica: an underestimated clinical entity, J Orthop Sports Phys Ther, 9(9):305, 1988.

Kendall FP and McCreary EK: Muscles testing and function, Baltimore, 1983, Williams & Wilkins.

Kennedy JC: The injured adolescent knee, Baltimore, 1979, Williams & Wilkins.

Kennedy JC et al: Anterolateral rotary instability of the knee joint, J Bone Joint Surg 60A(8):1031, 1978.

Kennedy JC and Hawkins RJ: Breast stroker's knee, Physician Sports Med 1:33, 1974.

Kerlan R and Glousman R: Tibial collateral ligament bursitis, Am J Sports Med 16(4):344, 1988.

Keskinen K et al: Breaststroke swimmer's knee, Am J Sports Med 8(4):228, 1980.

Kessler RM and Hertling D: Management of common musculoskeletal disorders, Philadelphia, 1983, Harper and Row.

King S, Butterick D, Cuerrier J: The anterior cruciate ligament, a review of recent concepts, J Sports Phys Ther 8(3):110, 1986.

Klein K: Developmental limb asymmetry: implications on knee injury, CATA Journal 6:9, 1979.

Knight Ken: Testing anterior cruciate ligaments, Physician and Sports Med 8(5):135, 1980.

Kosuke Ogata et al: Pathomechanics of posterior sag of the tibia in posterior cruciate deficient knees—an experimental study, Am J Sports Med, 16(6):630, 1988.

Larson R and Singer K: Clinics in sports medicine, vol 4 (2), #2 The knee, Toronto, 1985, WB Saunders.

Losee RE, Johnson T, Southwick W: Anterior subluxation of the lateral tibial plateau, J Bone Joint Surg 60A:1015, 1978.

Lysholm J and Wiklander J: Injuries in runners: J Sports Med 15(2):168, 1987.

Magee DJ: Orthopaedics conditions, assessments and treatment, vol II, Alberta, 1979. University of Alberta Publishing.

Magee DJ: Orthopaedic physical assessment, Toronto, 1987, WB Saunders.

Malek M and Mangine R: Patellofemoral pain sydromes: a comprehensive and conservative approach, J Orthop Sports Phys Ther 7:3, 108, 1981.

Malek M and Mangine R: Patellofemoral pain syndromes: a comprehensive and conservative approach, J Orthop Sports Ther 1981, 2:3, 108, 1981.

Mangine R (ed.): Physical therapy of the knee clinics in physical therapy, New York, 1988, Churchill Livingstone.

Mannheimer JS and Lampe GN: Clinical transcutaneous electrical nerve stimulation, Philadelphia, 1986, FA Davis Co.

Marshall J: Ligamentous injuries pose major diagnostic problem, Physician Sports Med 5:58, 1976.

Maitland GD: Peripheral manipulation, ed. 2, Boston, 1978, Butterworths.

McConnell J: Patellofemoral course notes, 1989.

McConnell J: The management of chondromalacia patellae: A long term solution, The Australian Journal of Physiotherapy, Vol 32 #4:215, 1986.

Medlar RC and Lyne ED: Sinding-Larsen-Johansson disease, J Bone Joint Surg 60(A)A:1113, 1978.

Nicholas J and Hershmann E: The lower extremity and spine in sports medicine, vols 1 and 2, St Louis, 1986, Mosby.

Nisonson B: Acute hemarthrosis of the adolescent knee, The Physician and Sportsmedicine 17(4):75, 1989.

Nitz A et al: Nerve injury and grades II and III sprains, Am J Sports Med, 13(3):177, 1985.

Noble CA: The treatment of iliotibial band friction syndrome, Br J Sports Med 13:51, 1979.

Noble HB et al: Diagnosis and treatment of iliotibial band tightness in runners, Physician Sports Med 10(4):67, 1982.

Norkin C and Levangie P: Joint structures and function—a comprehensive analysis, Philadelphia, 1983, FA Davis Co.

Nottage W et al: The medial patellar plica syndrome, Am J Sports Med 11(4):211, 1983.

O'Donaghue D: Treatment of injuries to athletes, Toronto, 1984, WB Saunders.

O'Donaghue D: Diagnosis and treatment of injury to the anterior cruciate ligament JOSPT 2(3):100-107, 1981.

Outerbridge R and Dunlop J: The problem of chondromalacia patellae, Clin Orthop 157:143, 1981.

Pappas A: Osteochondroses: disease of growth centers, Phys Sports Med 17(b):51, 1989.

Patee G et al: Four to ten year follow up on unconstructed anterior cruciate ligament tears, Am J Sports Med 17(3):430, 1989.

Peterson L and Renstrom P: Sport injuries, their prevention and treatment, Chicago, 1986, Year Book Medical Publishers.

Ray JM, Clancy W, Lemon R: Semimembranosus tendonitis: an overlooked cause of medial knee pain, Am J Sports Med 16(4): 347, 1988.

Reid DC: Functional anatomy and joint mobilization, Alberta, 1970, University of Alberta Publishing.

Reid DC: Sports injury assessment and rehabilitation, New York, 1992, Churchill Livingstone.

Reider B et al: Clinical characteristics of patellar disorders in young athletes, Am J Sports Med 9:4, #270, 1981.

Reuben J et al: Three-dimensional dynamic motion analysis of anterior cruciate deficient knee joint, Am J Sports Med 17(4):463, 1989.

Ritter M et al: Examination of the actively injured knee, The Physician and Sportsmedicine 8:10,41, 1980.

Round table discussion—injury to the anterior cruciate ligament, Physician Sports Med 10(11):47, 1982.

Rovere GD and Adair DM: Anterior cruciate-deficient knees: a review of the literature, Am J Sports Med 11(6):412, 1983.

Roy S and Irwin R: Sports medicine—prevention, evaluation, management, and rehabilitation, New Jersey, 1983, Prentice-Hall.

Schwarz C et al: The results of operative treatment of osteochondritis dissecans of the patella, Am J Sports Med, Vol 15, 15(6):622, 1987, (AOSSM abstracts).

Segal P and Jacob M: The knee, Chicago, 1983, Year Book Medical Publishers.

Seto Judy et al: Rehabilitation of the knee after anterior cruciate reconstruction, J Orthop Sports Physical Therapy 11(1):8, 1989.

Simons D and Travell J: Myofascial origins of low back pain. 3, Pelvic and lower extremity muscles Postgrad Med 73(2)99, 1983.

Simons D: Myofascial pain syndromes due to trigger points. 2, Treatment and Single Muscle syndromes, Manual Med 1:72, 1985.

Simons D: Myofascial pain syndromes. In Basmajian JV and Kirby RL (eds): Medical Rehabilitation, Baltimore, 1984, Williams & Wilkins.

Slocum DB and Larson RL: Rotatory instability of the knee, J Bone Joint Surg 50:211, 1968.

Smillie IS: Injuries of the knee joint, New York, 1978, Churchill Livingstone.

Subotnik S: Sports medicine of the lower extremity, New York, 1989, Churchill Livingstone.

Sutker AN et al. Iliotibial band syndrome in distance runners, The Physician and Sportsmedicine, 9(10):69, 1981.

Terry GC, Hughston J, Norwood L: The anatomy of the iliopatellar band and iliotibial tract, Am J Sports Med 14(1):39, 1986.

Torg J: Clinical diagnosis of anterior cruciate ligament instability in the athlete, Am J Sports Med 2:84, 1976.

Travell J and Simons D: Myofascial pain and dysfunction: the trigger point manual, vol 1, Baltimore, 1983, Williams & Wilkins.

Wenner K and McBryde A: Acute chondral and osteochondral fractures of the femoral condyles, Am J Sports Med 15(6):622, 1987 (AOSSM abstracts).

Williams PL and Warwick R: Gray's Anatomy, New York, 1980, Churchill Livingstone.

CHAPTER 4
Foot and Ankle Assessment

The foot and ankle are made up of several joints that must all function properly for normal walking and running. An injury to any one joint can lead to dysfunction in the other joints. Because most sports place tremendous demands on the lower extremity, the foot and ankle often take the brunt of the trauma or overuse. Sprains and fractures of the ankle and foot are common in sport because a great deal of torque is generated through the ankle and subtalar joint when the body or leg is twisted over the fixed foot. This occurs readily in sports and results in significant soft-tissue and boney injuries. Because most sports involve a great deal of repetitive trauma like running and jumping, these compressive forces and the repeated structural overuse can lead to stress fractures and stress-related soft-tissue damage.

TIBIOFIBULAR JOINTS

According to *Gray's Anatomy*, the inferior (distal) tibiofibular joint is a fibrous joint, and the superior (proximal) tibiofibular joint is a synovial articulation. The shafts of the tibia and fibula are connected by an interosseous ligament (membrane). With talocrural and subtalar movements there are slight accessory movements. With plantar flexion the fibula moves laterally, anteriorly, and inferiorly and the malleoli move closer together. With dorsiflexion the fibula moves medially, posteriorly, and superiorly and the malleoli separate. With subtalar inversion the head of the fibula slides inferiorly and posteriorly; with subtalar eversion the head of the fibula slides superiorly and anteriorly.

These joints have effects on both the knee and the ankle. The superior and inferior movement of the fibula is particularly important for normal ankle mechanics. If the fibula is fixed in a superior position, the ankle joint often compensates with overpronation; if the fibula is fixed inferiorly the ankle tends to compensate by staying in supination. Altered mechanics at the foot will affect the entire lower quadrant. Fibular movement can indirectly affect the knee through these altered foot mechanics but also its movement directly influences biceps femoris function where the muscle inserts. Instability of the superior tibiofibular joint will decrease the force generated by this muscle.

ANKLE OR TALOCRURAL JOINT

The ankle or talocrural joint (Fig. 4-1) is formed by the dome-shaped talus fitting within the mortise of the distal ends of the tibia and fibula. This joint allows plantar flexion and dorsiflexion. Dysfunction can result throughout the entire lower extremity if 10° of dorsiflexion does not exist during the midstance of the gait cycle. The medial and lateral collateral ligaments around the talocrural joint function to limit tilting and rotation of the talus within the mortise and to restrict forward and backward movement of the mortise over the talus. The anterior and posterior inferior tibiofibular ligaments and interosseous membrane hold the tibia and fibula together to form the mortise. If the mortise, formed by the tibia and fibula, is widened due to tibiofibular ligament or interosseous membrane tears, the joint breaks down and degenerative changes to the articular cartilage ensue.

During dorsiflexion there is posterior slide of the talus on the tibia and spreading of the inferior tibiofibular joint. During plantar flexion there is anterior slide of the talus on the tibia and approximation of the inferior tibiofibular joint.

The close-packed position of the joint is maximal dorsiflexion; the capsular pattern is limitation of plantar flexion and dorsiflexion (plantar flexion is usually slightly greater). The resting or loose-packed position of the joint is 10° to 20° of plantar flexion midway between maximum inversion and eversion.

SUBTALAR JOINT OR TALOCRURAL JOINT

The subtalar joint is made up of three articulations between the superior surface of the calcaneus and the inferior surface of the talus. The two

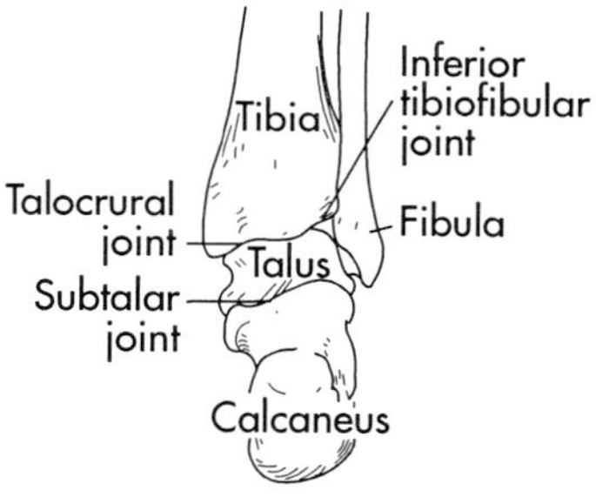

Fig. 4-1 Talocrural, subtalar, and inferior tibiofibular joints. Posterior view.

motions allowed by the subtalar joint are pronation and supination—pronation and supination are triplane movements. Normal pronation of the foot and subtalar joint is essential for normal adaptation to the terrain, shock absorption, and torque conversion, whereas supination is essential for propulsion with the foot and ankle as a rigid lever. Pronation is achieved in nonweight-bearing situations (open kinetic chain) with calcaneal eversion, abduction, and dorsiflexion. Supination is achieved in nonweight-bearing situations (open kinetic chain) with calcaneal inversion, adduction, and plantar flexion. Pronation is achieved in weight-bearing (closed kinetic chain) with calcaneal eversion, talar adduction, and plantar flexion. Supination is achieved in weight-bearing situations (closed kinetic chain) with calcaneal inversion, talar abduction, and dorsiflexion. The accessory movement of the posterior articulations of the subtalar joint during inversion is a lateral slide of the talus, and during eversion, a medial slide of the talus.

The posterior talocalcaneal articulation is the largest and is formed by a concave talar facet and a convex calcaneal facet. The anterior and medial articulations are between the convex facets of the body and neck of the talus and two concave facets in the calcaneus. Anatomically they are really part of the talonavicular joint. The posterior articulation has its own capsule, while the anterior and middle facets share a capsule with the talonavicular joint.

Prolonged pronation or supination during the stance phase of walking or running can cause foot, ankle, knee, hip, and even low-back dysfunction. The inversion and eversion components of movement are controlled mainly by the medial and lateral collateral ligaments. The interaction between the talus and calcaneus at the subtalar joint reduces the rotary stresses on the ankle joint. The close-packed position of the subtalar joint is eversion—the capsular pattern has inversion that is very restricted and eversion that is full. The resting or loose-packed position for the subtalar joint is midway between the extremes of range of motion.

TALOCALCANEONAVICULAR JOINT OR TALONAVICULAR JOINT (FIG. 4-2, *A*)

The talocalcaneonavicular joint includes the articulation between the medial and anterior facets for the talus on the calcaneus, the articulation between the talar head and spring ligament, and the articulation between the head of the talus and

the posterior surface of the navicular. These articulations control the longitudinal arch of the foot. The joint is reinforced by a capsule and ligaments, which include the talonavicular ligament, the bifurcate ligament (calcaneonavicular portion), and the plantar calcaneonavicular ligament (spring or short plantar ligament). This joint is capable of some sliding and rotational accessory movements. During inversion with supination and plantar flexion, the navicular slides in a plantar direction on the head of the talus. During eversion with pronation and dorsiflexion, the navicular slides in a dorsal direction on the head of the talus.

CALCANEOCUBOID JOINT (FIG. 4-2, *B*)

The calcaneocuboid joint is the articulation between the calcaneus and the cuboid bone. Its joint capsule is reinforced by the short (plantar calcaneocuboid) and long plantar ligaments and the calcaneocuboid portion of the bifurcate ligament, which help to maintain the normal arch of the foot. This joint is capable of accessory movements of gliding and rotation.

CUNEONAVICULAR JOINT (SEE FIG. 4-2, *A*)

The cuneonavicular joint is the articulation between the cuneiform and navicular bones. This joint is capable of the accessory movements of gliding and rotation.

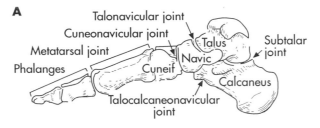

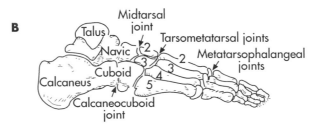

Fig. 4-2 Foot and ankle bones and joints. **A,** Medial aspect. **B,** Lateral aspect.

CUBOIDEONAVICULAR JOINT

The cuboideonavicular joint is the articulation between the cuboid and navicular bones and it permits the accessory movements of gliding and rotation. This joint is very important to the spring motion of the longitudinal arch.

CUNEOCUBOID JOINT

The cuneocuboid joint is the articulation between the cuneiform and cuboid bone in which there is some gliding and rotation.

The close-packed position for the midtarsal joints is supination; the resting or loose-packed position for the midtarsal joints is midway between the extremes of range of motion. The capsular pattern for the midtarsal joints is dorsiflexion, plantar flexion, adduction, and medial rotation.

TARSOMETATARSAL, INTERMETATARSAL, METATARSOPHALANGEAL, AND INTERPHALANGEAL JOINTS (SEE FIG. 4-2)

The tarsometatarsal, intermetatarsal, metatarsophalangeal, and interphalangeal joints allow forefoot mobility during subtalar pronation and forefoot rigidity during supination. During gait, this allows the foot to be a mobile adapter to the ground in midstance and a rigid lever during propulsion.

The close-packed position of the tarsometatarsal joints is supination. The resting or loose-packed position of the tarsometatarsal joints is midway between the extremes of the range of motion.

The close-packed position of the metatarsophalangeal and interphalangeal joints is maximal extension.

The resting or loose-packed position of the metatarsophalangeal and interphalangeal joints is neutral and one of slight flexion. (Kaltenborn believes the metatarsophalangeal resting position is at 10° of extension.)

The capsular pattern for the first metatarsophalangeal joint is limited extension and flexion. The pattern for the second to fifth metatarsophalangeal joint is variable. The capsular pattern for the interphalangeal joints is limited flexion and extension.

GRADING OF ANKLE LIGAMENTOUS INSTABILITY OR SPRAINS

There are many different methods of grading these sprains: some authors grade all the medial or lateral ligaments as a group; some authors grade each ligament individually. There are several terms used to name instability or sprains: grade I, II, and III instability: first-, second-, and third-degree sprains; mild, moderate, and severe sprains. Table 4-1 is condensed and combines mainly McConkey and Nicholas nomenclature in this area.

TABLE 4-1 McConkey and Nicholas Nomenclature

Sprain designation	Ligamentous pathology (Nicholas)	Clinical signs and symptoms (McConkey)
Grade I, first degree or mild	Microscopic tearing of the ligament with no loss of function	Shows minimal functional loss, little swelling, localized tenderness, and mild pain in response to stress. Pathologically there is a functional integrity with a minor ligamentous injury
Grade II, second degree or moderate	Partial disruption or stretching of the ligament with some loss of function	Shows moderate funtional loss with difficulty on toe raise and walking, diffuse tenderness, and swelling. Pathologically there is a near complete lateral complex injury
Grade III, third degree or severe	Complete tearing of the ligament with complete loss of function	Shows functional disability with marked tenderness and swelling, marked loss of range of motion, and a need for crutches. Pathologically it indicates a complete rupture

ASSESSMENT   INTERPRETATION

HISTORY

Mechanism of Injury
Overstretch

Was there such an overstretch?

Inversion (Fig. 4-3)

Lateral ankle sprains are very common in athletes, especially those who participate in jumping and running sports. In most sports, fractures only occur occasionally and are usually undisplaced fibular or avulsion fractures. Sports that can have more serious fractures include football, downhill skiing, and ice hockey; these sports cause comminuted fractures, fractures through articular surfaces, and widely displaced fractures, among others. Inversion injuries are not always attributable to a pure inversion mechanism; usually there is some plantar flexion and internal tibial rotation involved. Landing on an opponent's foot in basketball or the irregular surface of a football field are common causes of this injury.

Inversion can cause (in order of increasing damage):
- anterior talofibular ligament sprain, partial tear (most common), or complete tear
- anterolateral capsule sprain or tear
- calcaneofibular ligament sprain, partial, or complete tear
- posterior talofibular ligament sprain or tear

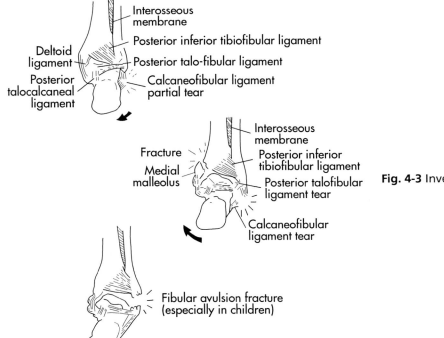

Fig. 4-3 Inversion injuries. Posterior view.

ASSESSMENT   INTERPRETATION

- undisplaced fracture of the lateral malleolus or malleolar epiphysis in the child or young athlete
- fracture of the medial malleolus (due to the talus being driven against the malleolus)
- bimalleolar fracture
- medial malleolar fracture and avulsion of the lateral collateral ligament

Secondary structure injury can be:
- peroneal tendons strain
- extensor digitorum brevis strain
- base of the fifth metatarsal fracture
- midtarsal joint sprain
- talar osteochondral fracture to the superomedial portion of the talus

Eversion (Fig. 4-4)

The lateral malleolus is longer and the talus cannot rock under it; therefore more stress is directed into the fibula before the medial ligaments are stressed. These eversion injuries are less common than inversion. Eversion forces are generated with tibial external rotation, foot abduction, and talocrural dorsiflexion. Fractures are more common in the medial aspect of the ankle than on the lateral aspect.

Eversion can cause a deltoid ligament sprain, which is the most common (either a partial tear or a complete tear). When the

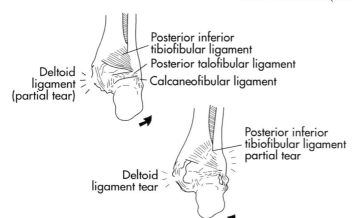
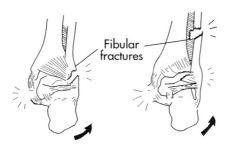

Fig. 4-4 Eversion injuries. Posterior view.

ASSESSMENT

INTERPRETATION

deltoid ligament was divided into its components, Siegler et al. found the following:

- The tibiocalcaneal ligament can only take negligible forces before tearing.
- The tibionavicular ligament is the longest and weakest of the medial collateral group, and when stressed to failure the ligament itself fails versus avulsing from the bone.
- The tibiospring ligament, which is rarely described in the anatomic literature but may be a very important medial ankle stabilizer, is a strong ligament with good elasticity, but one that failed through the ligament fibers. The tibiospring ligament as described by Siegler is the section of the tibiocalcaneal ligament that attaches to the spring ligament (plantar calcaneonavicular ligament).
- The posterior tibiotalar ligament is the shortest, thickest, and stiffest ligament of the collaterals, and failure occurred by boney avulsion.

Fracture of the lower third of the fibula is often accompanied by a torn deltoid ligament. This fracture separates higher up on the fibula if the deltoid and tibiofibular ligaments tear and may result in the following:

- avulsion of the medial malleolus
- bimalleolar fracture at or below the level of the lower end of the tibia

Plantar Flexion (Fig. 4-5)

Pure plantar flexion overstretch is very uncommon; what usually occurs is plantar flexion combined with an inversion. Pure plantar flexion overstretch can cause the following:

- anterior capsule sprain (this is the most common) or complete tear
- anterior talofibular ligament sprain or complete tear
- bifurcate ligament sprain
- posterior talar impingement of the lateral posterior tubercle of the talus between the tibia and calcaneus, resulting in soft-tissue compression or even fracture (this condition can occur if the athlete has a large posterior tubercle, os trigonum, or posterior process of the talus)
- midtarsal joint sprain

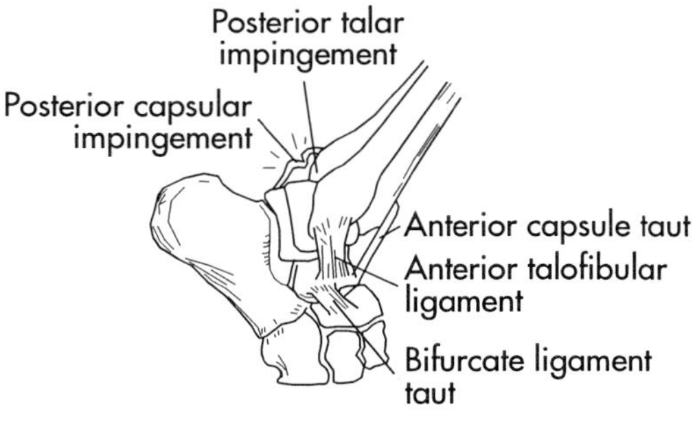

Fig. 4-5 Plantar flexion injuries.

Posterior talar impingement

Posterior capsular impingement

Anterior capsule taut

Anterior talofibular ligament

Bifurcate ligament taut

ASSESSMENT

INTERPRETATION

Plantar Flexion and Inversion

Of all ankle sprains, 80% to 85% occur to the lateral ligaments. Plantar flexion and inversion combination is the most common mechanism for ankle sprains. This mechanism occurs frequently in sport when a player lands on an opposing player's foot during rebounding under the net in basketball or returning from a block in volleyball. Uneven ground surfaces and rapid changes in direction that occur in sports like football and soccer also can cause this ankle mechanism. The structure damaged most often is the anterior talofibular ligament, which can sprain or partially tear. On occasion, it can completely tear. Siegler et al. found the anterior talofibular ligament the shortest and weakest of the collateral ligaments, with a tear occurring by bone avulsion (58% of the time). In plantar flexion the anterior talofibular ligament becomes the primary soft-tissue stabilizer of the lateral side of the joint. The anterolateral capsule can become sprained or torn and this may also include the retinaculum. The anterior tibiofibular ligament can also sprain or tear. Secondary structure injury (less common) can be:

- medial talar dome osteochondral fracture
- extensor digitorum brevis longus or tibialis anterior muscle strain
- peroneal tendon strain (brevis and/or longus)
- fifth metatarsal fracture at the base or shaft, or fifth metatarsal avulsion
- midtarsal joint sprain
- peroneal nerve damage with a severe sprain
- os trigonum or posterior lateral tubercle of the talus avulsion by the posterior talofibular ligament
- cuboid bone subluxation

Dorsiflexion (Fig. 4-6)

Because the talus is a bone that is wider anteriorly and narrower posteriorly it affects the stability of the talocrural joint during plantar and dorsiflexion. In plantar flexion the narrow posterior section of the talus is brought into contact with the anterior part of the malleoli and the joint has a great deal of extra joint play. In dorsiflexion, the wider section of the talus

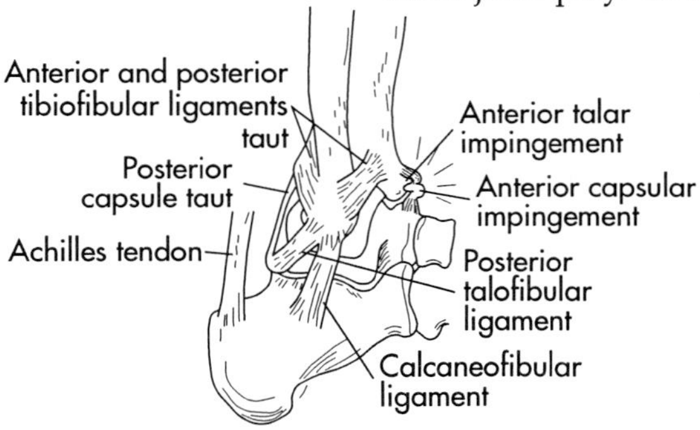

Anterior and posterior tibiofibular ligaments taut
Posterior capsule taut
Achilles tendon
Anterior talar impingement
Anterior capsular impingement
Posterior talofibular ligament
Calcaneofibular ligament

Fig. 4-6 Dorsiflexion injuries. Lateral view.

ASSESSMENT

INTERPRETATION

moves into the mortise like a wedge. If the foot is forced into dorsiflexion the talus acts like a wedge, separating the fibula from the tibia; therefore this dorsiflexion force can cause:
- inferior tibiofibular ligament sprain or tear (anterior and posterior)
- Achilles tendon strain, partial tear, or rupture
- posterior talofibular ligament sprain
- calcaneofibular ligament sprain
- posterior capsule sprain, tear, or rupture
- anterior talar impingement—Impingement of the anterior lip of the tibia on the talar neck, causing soft-tissue trauma (e.g., of the capsule or synovium). The impingement and trauma can be aggravated if there is an extra exostosis on the anterior talar neck or anterior lip of the tibia.
- fractured fibula
- fracture of the neck of the talus, with or without subtalar dislocation.

Dorsiflexion and Inversion

Dorsiflexion and inversion can cause:
- calcaneofibular ligament sprain or tear. Siegler et al. found the calcaneofibular ligament the longest and most elastic of the lateral collateral ligaments, with ligament failure occurring with boney avulsion (70% of the time).
- lateral talar dome lesions
- osteochondral fractures
- posterior talofibular ligament sprain or tear. Siegler et al. found that the posterior talofibular ligament was the thickest and strongest of the lateral collateral ligaments, with ligament failure by boney avulsion (70% of the time).

Dorsiflexion and Eversion

Most authors agree that a dorsiflexion and eversion position with a strong peroneal contraction can lead to an acute anterior dislocation of the peroneal tendons—that is commonly seen in downhill skiers. The injury usually occurs during a forward fall with the ankle dorsiflexing and the peroneals attempting to contract. The peroneals contract and are forced over the lateral malleolus, tearing the peroneal retinaculum. A dorsiflexion eversion mechanism can also damage the deltoid ligament and is often associated with a tibial or fibular fracture.

Hyperextension of the First Interphalangeal or Metatarsophalangeal Joint

Hyperextension of the first metatarsophalangeal or interphalangeal joint ("turf toe") is relatively common in football or baseball players who play on artificial turf. Often their shoes are too lightweight and flexible. Hyperextension to the first metatarsophalangeal joint can cause the following:
- capsuloligamentous sprain (this is the most common) or tear

ASSESSMENT   INTERPRETATION

- compression injury to the articular cartilage and underlying bone on the metatarsal head
- metatarsophalangeal dislocation (this is rare)

Dorsiflexion of the Forefoot (Fig. 4-7)

Dorsiflexion of the forefoot can cause the following:
- spring ligament sprain or tear
- plantar fascia sprain
- tibialis posterior muscle strain
- interphalangeal and metatarsophalangeal joint sprains

Direct Blow
Was there a direct blow?

Dorsum of the Foot

A direct blow to the dorsum of the foot is relatively common in sports; such an injury can be sustained when the player is struck by a hockey puck or is stepped on by another player. The skin and subcutaneous tissue is very thin, leaving the dorsum of the foot poorly protected from trauma. A direct blow to the dorsum of the foot can cause the following:
- contusion of the soft tissue of the forefoot or midfoot
- fracture of the forefoot or midfoot
- cuts (from spikes or cleats)
- sprains of the tarsometatarsal joints (this only happens occasionally)

Malleoli

A direct blow to the prominent medial or lateral malleoli can cause the following:
- contusion
- periosteitis
- fracture (this is rare)

A direct blow to the lateral malleolus, while the peroneals are taut with ankle dorsiflexion and eversion, can cause the peroneals to sublux or dislocate out of their groove.

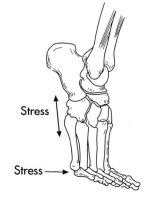

Stress

Stress

Fig. 4-7 Forefoot dorsiflexion stresses

ASSESSMENT   INTERPRETATION

Plantar Surface of the Foot

A direct blow to the plantar aspect of the foot is usually caused by the following:
- landing with the sole of the foot on a hard surface
- a faulty cleat
- stepping on a sharp or hard object

A direct blow to the plantar aspect of the foot can cause the following:
- contusion to the subcutaneous tissue
- sesamoiditis, which is contusion to the periosteum of the sesamoid bones of the great toe. (According to McBride, a direct blow to the sesamoid bones of the great toe will usually cause a transverse compression-type fracture of the tibial sesamoid.)
- laceration if the object is sharp
- occasionally, a sprain to the forefoot or midfoot ligaments, which may be forced apart on landing

Calcaneus

A direct blow to the calcaneus can cause the following:
- calcaneal heel pad contusion
- calcaneal periosteitis
- calcaneal compression fracture, which is usually the result of landing on the heel from a fall from a significant height

Repeated direct blows can be a predisposing factor to the development of Sever disease (calcaneal apophysitis) in the young athlete who is between the ages of 8 and 15 (Fig. 4-8).

Forced Muscle Contraction

Was there a forceful muscle contraction with the muscle on stretch (eccentric contraction) (Fig. 4-9)?

A forceful muscle contraction on landing or deceleration with the muscle on stretch can cause muscle strains or even tears. With the ankle joint in dorsiflexion and the Achilles (gastrocne-

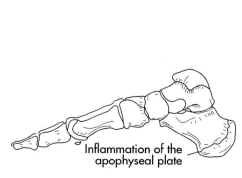

Inflammation of the apophyseal plate

Fig. 4-8 Calcaneal apophysitis—(Sever disease).

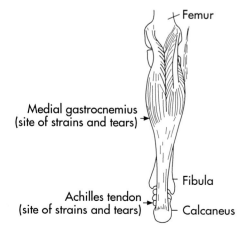

Femur

Medial gastrocnemius (site of strains and tears)

Achilles tendon (site of strains and tears)

Fibula

Calcaneus

Fig. 4-9 Posterior lower leg structures. Gastrocnemius and Achilles injury sites.

ASSESSMENT

Forceful plantar flexion or knee extension with the ankle joint dorsiflexed

Forceful dorsiflexion, subtalar eversion, and pronation when landing from a jump

INTERPRETATION

mius-soleus complex) on stretch, the eccentric forces through the muscle can cause the following:
- medial head of gastrocnemius strain, partial tear, or rupture
- Achilles tendon strain, partial tear, or rupture
- peroneal tendons subluxation

An Achilles tendon rupture tends to occur in middle-aged athletes between the ages of 30 to 50 years with a history of tendonitis or a previous strain, especially those who participate in sports that require quick forward and backward movements such as in tennis, squash, racquetball, or basketball. With the ankle joint in dorsiflexion and the subtalar joint in eversion, landing from a height can cause a tibialis posterior strain, especially if the arch collapses. This is a common injury because the muscle functions to maintain the arch as well as plantar flexing and inverting the foot.

Overuse

Was there an overuse or a repetitive mechanism? (Fig. 4-10)

Running, Jumping, Dancing

Overuse conditions in the lower extremity are most frequently caused by excessive running and some of the following variables:
- poor exercise surface (too hard or uneven)
- poor running technique
- inadequate shoe wear
- training errors
- muscle imbalances
- structural abnormalities such as compensated subtalar varus, compensated forefoot varus, compensated talipes equinnus, excessive tibial torsion, excessive tibial varum, or tarsal coalition

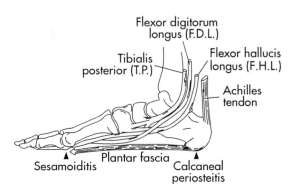

Fig. 4-10 Some foot structures stressed by overuse. Medial aspect.

ASSESSMENT   INTERPRETATION

Stress Fractures

Running, jumping, dancing, and some of the predisposing factors above can cause stress fractures to the following:
- tibia (this is more common in pronated feet)
- tarsal bones (talus, navicular)
- metatarsals, mainly the second and third (this is more common in cavus foot)
- fibula
- sesamoids
- calcaneus

Periosteitis or Stress Reaction

Overuse can also cause periosteitis or stress reactions of the:
- tibia (posterior or anterior)
- fibula
- calcaneus
- sesamoids (especially in the athlete with plantar-flexed first metatarsal or restricted dorsiflexion of the first MP joint)
- talus (talar compression syndrome)
- calcaneus (resulting in calcaneal spur or exostosis)

Tendonitis

Overuse can cause various types of tendonitis such as the following:
- Achilles tendonitis or peritendonitis
- peroneal tendonitis
- anterior and posterior tibial tendonitis
- flexor hallucis longus tendonitis
- flexor digitorum longus tendonitis

Blisters and Calluses

Blisters and calluses (plantar keratoses) of the posterior heel and under the metatarsal heads can result from overuse.

Compartment Syndromes

The following compartment syndromes can also be caused by overuse:
- anterior compartment
- posterior (deep or superficial) compartment
- lateral compartment
- tarsal tunnel syndrome

Synovitis

Overuse can irritate any of the foot and ankle joints, causing synovitis especially in the first metatarsophalangeal joint.

Calcaneal Irritations

Repetitive movements can cause irritation of tissue and structures in the heel area in particular. Structures in this area that can become irritated include:

ASSESSMENT

INTERPRETATION

- calcaneal nerves—lateral and medial
- calcaneal fat pad—Doxey describes a fat pad syndrome
- calcaneal bursa—retrocalcaneal bursitis
- calcaneus—can develop calcaneal exostosis and spurs
- plantar fascia—plantar fasciitis

Sport Related

Are the problems sport related?

Certain sports have inherent foot and ankle problems associated with them. For example, the repeated movements on the toes in ballet or gymnastics may cause a fracture of the posterior tubercle of the talus or a fracture of a steida process, which is a large tubercle on the posterior talus (Fig. 4-11). If an os trigonum is already present, this extreme position of plantar flexion will lead to its impingement and the resulting pain and inflammation.

For example, activities like basketball have a high incidence of ankle sprains due to the rebounding activities under the net, which cause players to turn their ankles when they land on an opposing player's foot.

Forces in the Sport

Determine the forces and nature of the sport.

Forces in each sport vary greatly. Contact sports such as hockey lead to more direct trauma or overstretch injuries. Solo sports that require repetitive movements lead to overuse injuries. A basic mechanical knowledge of the components of the sport is to understand the injury involved.

Body Position

Determine the body position and forces during injury.

The position of the athlete at the time of injury is important, especially the position of his or her foot and ankle in relation to the knee, hip, and body. If the athlete is weight-bearing when an impact is experienced, the ankle (and knee) can be traumatized more than if the athlete is nonweight-bearing on that limb. If the foot is fixed because of cleated footwear or a rubberized sole, more force is taken by the ankle and knee.When the athlete is weight-bearing, all the weight is transmitted through the talus to the other bones of the foot. The talus and calcaneus interaction (subtalar) reduces the rotary stresses through the ankle joint—these factors explain why the subtalar joint is often sprained in sport.

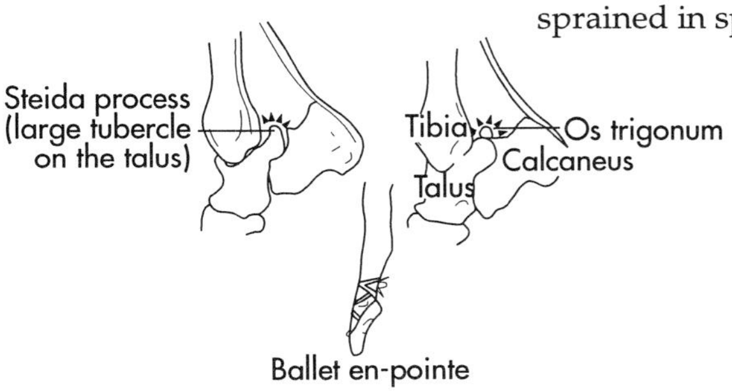

Steida process (large tubercle on the talus)

Tibia Os trigonum
Talus Calcaneus

Ballet en-pointe

Fig. 4-11 Posterior talar impingement in plantar flexion.

ASSESSMENT

INTERPRETATION

Demonstrate the Mechanism

Ask the athlete to demonstrate the mechanism with the opposite extremity.

Demonstrating the mechanism with the opposite limb clarifies the athlete's position, particularly when a verbal description is difficult to obtain. Demonstrating the mechanism that causes discomfort with the overuse injury may help determine the cause of the condition and which movements should be avoided.

Sport or Running Surface

Determine the sport or running surface (Fig. 4-12).

It is important to determine the sport surface to help determine the athlete's condition. Wood and spring floors absorb shock and reduce the forces of impact to the foot and ankle. Rug-covered concrete or other poor shock-absorbing floors lead to lower leg, as well as foot and ankle, overuse conditions, especially in aerobics, gymnastics, and dancing. This problem is increased when the athlete exercises on his or her toes. Synthetic surfaces such as all-weather tracks, asphalt, or concrete eliminate the skidding that can occur on surfaces of cinders or grass. The latter surfaces allow more efficient running but increase the friction that torque generates through the forefoot, and they lack shock absorbency.

Footwear

Determine the footwear worn and if it fits.

Footwear often influences the athlete's injury and may even cause it. Questions related to footwear are important. It is important to determine how the footwear fits and how well it serves the athlete's needs.

Toe Box

If the toe box is shallow, the great toe is subjected to toenail injury; if the toe box is narrow, the first or fifth metatarsal will develop problems.

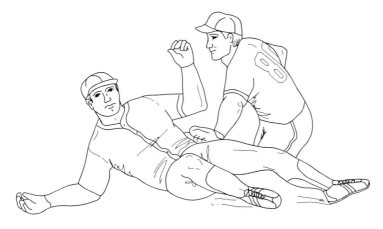

Fig. 4-12 The sport surface can cause lower leg, foot, and ankle problems.

ASSESSMENT

INTERPRETATION

Longitudinal Arch

If the longitudinal arch is inadequate the athlete can develop the following:
- pronation problems
- tibialis posterior tendonitis
- tibialis anterior tendonitis
- plantar fasciitis

Heel Counter

If the heel counter is inadequate, there can be ankle sprains and Achilles tendonitis. If the heel counter is rigid, retrocalcaneal blisters and exostosis can develop.

Sole
- Flexible
- Stiff
- Straight last
- Curved last

If the sole is too flexible it can lead to metatarsalgia or hyperextension of the first metacarpophalangeal joint. If the sole is too stiff at the metatarsophalangeal joint, it will place excessive strain on the Achilles tendon and will cause excessive force through the calcaneus. It is important to remember that straight-last soles are better for a pronating foot and curve-last soles are better for a supinatory foot.

Pain

Location

   Where is the pain located?

Local Pain

If the sole point tenderness comes usually from the more superficial structures. The anatomic structures that project localized areas of pain when injured include the following:
- skin
- fascia
- superficial muscle (e.g., peroneal muscles, tibialis anterior, gastrocnemius)
- superficial ligament (e.g., anterior talofibular, calcaneofibular, spring, bifurcate)
- periosteum (e.g., malleoli, tibia, calcaneus)

Referred Pain

Referred pain can come from the following structures:
- deep muscle—myotomal (e.g., tibialis posterior and soleus); this is often referred through the length of the muscle
- deep ligament—sclerotomal (e.g., posterior talofibular)
- bursa—sclerotomal (e.g., posterior calcaneal)
- capsule—myotomal or sclerotomal (e.g., talocrural joint capsule)
- bone—sclerotomal (e.g., tibia and fibula); this is often referred distally or proximally along the length of the bone

ASSESSMENT   INTERPRETATION

- nerve root (L4, L5, S1)—ventral (myotomal) and dorsal (dermatomal, radicular pain)
- superficial nerve (e.g., sural, deep or superficial peroneal); superficial pain is easy to localize; pain from deep somatic structures is more difficult to pinpoint.

Onset of Pain

How quickly did the pain begin?
- Sudden onsets
- After 24 hours
- Gradual or insidious onset

A quick onset of pain suggests a more severe problem than a gradual or insidious onset. A quick onset of pain occurs with a sprain, partial tear, strain, hemarthrosis, fracture, or contusion.

If the pain develops 24 hours after the blow, twist, or overuse, it is usually indicative of a gradual tissue response to trauma such as synovial swelling, tendonitis, a minor sprain, or capsulitis.

An insidious onset can suggest a systemic disorder. For example the following can occur:
- rheumatoid arthritis can initially present in the metatarsophalangeal joints of the feet, although it can arise in the subtalar or tarsal joints
- Reiter disease can cause collagen disorders in the tendons or synovium in the subtalar or talocrural joints
- psoriatic disease can cause discomfort in the connective tissue of the foot and ankle
- gout usually develops in the great toe, but also can predispose the foot and ankle to tendonitis or synovitis

Type of Pain

Describe the pain.

Different anatomic structures can elicit different types of pain.

Sharp

Sharp pain can be elicited from the following structures:
- skin (e.g., retrocalcaneal and metatarsal head blisters)
- superficial fascia (e.g., dorsal foot contusions)
- tendon (e.g., Achilles and peroneal tendonitis)
- superficial muscle (e.g., tibialis anterior or posterior)
- superficial ligament (e.g., anterior talofibular or calcaneofibular ligament sprain)
- bursa (e.g., retrocalcaneal bursitis—superficial)
- periosteum (e.g., anterior tibial periosteitis)

Dull

Dull pain is experienced from the following structures:
- tendon sheath (e.g., peroneal tendons)
- deep muscle (e.g., anterior, posterior, or lateral compartment syndrome)
- stress fractures (e.g., metatarsal, fibular, tibial)

ASSESSMENT

INTERPRETATION

Aching

Aching pain is experienced from an injury to the following structures:
- compact fascia (e.g., calcaneal fat pad contusion)
- deep muscle (e.g., compartment syndromes)
- tendon sheath (e.g., chronic peroneal tendonitis)
- deep ligament (e.g., anterior tibiofibular ligament sprain)
- fibrous capsule (e.g., talocrural joint capsular sprain)
- chronic bursa (e.g., retrocalcaneal bursitis)

Burning

Burning pain is elicited by an injury to the following structures:
- skin (e.g., blister on sole of foot)
- tendon sheath (e.g., acute extensor hallucis longus tendonitis)
- peripheral nerve (e.g., calcaneal or sural nerve entrapment)

Pins and Needles (Paresthesia)

Paresthesia is elicited by an injury to the following structures:
- peripheral nerve (e.g., lateral cutaneous nerve with paresthesia into the lateral thigh)
- nerve roots (e.g., L4, L5, and S1 nerve roots with paresthesia into the segmental dermatome)

Numbness (Anesthesia)

Numbness is attributed to the following structures:
- dorsal nerve root (e.g., herniated disc with L4, L5, or S1 nerve root compression)
- peripheral nerve (e.g., deep or superficial peroneal cutaneous nerve compression)

When Pain Occurs
When is it painful?

All the Time

Acute conditions and long-term chronic injuries, such as the following, can lead to continuous pain:
- acute bursitis
- acute ligament sprain
- osteoarthritis
- neoplasm

Only After Repeating the Injury Mechanism

Pain that occurs only when the causative mechanism is repeated suggests a very localized lesion. Pain that occurs only on certain joint movements suggests that the muscle, joint, or joint support structures (muscle, tendon, ligament, capsule) are injured. Pain in ligaments, capsules, and muscles increases

ASSESSMENT

INTERPRETATION

when these structures are stretched. Pain in bursae, synovial membranes, and nerve roots increases when these structures are compressed or pinched.

Only After Repeated Movement

Pain that occurs only after repeated movement suggests that overuse is the cause of the problem; the anatomic structures that usually suffer from overuse are one of the following:
- tendon
- bone
- muscle
- synovial membrane

Severity of Pain
How severe is the pain?
- Mild
- Moderate
- Severe

As a rule, the greater the pain the more severe the injury, but this is not always true; complete tears can be painless. For example, an S1 nerve root compression may cause painless weakness of the gastrocnemius, whereas a mild first degree anterior talofibular ligament sprain may be very painful. Another example is a partial Achilles tendon rupture that may be more painful than a complete rupture. Often, as the pain increases in severity, it becomes more difficult to localize the lesion site. The degree of pain is not a very accurate measurement because the perception of pain varies with the athlete's emotional state, cultural background, and previous painful experiences. The number of nociceptors in the injury tissue and surrounding structures can also influence the severity of pain. In general, structures that are highly innervated cause more discomfort than poorly innervated structures. For example, the articular cartilage has few nociceptors to elicit pain but the periosteum has many.

Swelling

Location
Where is the swelling located?

Local

Localized swelling can occur with extra-articular (outside the joint) swelling that accompanies lateral ankle sprains. The swelling localizes below the lateral malleolus, in the sinus tarsi, or in related traumatized soft tissue. Intra-articular swelling (inside the joint) appears below both malleoli. Localized swelling can also be a local bursitis. Bursitis, a small pocket of swelling, can develop in areas where there is increased friction. In the foot and ankle, tendons or skin that rub over boney prominences can develop bursitis (i.e., posterior calcaneal bursitis, retrocalcaneal bursitis).
Local swelling can occur over the following:
- stress fracture of the fibula

ASSESSMENT   INTERPRETATION

- stress fractures of the metatarsals (mainly the second, third, or fifth)
- peroneal tendons with peroneal strain or tendonitis
- Achilles tendon with Achilles strain or tendonitis
- flexor hallucis longus behind the medial malleolus
- extensor digitorum tendons with tendonitis or tenosynovitis

Diffuse

Diffuse swelling in the foot and ankle can occur as:
- generalized edema appearing over the soft tissue that is contused (especially on dorsum of foot)
- diffuse ecchymosis tracking down into the foot after an extra-articular injury
- intramuscular or intermuscular swelling in the surrounding muscle tissue, especially the peroneals, extensor digitorum brevis, or longus

Intermuscular swelling occurs in between the muscles involved, intramuscular swelling occurs within the muscle.

Time of Swelling
How quickly did the injury swell?

Immediately

Immediate joint swelling (hemarthrosis) indicates a severe injury with damage to a structure with a rich blood supply. The cause can be:
- severe ligament partial or complete tear
- acute osteochondral lesion of the talar dome
- calcaneal fracture of the anterior process
- talar fracture

After 6 to 12 Hours

Joint swelling that develops 6 to 12 hours post-injury is less severe and suggests a synovitis or irritation of the joint synovium. The cause can be:
- capsular sprain
- subtalar subluxation
- ligamentous sprain

After Activity

Joint swelling that develops after activity suggests that activity aggravates the condition. The cause can be:
- chronic ankle instability
- undetected osteochondral lesion
- irritation of subacute ankle injury
- joint irritation from a decreased dorsiflexion range of motion

ASSESSMENT	INTERPRETATION

Insidious Onset

Swelling without a mechanism can be caused by a collagen disorder (i.e., rheumatoid arthritis, Reiter syndrome, ankylosing spondylitis, gout, lupus) or osteoarthritic joint condition.

Amount of Swelling
How much did it swell?

Everyone's blood clotting time is different, but usually the more swelling present, the greater the severity of the injury (especially if the swelling occurs immediately after the injury).

Immediate Care
Was the injury given any immediate care?

If rest, ice, compression, and elevation were used immediately in the acute phase of the injury, the amount of swelling present may be reduced. If heat was applied or the injury site was not rested, compressed, or elevated, there can be significant swelling even with a minor injury.

When Does it Swell
How often and when does it swell?

Chronic joint swelling can develop after a cast has been removed, after repeated sprains, if full range of motion is not restored after injury, or if there is a bone chip or fracture in the joint. Also, if the activity level is too great to let the inflammation process subside, the swelling may persist. Joint swelling at the end of the day can indicate:
- chronic problem from scar tissue aggravation
- lack of elevation of an injured foot or ankle during the day
- osteochondritis dissecans (osteochondral lesion) of the joint, which is irritated by weight-bearing activities

Function

Could the athlete weight-bear immediately or only after several hours? How much movement was available at the time of the injury and now?
   Could the athlete carry on playing?
   Is there locking?
   Is there a feeling of weakness?
   Is there a capsular pattern of movement?

Inability to weight-bear immediately after injury suggests that a more severe injury has occurred. These injuries could be fractures or severe sprains, or the inability to weight-bear could be a hysterical reaction. The one exception is the athlete who has relatively little pain and full function after a complete rupture of a ligament because there are no ligamentous fibers intact to carry a pain message. If movement of the joints is less than 50% range of motion or strength, suspect a second-degree (or greater) problem. Recurring ankle sprains usually cause less pain and loss of function than the original episode. The ability to return to the game immediately after the injury usually indicates a first-degree problem in which the injured structure may be mildly sprained or strained but function of the foot and ankle is relatively complete. A locking of the joint is often the sign of a bone chip (osteochondritis dessicans of the talus or talar dome). Weakness when attempting movements immediately after injury can suggest the following:
- neural injury to the muscle allowing movement (i.e., peroneal nerve—peroneals)

ASSESSMENT

INTERPRETATION

- significant muscle injury
- reflex muscle inhibition due to the immediate swelling or pain
- fracture

A capsular pattern will cause decreased range of motion in plantar flexion and dorsiflexion. A capsular pattern is caused when the entire joint capsule is irritated and a pattern of limitation occurs. There is a total joint reaction and muscle spasm limits the normal joint movements. Each joint has its own pattern of limitation; to determine what is causing the capsular pattern, full testing noting the end feels is necessary.

Instability

Is there a feeling of insecurity?
- Occasionally
- Always
- Immediately after injury

Are there lumbar spine symptoms and ankle instability?

Chronic ankle sprainers have very lax ligaments and joint capsules, which can result in the ankle giving way or turning over very easily.

If the ankle is unstable immediately after injury, this is a sign of a significant ligament tear with capsular and soft-tissue damage. A fracture can cause gross instability. Long-term lumbar spine problems with an L5-S1 nerve root irritation can cause weakness in the peroneals and result in recurring lateral ankle sprains. There are usually lumbar symptoms as well (e.g., radicular pain, paraspinal spasm, and reflex changes).

Sensations

Type of Sensation

Describe the sensations felt at the time of injury, and now.

Warmth

Warmth can indicate active inflammation, infection, or gout.

Numbness

Numbness can indicate local neural involvement. Occasionally, nerve injuries are associated with inversion ankle sprains, especially with severe sprains involving the lateral and medial collateral ligaments. The nerves most commonly involved are the peroneal or the posterior tibial nerves.

Local cutaneous nerves can be involved secondarily with foot or ankle injuries. They include the following:
- sural nerve
- interdigital nerve with Morton neuroma (Fig. 4-13)
- calcaneal nerves

Lumbar spine nerve root problems can cause numbness in the lower leg, foot, and ankle.

Lower leg anterior compartment syndrome or overuse can lead to nerve compression and numbness in the dorsal web between the great and second toes.

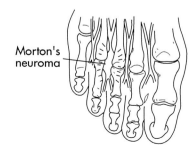

Morton's neuroma

Fig. 4-13 Morton neuroma.

ASSESSMENT

INTERPRETATION

Tingling

Tingling usually indicates a neural or circulatory problem. Nerve root pain can be referred to the foot and ankle. Circulatory problems can be caused by a fracture or lower-leg anterior, posterior, or lateral compartment trauma or overuse. With a lower limb compartment syndrome, there is a history of muscle overuse or direct trauma that can cause this paresthesia in the following locations:

- along the longitudinal arch of the foot (deep posterior compartment)
- in the dorsal first web space (anterior compartment)
- in the anterolateral aspect of the leg (lateral compartment)

Clicking and Catching

Clicking and catching usually indicate an osteochondral lesion of the talus.

Snapping

Snapping usually indicates:

- subluxing peroneals (if the snapping is felt at the lateral malleolus)
- tendons snapping over boney prominences (i.e., extensor tendons)

Popping or Tearing (At Time of Injury)

Popping or tearing at the time of injury can indicate a significant muscle or ligament tear.

Grating

Grating during ankle movements can indicate:

- osteoarthritic changes
- osteochondral lesion of the talus
- lateral talar chondromalacia

Crepitus

Crepitus in a tendon can be caused by an inflammation or any of the following:

- Achilles tendon
- peroneal tendon
- extensor tendon (tenosynovium)
- flexor hallucis longus tendon

Particulars

Chronic

Has this happened before?
Is it chronic?
How many times has it recurred?

Repeated trauma, sprains, tendonitis, or subluxations are important to record. Common ongoing problems at the foot and ankle include the following:

- stress fractures

ASSESSMENT

INTERPRETATION

- tendonitis (Achilles, peroneals, flexor hallucis longus)
- peroneal dislocations
- repeated ankle sprains
- anterior capsule impingement (Mandelbaum et al.) from repeated lateral ankle sprains (may be due to osteophytes on the neck of the talus or tibia)

Other chronic problems that may exist here are:
- arthritis
- osteochondral damage (usually at the dome of the talus)
- painful tarsal coalition when there is an absence or restriction of movement between two or more bones of the foot (Percy and Mann). The usual cause is a congenital abnormality with cartilage, fibrous, or boney union. The most common sites are the calcaneonavicular and talocalcaneal areas and, occasionally, the talonavicular area. The coalition may only become obvious after an ankle or foot injury occurs.

Other Limb Problems

Are there any other limb problems?
- Leg-length difference
- Knee problem
- Unrelated previous tibia, foot, or ankle injuries

A leg-length difference can cause more force to be exerted through the short leg and more stress to be experienced in the case of an overuse injury.

A knee problem can cause the athlete to favor that leg and put extra stress through the opposite leg. This has potential for altered mechanics on the foot and ankle, especially when it is a chronic knee problem.

Unrelated previous injuries to the tibia, foot, or ankle can cause atrophy or altered mechanics and should be investigated before the observations and functional tests are carried out.

Previous Care

Has a family physician, orthopedic surgeon, osteopath, physiotherapist, physical therapist, athletic therapist, athletic trainer, or other medical personnel assessed the injury this time or previously?

Were X-rays taken?

What were the results?

Was treatment administered previously?
- Prescriptions
- Physiotherapy

Was physiotherapy successful?

It is important to (1) record the physician's diagnosis, prescriptions, and treatment, as well as previous x-ray results and previous rehabilitation, and (2) the treatments or rehabilitative techniques that helped and those that did not help, because this information will be an aid when assessing the injury and when designing a rehabilitation program.

ASSESSMENT

INTERPRETATION

OBSERVATIONS

The lumbar spine, pelvis, and entire lower limb should be observed from the anterior, posterior, and lateral views while weight-bearing and nonweight-bearing. The low back, pelvis, hip, knee, ankle, and foot must be exposed as much as possible—the athlete should wear shorts or a swimsuit.

Prolonged Pronation

Pronation during weight-bearing (closed kinetic chain) is defined as movement in three planes that include forefoot abduction, talar adduction and plantar flexion, and talar adduction and subtalar eversion (Table 4-3). It is also suggested that prolonged pronation can even lead to thoracic kyphosis, forward head, and malocclusion. Pronation can be excessive, it can occur when supination should occur, or can occur to compensate for bony or soft-tissue abnormalities.

Fixed Supination

During weight-bearing (closed kinetic chain) fixed supination is defined as movement in three planes that includes forefoot adduction, dorsiflexion, talar abduction, and subtalar inversion (Table 4-4).

Supination can be excessive, can occur when pronation should occur, or can occur because of a boney or soft-tissue abnormality that restricts function.

Weight-bearing

It is important to view the athlete in weight-bearing because this shows how the body compensates for structural abnormalities and how many normal structures can become abnormal with weight-bearing forces (Table 4-2).

Anterior View
Lumbar Lordosis

Excessive lumbar lordosis can be associated with facet dysfunction and intervertebral disc herniations that can radiate pain or numbness into the lower leg, ankle, and foot.

Anterior Pelvic Tilt

Excessive anterior pelvic tilt is often associated with foot pronation problems in weight-bearing. If the anterior superior iliac spine is lower on one side, it can suggest a structural or

ASSESSMENT   INTERPRETATION

TABLE 4-2   Nonweight- bearing to Weight- bearing chart

Nonweight-bearing	Weight-bearing	Possible problems

Talipes Equinus
   <10 degrees dorsiflexion
   in talocrural joint
	Compensated talipes equinus
	 Uncompensated talipes equinus
		Prolonged pronation problems
		   (rocker-bottom foot)
		 Metatarsal problems

Subtalar Varus
   increased subtalar inversion
	Compensated subtalar varus
	
	 Uncompensated subtalar varus
		Prolonged pronation problems
		   (common)
		 Fixed supination problems

Subtalar Valgus increased subtalar eversion	Compensated subtalar valgus Uncompensated subtalar valgus	Pes planus (rare) Prolonged pronation prblems

Forefoot Varus,
   forefoot angled,
   fifth toe lower than first
	Compensated forefoot varus
	
	 Uncompensated forefoot varus
		Prolonged pronation problems
		   (common)
		 Fixed supination and/or first
		   ray problems (rare)

Forefoot Valgus,
   forefoot angled,
   first toe lower than fifth
	Compensated forefoot valgus
	
	 Uncompensated forefoot valgus
		Flexible cavus foot problems;
		   fixed supination problems
		 Rigid cavus foot problems
		   (forefoot); fixed supination
		   problems

functional leg-length discrepancy or that one ilium may be rotated or shifted in relation to the other ilium (anterior or posterior iliac rotation).

Leg-length Discrepancy

In weight-bearing, a leg-length discrepancy can be created when one foot is pronated and the other is supinated. Overuse conditions in the tibia, ankle, subtalar joint, and forefoot can develop with excessive pronation. In nonweight-bearing, determine if the arches remain pronated or supinated. A previous femoral or tibial fracture can cause a structural leg-length difference if the bone did not heal to its correct length.

Femoral Anteversion (Increased Femoral Medial Rotation) (see Fig. 3-15)

Femoral anteversion can cause foot pronation during gait, which will lead to pronatory overuse conditions.

Previous Knee Injury

The athlete may rely on ankle power to overcome knee weakness caused by a previous knee injury. The entire limb, including the foot and ankle, may be weaker if there was significant knee damage or if the athlete was nonweight-bearing for a long period of time—this weakness may have contributed to the foot, subtalar, or ankle injury.

Genu Varum (see Fig. 3-14)

This knee alignment is usually associated with a cavus foot (supinated subtalar joint) with more weight-borne forces

ASSESSMENT	INTERPRETATION

through the lateral side of the foot. This can cause ankle sprains and peroneal tendonitis (see Fixed Supination Problems).

Genu Valgum

This knee alignment is usually associated with an overpronated foot (pronated subtalar joint). More weight is transferred through the medial part of the foot (see Prolonged Pronation Problems; Table 4-3).

Tibial Internal Torsion

Tibial internal torsion usually creates pronation problems with weight-bearing, walking, and running. Excess forces go

TABLE 4-3 Prolonged Pronation Problems

Structure	Mechanism	Conditions
Hindfoot	Calcaneal stays everted	Achilles tendonitis Medial calcaneal compartment syndrome (Calcaneal—posterior tibial N, medial calcaneal N compression) Heel spur Peroneal tendonitis Navicular stress fracture
Midfoot	Longitudinal arch depresses, talus abducts, and plantar flexes	Spring ligament sprain Tibialis posterior strain Tibialis posterior tendonitis Flexor digitorum longus tendonitis Flexor hallucis longus strain Flexor hallucis longus tendonitis Peronei and toe extensor spasms Plantar fasciitis
Forefoot	Hypermobile first ray	Second metatarsal calluses and fractures Hallux valgus Metatarsalgia (II and III) Sesamoiditis Tailor's bunions Hammer toes Dislocated first ray (metatarsus, adductors)
Tibia	Excessive internal rotation Tibial varum	Stress reactions and stress fractures of tibia and fibula
Knee	Excessive internal rotation	Knee Joint Capsulitis Patellar alignment syndromes Chondromalacia Pes anserine bursitis
Hip	Internal rotation	Hip Joint Capsulitis Greater trochanteric bursitis Tensor fasciae lata strains Piriformis overstretch
Pelvis	Anterior pelvic tilt	Excessive lumbar lordosis pain Hip flexor strains Hip adductor strains Sacroiliac joint problems

ASSESSMENTINTERPRETATION

through the medial aspect of the foot and ankle. To keep the center of gravity over the foot, the forefoot abducts on the rear foot or the foot abducts on the leg, causing problems.

Tibial External Torsion

Tibial external torsion often leads to high-arched cavus foot and its related supination problems when walking and running. It may be compensated for in some athletes by overpronation of the subtalar joint.

Tibial Varum

This alignment causes foot pronation problems because the foot pronates to compensate for the angle of the tibia.

Tibial Localized Swelling or Enlargement

Localized tibial swelling can be periosteitis from overuse or ecchymosis from direct trauma.

TABLE 4-4   Fixed Supination Problems

Structure	Mechanisms	Conditions
Hindfoot	Calcaneus stays inverted	Plantar calcaneal contusions Medial calcaneal nerve entrapment Retrocalcaneal exotosis Achilles tendonitis Heel spurs
Midfoot	Center of gravity laterally over base of support (no arch depression); talus abducts and dorsiflexes	Inversion ankle sprains Plantar fasciitis Peroneal tendonitis Cuboid subluxation or dislocation
Forefoot	Rigid inverted forefoot with push off lateral aspect of foot	Neuromas Hypomobile first ray Fourth and fifth metatarsal calluses and stress fractures Peroneal tendonitis Plantar keratomas under metatarsal heads Metatarsalgia (overuse) Hammer toes
Tibia	Stresses through lateral tibia and compression forces (not absorbed through pronation); external rotation	Fibular stress fractures Tibial stress fractures
Knee	Torque and compression forces	Knee capsular pain Undue compressing forces transmitted into knee joint
Hip	Compression forces	Compression hip joint capsulitis
Sacroiliac joint	Compression forces	Sacroiliac joint irritation
Lumbar spine	Compression forces	Facet irritations

ASSESSMENT

INTERPRETATION

Foot

LONGITUDINAL ARCH

Is this arch depressed (pronated) or elevated (cavus in weight-bearing)?

Observe the arch in a nonweight-bearing position later to see if it is still depressed or elevated. If the talus is prominent on the medial side of the foot (talus slides forward and medially), the arch is depressed—this can be graded as mild, moderate, or severe (see Prolonged Pronation; Table 4-3). If the arch stays high and does not depress in weight-bearing (there may be Fixed Supination Problems; Table 4-4).

TRANSVERSE ARCH

If the transverse arch is depressed in weight-bearing, it can lead to metatarsalgia, Morton neuroma, or digital nerve problems. Compare the transverse arch later to see if it is elevated or depressed in a nonweight-bearing position. When the arch is depressed the metatarsal heads bear too much weight.

SUBUNGUAL HEMATOMAS

Subungual hematomas can occur in the toes, especially the great toe. These hematomas are common in athletes involved in repetitive-action sports (such as running and tennis) when the shoe toe box is not deep enough. The athlete often has a problem with hyperextending toes that make contact with the shoe box and cause bleeding under the toe nails.

TOE ALIGNMENT
- Hallux valgus (Fig. 4-14)
- Morton's foot (Greek foot)
- Swelling (local)

Hallux valgus is a valgus angulation of the proximal phalanx of the great toe. Hallux valgus leads to pronation problems and bunion development on weight-bearing. The basic underlying predisposing factor according to Subotnik is a hypermobile first ray. Research has also indicated that a varus angle of the metatarsals and shoe wear (high heels, pointed-toe shoes) may also be causes of this deformity. This is a progressive deformity. The great toe will angle toward the second toe and may even disrupt its function. If left unattended, the great toe can move over the top of the second toe, the medial portion of the first metatarsal head enlarges (metatarsus primus varus), and extra forces go through the medial sesamoid bone. This condition is often compounded by a fallen transverse arch as well. Often the great toe will have ingrown nail problems at the lateral border of the hallux because of the valgum deviation and the friction of this toe on the inside of the shoe. During walking and running, the second metatarsal will bear most of the body weight because the unstable hallux valgus will dorsiflex and invert during midstance. The second metatarsal head can develop callus and stress fractures; the second metatarsophalangeal joint can develop synovitis. Bursitis at the medial aspect of the first metatarsal head is a frequent development in the athlete with hallux valgus

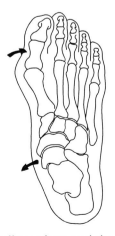

Fig. 4-14 Hallux valgus and the resulting pronation.

ASSESSMENT	INTERPRETATION

because of the toe's hypermobility and the increased friction in this area. This can create problems for athletes who wear ski boots, skates, or other tight footwear. The first metatarsophalangeal joint can also develop synovitis due to the hypermobility of the joint and excessive pressure on this area. Eventual arthritic and degenerative changes will develop on this joint surface.

Morton's foot (Greek foot) where there is a shorter big toe than the second toe leads to more weight-bearing forces through the second toe and hypermobility in the first ray. Metatarsalgia can occur in the runner who has this long second metatarsal. A shorter first metatarsal occurs in about 50% of the population. Local swelling helps determine the location of the lesion but it can also track into the forefoot from the tibia, ankle, or subtalar joints because of the pull of gravity.

ANKLE AND FOOT
- Boney contour deformities
- Muscle atrophy

Boney contour deformities with a history of trauma can suggest fracture of any of the following: talus, tarsals, metatarsals, or phalanges, or a medial or lateral malleolus avulsion.

Muscle atrophy may indicate a previous nonrehabilitated sprain, a fracture, neural problems, or a nerve impingement.

Lateral View
Anterior Pelvic Tilt

This is usually associated with pronated foot problems (see Prolonged Pronation Problems; Table 4-3).

Genu Recurvatum (Hyperextension) (Fig. 4-15)

This knee position usually results in plantar flexion of the ankle joint even in the normal standing position. If the Achilles tendon is shortened, this can cause problems during midstance of gait when the talocrural joint cannot attain the necessary 10° of dorsiflexion. This may result in pronation problems.

Ankle Swelling, Discoloration, Deformity

Ankle swelling, discoloration, and deformity pinpoint the location of the injury and the amount of bleeding (lateral ligament, medial ligament, capsule, general ecchymosis).

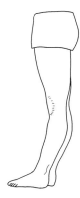

Fig. 4-15 Genu recurvatum.

ASSESSMENT   INTERPRETATION

Forefoot Swelling

Forefoot swelling is due to injury of the tarsals, metatarsals, or phalanges. Swelling can also track into the forefoot from an injury above.

Longitudinal Arch

If the longitudinal arch is depressed, it can result in pronation problems; if it is elevated, it can lead to supination problems. The arch should be measured later in special tests if it seems depressed. The height of the arch should be recorded and it should be re-examined during gait to determine its dynamic position.

Claw Toe

Claw toe is defined as a toe with a hyperextended metatarsophalangeal joint, with the proximal interphalangeal and distal interphalangeal joints flexed. It will often result in callus formation over the proximal interphalangeal joint dorsally, and an associated plantar keratoma under the involved metatarsal head. The proximal phalanx may sublux dorsally. Several mechanisms have been suggested for this deformity:
- restrictive effect of poorly fitted shoes
- weakness of foot intrinsics
- muscle imbalances
- deficiencies in plantar structures, such as weak flexors or joint capsule shortening

Hammer Toe

Hammer toe is defined as a toe with a hyperextended metatarsophalangeal joint, a flexed proximal interphalangeal joint, and an extended distal interphalangeal joint. It indicates muscle imbalances, poorly fitting shoes, or a hereditary component. Calluses form over the raised proximal interphalangeal joint. This deformity is most common in the fifth toe, with an associated dorsolateral callus.

Mallet Toe

An extensor tendon rupture or a flexion deformity of only the distal interphalangeal joint results in the distal interphalangeal joint remaining flexed. The mallet toe will often have a distal lesion due to abnormal pressure on the tip of the toe at the dorsal distal interphalangeal joint.

Enlarged Malleoli

Malleoli that are enlarged with a callus formation can be caused by a previous fracture.

Lateral Calcaneal Exostosis (Pump Bump)

Lateral calcaneal exostosis is common in the overpronating

ASSESSMENT   INTERPRETATION

foot with a compensated subtalar varus foot and the resulting hypermobile foot.

Fifth Metatarsophalangeal Exostosis (Tailor's Bunion)

Fifth metatarsophalangeal exostosis is commonly the result of a fallen metatarsal arch in the pronated foot and is common in individuals with hallux valgus deformities in which the bunion increases the width of the foot and the fifth toe then rubs on the shoe.

Talar Exostosis
- Anterior
- Posterior

Anterior talar exostosis is a dorsal spur on the neck of the talus. It can cause impingement problems when the talar neck impinges on the anterior lip of the tibia during forced or repeated dorsiflexion—soft-tissue (i.e., capsule, extensor tendons) or boney damage can result. This is common in the high-arched cavus foot. This exostosis can restrict midfoot movements and can rub in the shoe or skate, causing pain. Posterior talar exostosis is an enlargement of the posterior lateral tubercle of the talus or an os trigonum. Posterior impingement can occur between this talar tubercle or os trigonum and the posterior inferior surface of the tibia with excessive or forced plantar flexion (Fig. 4-11) (i.e., ballet en pointe position, soccer player with frequent kicking, basketball player with jumping). It can result in soft-tissue or boney damage (i.e., flexor hallucis tenosynovitis, synovium capsule).

First Metatarsal-Cuneiform Exostosis (Fig. 4-16)

First metatarsal-cuneiform exostosis develops from excess force going through the first metatarsal head. This exostosis can restrict forefoot movements and also can rub in the shoe or skate.

Os Navicularis

This extra bone may cause the tibialis posterior to attach to the medial side of the foot and therefore not support the longitudinal arch, which therefore can lead to overpronation problems. This prominent bone can also cause problems when it rubs on the inside of the shoe, skate, or boot. If the bone is attached to

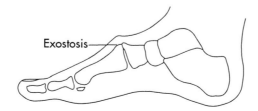

Fig. 4-16 First metatarsal-cuneiform exostosis.

ASSESSMENT

INTERPRETATION

the navicular it can be avulsed with a violent contraction of the tibialis posterior or from repeated trauma. An overlying callus or bursa can develop.

Posterior View
Pelvis
- Level of the pelvis, iliac crest, and posterior superior iliac spines
- Muscular symmetry
- Gluteal, calf, and hamstring development symmetry

The pelvis, iliac crest, and posterior superior iliac spines should be level and symmetrical. Any difference in the level of the pelvis from one side to the other can indicate a leg-length difference, a pelvic rotation, or a pelvic shift upward or downward.

These asymmetries can lead to altered forces through the entire quadrant.

Atrophy of the gluteal, hamstring, and calf musculature on one side can indicate an S1 nerve root irritation. Atrophy of the gluteals or hamstrings can indicate hip or knee dysfunction or a local muscle or nerve injury. Atrophy of the calf can indicate a local nerve or muscle injury or dysfunction at the ankle joint.

Ankle

SUBTALAR VARUS (INVERTED CALCANEUS)

Subtalar varus can be associated with a fixed cavus foot (uncompensated subtalar varus) or a pronating foot with gait (compensated subtalar varus); to determine if it is compensated or not requires observing the athlete's gait.

SUBTALAR VALGUS (EVERTED CALCANEUS)(FIG. 4-17)

Subtalar valgus usually causes overpronation problems; if severe, the foot may already be fully pronated (pes planus).

ACHILLES TENDON ALIGNMENT

An uncompensated subtalar varus position will cause the Achilles tendon to bow, which will result in a shortened or tight gastrocnemius/soleus complex that, in turn, can pull the calca-

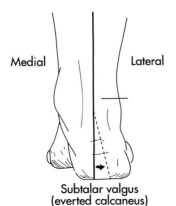

Medial   Lateral

Subtalar valgus
(everted calcaneus)

Fig. 4-17 Posterior aspect of the right ankle.

ASSESSMENT

INTERPRETATION

neus upward and stress the plantar fascia. The Achilles tendon will be susceptible to strain or tendonitis and the plantar fascia will be susceptible to fasciitis. When the athlete runs, the Achilles tendon will not track up and down in a straight line but will work over the calcaneus at an angle. This can also result in Achilles tendonitis.

ACHILLES TENDON ENLARGEMENT

Achilles tendon enlargement suggests present or previous Achilles tendonitis, strain, or partial tear.

INTRACAPSULAR SWELLING

Intracapsular swelling causes swelling on both sides of the ankle joint, under the malleolus. This swelling within the capsule indicates a significant sprain or even fracture. If the swelling developed immediately after injury, the swelling is a hemarthrosis and is caused by damage to a structure within the joint with a rich blood supply. Gradual swelling in the capsule usually indicates a synovitis type swelling with less severe damage.

EXTRACAPSULAR SWELLING

Extracapsular swelling causes swelling on one side of the ankle only—under the malleolus (usually lateral) because of the higher incidence of inversion sprains. This swelling is usually caused by soft-tissue damage outside the joint capsule. Ligamentous, tendinous, or muscular damage can cause this localized swelling.

ACHILLES BURSA SWELLING

Superficial retrocalcaneal or posterior calcaneus bursitis occurs between the tendon and the skin, usually from poorly fitting shoes. Deeper swelling between the tendon and calcaneus suggests a deep retrocalcaneal bursitis, which is more severe and has various overuse causes.

SWELLING AROUND THE CALCANEUS

Swelling that causes a wider calcaneus and swelling under both malleoli can be caused by a calcaneal fracture or apophysitis in the young athlete.

RIGID PES PLANUS (FLAT FOOT)

According to Percy and Mann, rigid pes planus can be caused by a tarsal coalition. The calcaneus has excessive valgus associated with forefoot abduction and there may also be peroneal shortening or spasm. The most common site of these conditions, as reported in the literature, are the calcaneonavicular and the talocalcaneal joints, and, less commonly, the talonavicular joint (Percy and Mann; Elkus; Olney and Asher; Scranton).

ASSESSMENT

INTERPRETATION

Nonweight-bearing

Ask the athlete to sit down.

It is important to observe the foot and ankle in nonweight-bearing situations to see the structure of the joints when there is no weight through them.

Foot and Ankle
Plantar Aspect of the Foot (Fig. 4-18)
- Calluses, blisters
- Corns
- Plantar warts
- Tight plantar fascia
- Nodes in the fascia

In the normal foot the skin should be thicker at the heel. The presence of blisters, calluses, and corns indicates a mechanical dysfunction with excessive pressure or friction. Calluses (plantar keratosis) are protective and develop in response to repetitive mechanical stress. They often develop under the stressed second metatarsal with Morton's foot or hallux valgus. Calluses under the third, fourth, or fifth metatarsal show excess weight through this area in the uncompensated subtalar varus or forefoot varus foot. Calluses on the lateral side of the foot can indicate an uncompensated subtalar varus foot. Calluses develop under the transverse metatarsal arch when it collapses or in a high-arched cavus foot with claw toes. Calluses develop on the medial border of the great toe if hallux valgus exists because the weight rolls off the toe on that angle. Coin-shaped circular calluses develop in the high-arched cavus foot from direct force through the rigid foot. Long calluses develop in the pronating foot because when the foot pronates it lengthens and the stress moves with the lengthening of the foot. Soft corns (hyperkeratosis) develop interdigitally and often occur between the fourth and fifth toe. Tight footwear is the chief cause. A short fifth toe will result in extra force between it and the fourth toe resulting in a corn formation. Plantar warts (verrucae plantaris) are caused by papovavirus and are associated with areas of mechanical stress. A tight plantar fascia can lead to plantar fasciitis or even Achilles tendonitis. Pea-sized nodes in the fascia can suggest the presence of Dupuytren's contracture.

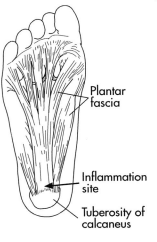

Plantar fascia

Inflammation site

Tuberosity of calcaneus

Fig. 4-18 Plantar aspect of the foot showing plantar fascia.

ASSESSMENT

INTERPRETATION

Dorsum of the Foot
- Tendons
- Skin color and its changes: red rubor or cyanosis with changes in elevation or weight-bearing

If the extensor tendons are prominent they may be tight, which suggests a muscle imbalance between the flexors and extensors.

Skin color and changes indicate the presence of circulatory or neural problems. If the foot color becomes red or blue (cyanotic) when lowered, there may be small-vessel vascular disease or arterial insufficiency.

Longitudinal Arch of the Foot

If the longitudinal arch was depressed in a weight-bearing position, determine if it is still lower when in a nonweight-bearing position. If the arch is elevated in a nonweight-bearing position and depresses on weight-bearing, the athlete may have a compensated foot type that is over pronating during gait (see Prolonged Pronation Problems; Table 4-3). Does the longitudinal arch rise into a cavus position with the toes clawed mildly, moderately, or severely when in a nonweight-bearing position? Knowing the answer to this question can help determine the type of cavus foot that is being dealt with. If the toes stay clenched and the arch high in weight-bearing and nonweight-bearing positions, the athlete has a severe inflexible cavus deformity. If the arch lowers on weight-bearing, it is a flexible mild or moderate cavus foot (see Fixed Supination Problems; Table 4-4).

Metatarsal Arch (Fig. 4-19)

If the metatarsal arch is collapsed on weight-bearing and rises on nonweight-bearing, the architecture of the arch has not collapsed completely and restorative measures can be taken. All the metatarsal bones should be parallel to each other. A dropped metatarsal head should be looked for, since a callus and pain can develop under the dropped head because of the shearing forces.

First Ray
- Plantar flexed or dorsiflexed
- Rigid or flexible

Normally the first metatarsal should be parallel to the other metatarsal heads. If a problem exists the first ray may be plantar flexed or dorsiflexed (can be flexible or rigid). If it is plantar flexed and flexible, the weight-bearing forces are shifted to the second metatarsal during gait while the first ray will dorsiflex and invert. If it is plantar flexed and rigid, the first metatarsal will take the brunt of the force and may prevent the subtalar joint from achieving normal pronation during gait. Dorsiflexed,

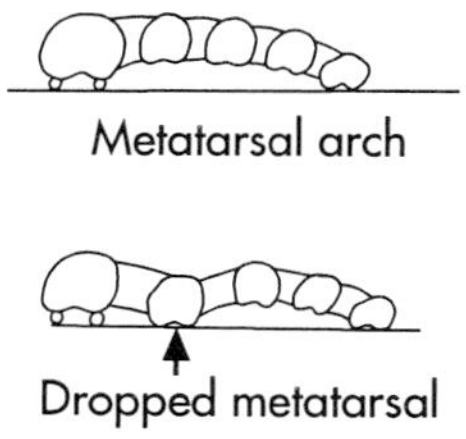

Metatarsal arch

Dropped metatarsal

Fig. 4-19 Metatarsal arch of the foot.

ASSESSMENT   INTERPRETATION

flexible, and rigid first rays will cause overpronation during gait. If the athlete has a degenerative arthrosis of the first metacarpophalangeal joint (hallux rigidus), then during weight-bearing the forces are shifted to the lateral side of the foot and up the lateral side of the limb.

Walking

Normal

Watch the lumbar spine, pelvis, and entire lower limb during the stance phase (heel strike, foot flat, midstance, push off) and the swing phase (acceleration, midswing, and deceleration). Look at the tibia, ankle, and foot specifically. Look for excessive tibial rotation, foot pronation, supination, forefoot collapse, and toe alignment during push off. Watch for antalgic gait and the degree of pain that exists—this will help determine what kind of functional testing needs to be done.

Stance Phase (Fig. 4-20)
Heel Strike

The calcaneus is inverted to an angle of 2° to 4° of varus dur-

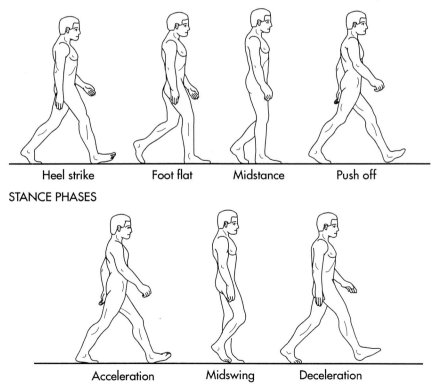

| Heel strike | Foot flat | Midstance | Push off |

STANCE PHASES

| Acceleration | Midswing | Deceleration |

SWING PHASES

Fig. 4-20 Walking phases or gait.

ASSESSMENT

INTERPRETATION

ing heel strike. The subtalar and midtarsal joints are supinated at heel strike and start to move toward pronation. The tibia, talus, and calcaneus must be aligned to absorb the vertical force (80% of the body weight). The ankle dorsiflexors contract eccentrically to lower the foot to the ground and to control the amount of pronation. The knee moves into slight flexion to absorb the body weight. The hip extensors and lateral rotators contract to move the body forward and to stabilize the hip and pelvis.

Foot Flat

The tibia medially rotates to allow the subtalar joint to pronate, the talocrural joint continues to dorsiflex, and the talus rolls medially (plantar flexes and adducts) to fully articulate with the medial facet of the calcaneus. This rotation has been described as the "torque converter" for the medial rotation of the entire lower limb. The midtarsal joint, which consists of the talonavicular and the calcaneocuboid articulations, unlocks when the subtalar joint pronates. The longitudinal arch depresses, the cuboid and the navicular alignment become more parallel (allowing the forefoot to release), and the forefoot becomes mobile, absorbs shock, and accommodates to the terrain.

Midstance

In midstance, the knee moves into extension, the tibia rotates laterally, the subtalar joint supinates (the calcaneus inverts), and the midtarsal joints lock to make the foot a rigid lever with which to push off. The midtarsal joint, the cuboid, and the navicular set up a pulley system for the peroneus longus and tibialis posterior. These muscles pull the foot up into a close-packed position and stabilize the first ray to allow the hallux to dorsiflex before push off.

The abductor digiti minimi, flexor hallucis brevis, flexor digitorum brevis, abductor hallucis brevis, dorsal interossei, and the extensor digitorum brevis all contract during midstance and push off for stabilization of the midtarsal joints.

Heel Rise and Push Off

The resupination of the foot as the athlete pushes off is not an active movement but is initiated by the lower limb lateral (external) rotation. The lateral rotation of the tibia causes subtalar supination (calcaneal inversion). The talus is pushed into a lateral position (abducted and dorsiflexed). The cuboid and navicular bones move more perpendicular, causing the midtarsal joints to lock up. These bones now act as rigid levers for the peroneus longus and tibialis posterior muscles. These muscles also stabilize the first ray for push off. When the foot starts to push off, the toes extend and the aponeurosis, which wraps around the metatarsophalangeal joints, becomes taut, assisting in subtalar

ASSESSMENT

INTERPRETATION

supination (windlass effect). The increasing tension allows the aponeurosis to absorb a great deal more stress. The ankle plantar flexes to propel the body forward with the foot pushing straight backward. The hallux and toe metatarsophalangeal joints must be able to extend and even hyperextend to get the windlass effect and to allow an even push off. The first metatarsophalangeal joint's mobility influences this supination. The foot acts as a rigid lever.

Swing Phase
Acceleration, Midswing, Deceleration

The lower extremity is brought forward by the hip flexors while the knee is flexed, the ankle dorsiflexed, and the metatarsophalangeal joints extend. All these joints contract to allow the foot to clear the ground.

Problems
Stride Length
Stride length is determined by measuring the distance from the heel strike of one limb until the heel strike of the same limb.

The average stride length should be the same bilaterally. Stride length varies according to the athlete's leg length, height, age, and sex. With low back or limb pain or fatigue, the stride length may decrease.

Step Length (Fig. 4-21)
Step length is the linear distance between two successive points of contact of opposite limbs. It is usually measured from heel strike of one foot to heel strike of the opposite foot.

Step length measurement is used to analyze gait symmetry. The more equal the step length, the more the gait symmetry and, usually, the less the lower limb dysfunction.

Degree of Toe Out
The degree of toe out is determined by the angle of foot placement. The angle can be measured by drawing a line from the center of the heel to the second toe.

The angle of foot placement is normally 7° from the sagittal plane. An angle of toe out greater than 7° can cause the following:
- excessive pronation problems
- longitudinal arch collapse
- decreased stride length
- rotational torsion through the entire lower limb

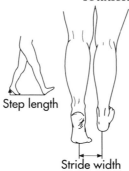

Step length

Stride width

Fig. 4-21 Gait.

ASSESSMENT

INTERPRETATION

Stride Width (Fig. 4-21)
Stride width is the distance from the midpoint of one heel to the midpoint of the opposite heel.

The width of the stride is usually 2 to 4 inches—the base is widened if the athlete has heavy thighs, balance or proprioception problems, or decreased sensation in the heel or sole of the foot.

Rhythm of the Gait
- Weight distribution
- Antalgic gait (limp)
- Ability to lock knee in midstance

Rhythm of the gait indicates the coordination between the limbs and the weight distribution on each limb. An antalgic gait occurs when the time spent on the injured limb is shortened because a structure in the lower quadrant is painful.

The knee should go into full extension and lock in midstance.

The upper body movements should be opposite to the lower limb movements and move smoothly in the sagittal plane. For example, the right arm swings forward as the left leg swings forward. Any swinging of the arm across the body increases the horizontal torque and results in lower limb compensatory rotation.

Heel Strike

To determine the lesion site, functional structure testing must be done before palpation and before a decision is reached on the possible condition. A shortened period of time or foot pain in heel strike usually indicates heel pain and can be caused by the following:
- calcaneal spur
- plantar fasciitis
- calcaneal periosteitis
- calcaneal apophysitis
- calcaneal medial entrapment problems

Foot Flat

Pain during the foot flat phase can be caused by an anterior compartment syndrome or a dorsiflexor muscle strain (tibialis anterior, extensor digitorum brevis).

Midstance

Shortened time in midstance with foot pain can be caused by an injury to any of the foot or ankle joints (talocrural, subtalar, midtarsal, metatarsal) or an injury to any of the bones or soft tissue of the foot or ankle.

PROLONGED PRONATION DURING MIDSTANCE

The time spent in pronation and supination is important—pronation should take 33% and supination 67% of the time. An athlete who pronates for more than 50% of the stance phase is an abnormal pronator, according to Donatelli. If the resupination is too late, pronation problems can also develop. Prolonged subtalar pronation without supination at the end of midstance

ASSESSMENT

INTERPRETATION

can cause overpronation conditions in the foot and ankle (see Prolonged Pronation Problems; Table 4-3). The first ray (first metatarsal and first cuneiform) needs to be stable for normal resupination to be possible—this ray is stabilized by the peroneals and the tibialis posterior. These muscles rely on stable bones to operate as pulleys. If the subtalar joint does not resupinate and lock the cuboid and navicular in place, these muscles cannot stabilize the first ray.

NO PRONATION DURING MIDSTANCE

No pronation in the midstance (or if the subtalar joint remains supinated throughout the gait) can cause supinatory conditions in the foot and ankle. These include peroneal tendonitis and fifth metatarsal and fibular stress fractures (see Fixed Supination).

Heel Rise

The heel rise time should be carefully observed. Normally the heel rise should occur just as the opposite leg swings by the stance leg. If the triceps surae is tight the heel rise will occur prematurely, leading to excessive forces through the forefoot. If the heel rise is delayed, there may be a triceps surae weakness or previous rupture.

Push Off

Uneven forces on push off can occur when forefoot valgus, forefoot varus, or hallux valgus is present. Pressing mainly through just the first toe can cause sesamoiditis or calluses. Pushing the foot at an increased toe-out angle-abducted causes shearing forces under the metatarsal heads. These can cause the following:
- calluses
- metatarsalgia
- forefoot sprains
- transverse arch collapse

If the athlete is unable to push off with the plantar flexors it may be because of the following:
- gastrocnemius or soleus muscle strain or tear
- S1 nerve root irritation (L5, S1 disc herniation)
- Achilles tendon rupture
- Achilles tendonitis

If the athlete is not able to hyperextend (dorsiflex) the forefoot or toes during the late phases of push off, it may be because of the following:
- plantar fasciitis
- metatarsophalangeal joint sprain or tear
- metatarsal flexor strain
- hallux rigidus

ASSESSMENT   INTERPRETATION

Swing Phase Problems
- Acceleration
- Midswing
- Deceleration

Any injury to the anterior tibial group or toe extensors will cause pain as the ankle and foot are dorsiflexed to clear the ground. There are rarely any injuries during the swing phase because there are no weight-bearing forces through the lower limb.

Running

If the athlete is a runner with an overuse condition, observing the running is important. Look at the entire lower quadrant. Look for overpronation, no supination, lower leg rotation, and foot and toe alignment. Look for upper body and upper extremity rotation.

Stance Phase Problems in Runners
Prolonged Pronation

During running gait, pronation problems that were not present during normal walking gait may show up. The extra body weight and force can cause longitudinal arch collapse.

No Supination

If the subtalar joint stays supinated the lack of shock absorption can cause overuse problems (see Fixed Supination Problems; Table 4-4).

Rotation

Good mechanics in running allow the knee and talocrural joint to function mainly in the sagittal plane without rotation. If the lower leg kicks outward to the side during the swing phase or if the foot, pelvis, or upper body rotate, rotational forces can cause overuse problems.

Footwear (Fig. 4-22)

Upper

With excessive pronation the upper of the shoe will bend medially; with supination the upper will bend laterally. If there is excessive wear in the upper, it will no longer give the necessary support and can even lead to overuse problems.

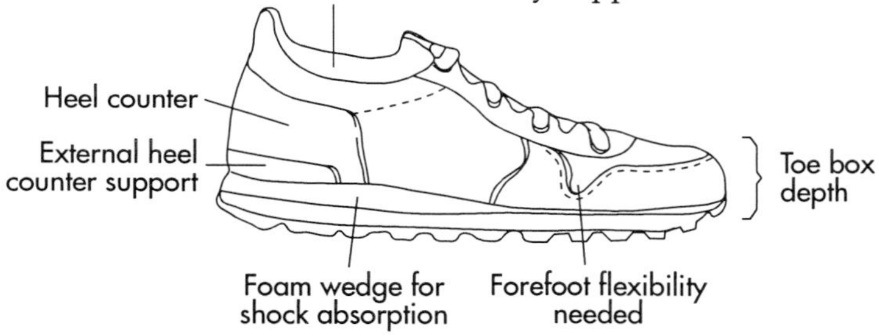

Padded collar

Heel counter

External heel counter support

Foam wedge for shock absorption

Forefoot flexibility needed

Toe box depth

Fig. 4-22 The athletic shoe.

ASSESSMENT   INTERPRETATION

Sole

The lateral edge of the sole of the heel should be slightly worn, as should the sole under the metatarsal heads. If it is too worn, the shock-absorbing properties of the shoe may be lost. A wear bar under the metatarsal heads indicates a rotation of the foot prior to take off.

Heel Counter

If the heel counter is too loose, it can no longer support the subtalar joint and may allow overpronation. If it is too tight, it can cause blisters and problems of skin abrasion.

Toe Box

If the toe box is creased on an angle, hallux rigidis may be the cause; if it is inflexible, it can cause midfoot problems. The shoe must flex at the metatarsophalangeal joints of the toes. If the toe box is too narrow, problems can develop between the toes. If the tip of the toe box is worn, the athlete may not have full dorsiflexion to allow the foot to clear the ground.

Arch Support

An arch support is needed for good shock absorption and the shoe's arch should fit correctly under the athlete's longitudinal arch.

Heel

Running in a shoe with excess wear on the lateral side of the shoe's heel can increase the chance of ankle sprain, Achilles tendonitis, and peroneal tendonitis. Wear medially on the heel of the shoe is a sign of calcaneal valgus problems and overpronation. According to Nigg and Morlock, an increased lateral heel flare can increase the amount of initial pronation by as much as 40%; therefore the authors conclude that shoes without a heel flare could be used to reduce the initial pronation during running to help prevent overuse injuries.

Last (Curved or Straight)

A curved last shoe is best for a rigid cavus foot; a straight last shoe is better for supporting the overpronating foot.

Flexibility

Lightweight flexible shoes must have enough support to help support the arches of the foot and stabilize the subtalar joint. Shoes that are too flexible may permit hyperextension injuries to the metatarsophalangeal joints.

FUNCTIONAL TESTING

General ankle and foot movements involve combinations of

ASSESSMENT	INTERPRETATION

movements:
- ankle movements (talocrural)—plantar flexion, dorsiflexion
- subtalar movements—inversion, eversion
- midtarsal movements—forefoot adduction, abduction
- toe motion—flexion, extension

SUMMARY OF TESTS

Rule Out
  Inflammatory Disorders
  Lumbar Spine
  Knee Joint
  Superior Tibiofibular Joint
  Fracture

Tests in Long Sitting
  Active talocrural plantar flexion
  Passive talocrural plantar flexion
  Active talocrural dorsiflexion
  Passive talocrural dorsiflexion (knee extended and knee flexed)
  Resisted talocrural dorsiflexion
  Active subtalar inversion
  Passive subtalar inversion
  Passive plantar flexion and subtalar inversion
  Passive dorsiflexion and subtalar inversion
  Resisted subtalar inversion
  Active subtalar eversion
  Passive subtalar eversion
  Resisted subtalar eversion
  Resisted talocrural plantar flexion
  Active toe flexion
  Great toe (Hallux) flexion and extension
  Passive toe flexion (I to V)
  Resisted toe flexion (I to V)
  Active toe extension (I to V)
  Passive toe extension (I to V)
  Resisted toe extension (I to V)

Special Tests
  Drawer sign
  Posterior talofibular ligament test (Lapenskie)
  Talar tilt
  Wedge test
  Inferior tibiofibular joint stability test (Lapenskie)
  Anterolateral subluxation of the talus (Lapenskie)
  Subtalar joint irritation (Lapenskie)
  Homan's sign
  Thompson Test (Achilles tendon rupture)

ASSESSMENT   INTERPRETATION

Longitudinal arch mobility tests
  Toe raise
  Squat
  Legs-crossed weight transfer
Standing superior tibiofibular mobility (Lapenskie)
Mobility of the tibia and fibula around the X-axis (Lapenskie)
Swelling measurements
Longitudinal arch height measurement (Feiss line)
Proprioception testing
Neurological scan
  Dermatomes
  Cutaneous nerve supply
  Achilles tendon reflex
Circulatory scan
  Posterior tibial artery
  Dorsal pedis artery

Biomechanical Analysis
Nonweight-bearing
  Talocrural joint range
  Subtalar joint range
  Midtarsal relation of forefoot to hindfoot
  Mobility of first ray

Weight-bearing
  Tibial Varum
  Talocrural joint
  Subtalar joint
    Compensated subtalar varus
    Uncompensated subtalar varus
    Subtalar valgus
  Forefoot
    Compensated forefoot varus
    Uncompensated forefoot varus
    Uncompensated forefoot valgus
    Compensated forefoot valgus

Accessory Movement Tests
  Superior tibiofibular joint
    Anterior-posterior glide
  Inferior tibiofibular joint
    Anterior-posterior glide
    Superior-inferior glide
  Talocrural joint
    Posterior glide of tibia on talus
    Anterior glide of talus on tibia
  Subtalar joint
    Distraction
    Distraction with passive inversion and eversion

ASSESSMENT   INTERPRETATION

Calcaneotalar dorsal rock
Calcaneoplantar rock
Midtarsal and tarsometatarsal joints
Dorsal-plantar midtarsal glide
Dorsal-plantar tarsometatarsal glide
Tarsometatarsal rotation
Metatarsophalangeal, proximal interphalangeal, and distal interphalangeal joints

Rule Out

Inflammatory Disorders

Test for inflammatory disorders if any of the following are true:
- insidious onset of pain
- other joints or joints bilaterally are painful
- athlete feels unhealthy or overly fatigued
- athlete experiences repeated joint discomfort without a predisposing cause

Test the joints as usual, but if you suspect an inflammatory disorder, refer the athlete to his or her family physician for a complete check-up, including x-rays and blood work.
- Rheumatoid arthritis
- Reiter disease
- Psoriatic arthritis
- Ankylosing spondylitis
- Gouty arthritis

Rheumatoid arthritis can be initially present with subtalar and talocrural pain in 15% to 30% of the population. Erosion can occur to the posterior aspect of the calcaneus.

Reiter disease can cause conjunctivitis, arthritis, and foot and ankle pain.

Psoriatic arthritis can cause foot and ankle pain, especially on the posterior aspect of the calcaneus and into the plantar fascia.

Ankylosing spondylitis can also cause foot or ankle pain but this usually appears in the sacroiliac joints first.

Gouty arthritis can cause discomfort in the first metatarsophalangeal joint and occasionally in the ankle or talar joints.

Lumbar Spine

Test the lumbar spine if the following are true:
- history includes low-back symptoms
- athlete indicates an insidious onset of symptoms
- sensations felt in the lower leg, foot, or ankle include numbness or tingling (especially if these sensations are within a specific dermatome area)
- history suggests low-back involvement and the observations indicate lumbar lordosis, myotome atrophy, or multiple lower limb joint dysfunction

Lumbar spine nerve-root irritation can cause myotome and dermatome problems into the lower extremity.

ASSESSMENT

INTERPRETATION

The athlete actively forward bends, backward bends, side bends right and left, and rotates right and left (with you stabilizing the athlete's pelvis). If any of these movements are limited or elicit pain in the lumbar spine or lower extremity, a full lumbar assessment should be carried out (see Lumbar Assessment).

Myotomes (Gray's Anatomy)

- L4 can cause weakness with ankle dorsiflexion.
- L5 can cause weakness with great toe extension.
- S1 can cause weakness with ankle plantar flexion and eversion.
- S2 can cause weakness with toe flexion.

Dermatomes (Gray's Anatomy)

- L4 affects skin sensation over the dorsal medial surface of the tibia and the plantar and dorsal surface of the foot and great toe.
- L5 affects the skin sensations over the dorsal lateral surface of the tibial area and the plantar and dorsal surface of the foot and middle three toes.
- S1 affects the skin sensations on the plantar and dorsal surface of the lateral ankle and foot.
- S2 affects the skin sensations on the posterior surface of the upper tibial area.

Knee Joint

Test the knee joint if the history includes knee symptoms, knee surgery or pain referred from the knee. Test the active ranges of motion of the knee joint. The athlete flexes and extends the knee joint actively through the full range of motion. Apply an overpressure in flexion and extension at the end of the range of motion. If these movements are limited or elicit pain in the knee or down the leg, foot, or ankle, a full knee assessment is necessary (see Knee Assessment).

Because the gastrocnemius works over the knee and ankle joint, it should be tested for knee involvement. Weakness or pain in the gastrocnemii during active knee flexion and a decreased range of motion with terminal extension may demonstrate a muscle strain, a partial tear, or an Achilles tendon problem. Ankle and/or foot pain can be referred from the knee and therefore it must be ruled out.

Superior Tibiofibular Joint

Test this joint if the history or your observations suggest that the superior tibiofibular joint or the peroneal nerve at this location is involved.

An injury to the superior tibiofibular joint can limit fibular movement, which will limit talocrural dorsiflexion and plantar flexion and can cause ankle joint dysfunction. During plantar flexion, the fibula moves inferiorly, laterally, and anteriorly.

ASSESSMENT

INTERPRETATION

Rule out this joint through your history-taking and observations.

Rule out this joint with passive anterior and posterior glides and superior and inferior glides of the fibula on the tibia.

During dorsiflexion, the fibula moves superiorly, medially, and posteriorly.

If the fibula is fixed superiorly, the foot and ankle may accommodate by allowing overpronation. If the fibula is fixed inferiorly, the foot and ankle may not be able to pronate and will stay in a supinated position.

A direct blow or fibular subluxation can injure the peroneal nerve with resulting neural problems extending into the ankle and foot.

Fracture

Test for a fracture if in the history a fracture is suspected (i.e., forced eversion) or your observations show deformity, then do the following fracture tests and do not carry out any further functional tests. Tap the involved bone along its length but not over the fracture site; i.e., tap the head and shaft of the fibula if a lateral malleolus fracture is suspected. Gently palpate the suspected fracture site for specific boney point tenderness or deformity.

If a fracture is suspected the athlete should be immobilized and transported. Treat the athlete for shock and monitor pulses into the foot and ankle (posterior tibial and dorsal pedal arteries).

Suspect a fracture if the following are true:
- the mechanism indicated sufficient force
- athlete felt or indicated a fracture
- athlete is reluctant to move the neighboring joints
- tapping the bone above and below the suspected site elicits pain at the fracture site
- there is deformity in the boney or soft-tissue contours
- athlete shows signs of sympathetic involvement or shock such as sweating, paleness, or a rapid pulse.

Fracture tests
Fibula

Percuss the fibula at the lateral malleolus and the head of the fibula. If the athlete feels pain along the fibula, the bone may be fractured.

A varus force with one hand and a valgus force with the other, above and below the suspected fracture site, can also be done (gently). If there is an obvious fracture or deformity, this should not be done. Crepitus and local point tenderness indicate a positive test.

The fibula is often fractured or the tip avulsed from an inversion ankle sprain. This fracture test is imperative when any inversion sprain has occurred. Percussion sends vibrations along the fibula and pain occurs at the fracture site. Stressing the fracture site will cause pain and maybe crepitus.

Fractures through the lower fibula's growth plate should always be suspected in children. Children's ligaments are stronger than their epiphyseal plates.

The fibula is important to the stability of the ankle mortise. It can be fractured at, above, or below the joint line. Fractures above the joint line are very severe and unstable.

Tibia

Percuss the tibia anywhere along its length if a stress or other fracture is suspected.

A varus and valgus force can be gently applied above and below the suspected fracture site—this is not done if a fracture is obvious or if a deformity exists.

Crepitus and local point tenderness indicate a positive test.

Percussion and stress to the tibia will cause pain if there is a fracture. The tibia is occasionally fractured with an eversion sprain mechanism.

Stress fractures or periostitis can cause pain during this test. Tests for fractures through the lower tibial growth plate should be done in children.

ASSESSMENT

INTERPRETATION

Tibia and Fibula

Fractures of both bones at the ankle joint can occur. Often a major fracture of one bone causes a small avulsion fracture of the opposite malleolus.

Talus

Tap the calcaneus up into the talus if a fracture of the talus (or its dome) is suspected. Pain can indicate a fracture.

A talus fracture causes pain during this test, but pain may also be experienced with a sprain, joint effusion, or an injury to the inferior tibiofibular ligament.

Calcaneus

Percussing and compressing the calcaneus can reveal the presence of a calcaneal fracture or periostitis.

Percussion or calcaneal compression will cause pain if there is a fracture or periosteal contusion. Adolescents may have epiphyseal plate pain in the heel.

Tests in Long Sitting

Tests in long sitting are done with the athlete's feet over the end of the plinth.

Active Talocrural Plantar Flexion (50°) (Fig. 4-23)

Ask the athlete to actively plantar flex the ankle as far as possible.

Pain, weakness, or limitation of range of motion can be caused by an injury to the prime movers or to their nerve supply. The prime movers and their nerve supply are:
- Gastrocnemius—tibial N. (S1, S2)
- Soleus—tibial N. (S1, S2)

The accessory movers are:
- Tibialis posterior and peroneus longus and brevis (forefoot and ankle joint flexors and plantar flexors).
- Flexor hallucis longus and flexor digitorum longus (great toe flexor, forefoot flexors, and ankle joint plantar flexors).

Achilles or peroneal tendonitis may cause pain at the injury site during active movement. With a totally ruptured Achilles tendon the athlete can often still plantar flex because a few fibers

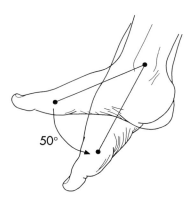

Fig. 4-23 Plantar flexion.

50°

ASSESSMENT

INTERPRETATION

of the soleus or gastrocnemius will fire, or because the plantaris, flexor hallucis longus, tibialis posterior, peroneus longus and brevis, and flexor digitorum are all intact and allow active plantar flexion to take place. The accessory muscles provide 15% to 30% of plantar flexion strength needed for push off during gait. Intracapsular and extracapsular ankle swelling can limit movement, especially if intracapsular fluid is present. Post-cast adhesions can also limit movement.

Passive Talocrural Plantar Flexion (50°)

Stabilize the subtalar joint by holding the calcaneus; the other hand holds the forefoot close to the talocrural joint. Invert the forefoot slightly to lock it into the hindfoot. The foot is plantar flexed through the full range of motion until an end feel is felt or movement is limited by pain. Do not force plantar flexion of the forefoot because midtarsal joint play may allow excessive range of motion.

There will be some joint play of the talus in full plantar flexion because the narrower posterior part of the talus is in the mortise. There is slight lateral mobility but excessive joint play should *not* exist. The passive range of motion may be limited and/or painful because of the following:
- tight or shortened ankle or foot dorsiflexors
- tight or adhesed anterior joint capsule
- an extra accessory bone (os trigonum or a steida process) located behind the talus above the calcaneus that limits plantar flexion when pinched in extreme plantar flexion
- intracapsular swelling
- extracapsular swelling
- anterior talofibular ligament sprain or tear
- posterior talofibular ligament sprain or tear
- tibialis anterior muscle tendonitis, strain, or tear
- tibialis posterior muscle tendonitis, strain, or tear
- extensor digitorum muscle tendonitis strain or tear
- sprain or tear of the anterior fibers of the deltoid ligament.

The end feel should be boney contact of the talus in the mortise or a soft-tissue stretch of the dorsiflexor muscles and the anterior fibers of the collateral ligaments.

Active Talocrural Dorsiflexion (20°) (Fig. 4-24)

Ask the athlete to actively dorsiflex the ankle through the full range of motion.

Pain, weakness, or limitation of range of motion can be caused by an injury to the prime movers or to their nerve supply. The prime movers and their nerve supply are the following:

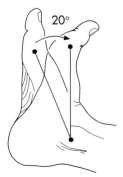

20°

Fig. 4-24 Dorsiflexion.

ASSESSMENT

INTERPRETATION

- Tibialis anterior—deep peroneal N. (L4, L5, S1)
- Extensor hallucis longus—deep peroneal N. (L4, L5, S1)
- Extensor digitorum longus—deep peroneal N. (L4, L5, S1)
- Peroneus tertius—superficial peroneal N. (L4, L5, S1)

Intermittent claudication after repeated dorsiflexion (such as after a long walk or run) from a tight anterior fascial compartment can cause an inability to actively dorsiflex the ankle. This anterior compartment syndrome can be very severe if it occurs from swelling. It can occur from a fracture, direct trauma, or from a cast that is too tight. Foot drop can occur if the peroneal nerve is damaged or if an L4 neurological problem exists.

Passive Talocrural Dorsiflexion (Knee Extended and Knee Flexed; 20°)

Stabilize the athlete's subtalar joint by holding the upper tibia and fibula with one hand while the other hand on the plantar aspect of the foot moves the foot into full dorsiflexion. Pressure is applied until an end feel is reached or until the athlete indicates pain. Perform this test with the athlete's knee flexed and then repeat it with the knee extended. Do not force the collapse of the forefoot to gain dorsiflexion range.

The passive range of motion may be limited and/or painful because of a tight gastrocnemius (when knee is extended during testing) or soleus (when knee is flexed during testing). This tight triceps surae may be attributable to an inherited talipes equinus or a functional talipes equinus. Moderate talipes equinus individuals are toe walkers and, to get the heel down, may cause a midtarsal collapse resulting in a pes planus or rocker-bottom foot. Functional talipes equinus develops in athletes (particularly sprinters who run on their toes) in which a muscle imbalance is created. Overwork of the plantar flexors without stretching them leads to shortening of this muscle group. If the dorsiflexors are not strengthened, a muscle imbalance can develop—this will limit passive dorsiflexion. The midstance of normal gait requires 10° of dorsiflexion; if 10° does not exist, the midtarsal joint collapses to get the necessary range of motion. This collapse will lead to subtalar pronation and its related pronation problems (see Prolonged Pronation Problems; Table 4-3). Passive talocrural dorsiflexion can also be limited by:

- gastrocnemii, soleus, or plantaris muscle strain or tear
- medial head of a gastrocnemius strain or rupture
- posterior joint capsule sprain or tear
- posterior talofibular ligament sprain or tear
- sprain or tear of the posterior fibers of the deltoid ligament
- intracapsular joint swelling
- posterior joint contracture
- the anterior inferior tibiofibular ligament can limit dorsiflexion when it is thickened because of previous injury (Bassett et al.)
- an anterior talar exostosis can limit full dorsiflexion as the talus abuts the tibia, which occurs in the high-arched cavus foot

If full dorsiflexion is restricted, metatarsalgia often develops in the forefoot.

Passive dorsiflexion at the end of range will open the mortise excessively if the ankle and tibiofibular diastasis is torn. This

ASSESSMENT

INTERPRETATION

may be missed, since the ankle joint will dislocate and spontaneously reduce. An x-ray will show a widened mortise.

The normal end feel is a soft-tissue stretch of the triceps surae or a capsular end feel if the triceps surae are flexible.

Resisted Talocrural Dorsiflexion (Fig. 4-25)

Resist with all four fingers against the athlete's proximal forefoot while the other hand stabilizes the tibia. The athlete attempts to dorsiflex his or her ankle. If dorsiflexion is weak, test inner, middle, and outer ranges. To determine which muscle is involved, test dorsiflexion with inversion (tests tibialis anterior)—the resisting hand should move medially. Also test dorsiflexion with eversion (test peroneus tertius)—the resisting hand should move laterally.

Normal dorsiflexion can easily overcome your resistance. Weakness, pain, or limitation of range of motion can be caused by:

- injury to the prime movers or their nerve supply (see Active Talocrural Dorsiflexion)
- L4 nerve root injury
- tibialis anterior tendonitis—pain develops where it crosses the tibia or the ankle joint
- tibialis anterior periosteitis (shin splints)—pain develops where it originates on the tibia
- anterior compartment syndrome problems
- extensor digitorum longus tendonitis, especially in race walkers and backstroke swimmers (flutter kick)

Dorsiflexion with inversion weakness or pain suggests a tibialis anterior problem. Dorsiflexion with eversion weakness or pain suggests a peroneus tertius problem.

Active Subtalar Inversion (Fig. 4-26)

Stabilize the athlete's tibia and describe the inversion mechanism to the athlete—you may need to move the joint to show the athlete the action in the first attempt. Then ask the athlete to actively invert the foot as far as possible.

This is a subtalar movement but the talocalcaneal, talonavicular, and calcaneocuboid joints all assist in the movement. Pain, weakness, or limitation of range of motion can be caused by an injury to the prime movers or to their nerve supply. The prime movers and their nerve supply are:

- Tibialis anterior—deep peroneal N. (L4, L5, S1)
- Tibialis posterior—tibial N. (L5, S1)

The accessory movers are:

- Flexor digitorum longus
- Flexor hallucis longus
- Extensor hallucis longus

A peroneal tendonitis or lateral ankle sprain may cause pain when on stretch at the end of active range of motion. Subtalar joint swelling can limit active range of motion.

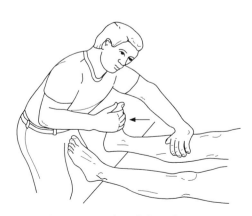

Fig. 4-25 Resisted dorsiflexion.

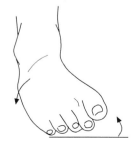

Fig. 4-26 Active subtalar inversion.

ASSESSMENT   INTERPRETATION

Passive Subtalar Inversion (Talocrural Joint in Neutral)

This must be done very gently. If an inversion sprain is suspected, this test should be performed at the end of the assessment. Have one hand on the athlete's tibia while the other hand gently swings the calcaneus into inversion until an end feel is reached or until the movement is limited by pain.

The passive range of motion may be limited and/or painful because of the following:
- anterior talofibular ligament sprain or tear
- lateral capsule sprain or tear
- subtalar joint effusion
- calcaneal fracture
- calcaneofibular ligament sprain or tear
- bifurcate ligament sprain or tear (the calcaneocuboid part)
- peroneal tendonitis
- fracture of the fifth metatarsal

There should be a boney end feel with contact of the sustentaculum tali and the posterior medial portion of the talus. There may be a soft-tissue stretch of the peroneals and capsular stretch of the lateral ligaments.

Passive Plantar Flexion and Subtalar Inversion (Fig. 4-27)

If an inversion sprain is suspected, this test should be performed at the end of the assessment. Stabilize the lower tibia with one hand while the other hand swings the foot into inversion and plantar flexion until an end feel is reached or the movement is limited by pain.

Passive plantar flexion and subtalar inversion tests the anterolateral structures of the subtalar joint and ankle joint. The passive range of motion may be limited and/or painful because of the following:
- anterior capsule sprain or tear
- anterior talofibular ligament sprain or tear
- calcaneocuboid ligament sprain or tear
- extensor digitorum longus or brevis strain or tear
- peroneal tendonitis or strain

Passive Dorsiflexion and Subtalar Inversion (Fig. 4-28)

Perform this test at the end of the assessment if you suspect a lateral ankle sprain. Stabilize the lower tibia with one hand while the other hand dorsi

Passive dorsiflexion and subtalar inversion tests the posterolateral structures of the subtalar joint and the ankle joint. The passive range of motion may be limited and/or painful because of the following:

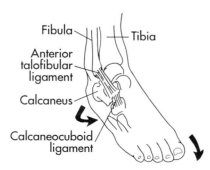

Fig. 4-27 Passive plantar flexion and inversion stress to the anterolateral structures.

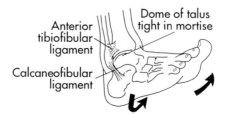

Fig. 4-28 Passive dorsiflexion and inversion stress to the posterolateral structures.

ASSESSMENT

INTERPRETATION

flexes and inverts the foot until an end feel is reached or the movement is limited by pain.

- calcaneofibular ligament sprain or tear
- posterior talofibular ligament sprain or tear
- osteochondral dome of talus lesion
- anterior and posterior tibiofibular ligament sprain or tear
- fibular stress fracture
- lateral malleolus fracture

Resisted Subtalar Inversion

The athlete is in the supine position with feet over the end of the plinth. The athlete attempts to invert his or her foot. Resist inversion with one hand beside the length of the foot while the other hand rests on the tibia and supports the talocrural joint.

This test can be done in plantar flexion or dorsiflexion to isolate the tibialis posterior or anterior respectively.

Pain or weakness can be caused by an injury to the muscle or to its nerve supply (see Active Subtalar Inversion). Tibialis posterior tendonitis or deep posterior compartment syndrome can occur from overpronation, overuse, or direct trauma and will be painful with this resisted test. Plantar flexion and inversion tests the tibialis posterior; dorsiflexion and inversion tests the tibialis anterior.

Active Subtalar Eversion (Fig. 4-29)

Ask the athlete to evert the foot fully. You may have to move the athlete's uninjured foot passively through eversion to show the athlete the correct action. The athlete then repeats it actively.

Pain, weakness, or limitation of range of motion can be caused by an injury to the prime movers or to their nerve supply. The prime movers are:
- Peroneus longus—superficial peroneal N. (L4, L5, S1)
- Peroneus brevis—superficial peroneal N. (L4, L5, S1)
The accessory movers are:
- Peroneus tertius
- Extensor digitorum longus
Active subtalar eversion can be limited by joint swelling.

Passive Subtalar Eversion

Passive subtalar eversion must be done last if an eversion sprain is suspected. It need not be done at all if a fracture is suspected (the incidence of fractures with eversion sprains is high).

The passive range of motion may be limited and/or painful because of an injury to any of the following:
- invertors (tibialis anterior, tibialis posterior, flexor digitorum longus, flexor hallucis longus, and extensor hallucis longus)

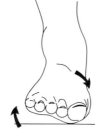

Fig. 4-29 Active subtalar eversion.

ASSESSMENT

One hand stabilizes just above the athlete's talocrural joint while the other hand everts the joint through the full range of motion until an end feel is reached or until pain limits range of motion.

Resisted Subtalar Eversion

The athlete should be in the supine position with his or her feet over the end of the plinth. The athlete attempts to evert the foot. Resist eversion with the ankle in neutral position (midposition between plantar flexion and dorsiflexion). Stabilize the athlete's tibia with one hand while the other hand resists the lateral border of the foot. Resist the foot downward and inward.

Resisted Talocrural Plantar Flexion

The athlete with a significant injury who is nonweight-bearing can be tested manually, but once the athlete can weight-bear the resisted test for plantar flexion must be done while the athlete is standing.

Manual Resistance

Place one hand on the athlete's tibia while the other forearm resists the length of the foot. This test should be done with the athlete's knee flexed and extended.

INTERPRETATION

- deltoid ligament sprain or tear
- bifurcate ligament sprain (calcaneonavicular part)

The normal end feel is boney, with the lateral articular process of the talus into the anterior lateral process of the calcaneus.

Pain and/or weakness can be caused by the following:
- injury to the muscle or to its nerve supply (see Active Subtalar Eversion)
- tendonitis in the peroneal muscles, which can occur anywhere from the lower fibula to the cuboid and fifth metatarsal base (the most common site is behind the lateral malleolus)
- peroneal tendon subluxations that may slip out of their groove behind the lateral malleolus from one traumatic incident or from a gradual onset—this often occurs with the ankle in a plantar flexed position with a sudden inversion or forefoot twist
- Chronic subluxing peroneal tendons that give rise to a "snapping ankle," usually not painful or disabling when the tendons slip forward over the malleolus.

Weakness of the peroneals can be caused by the following:
- disc protrusion at the fifth lumbar level with nerve root irritation
- repeated ankle sprains
- peroneal strains, partial tears, or tendonitis
- lateral compartment syndrome from peroneal overuse or trauma

Any weakness in the peroneals makes the ankle more susceptible to inversion sprains.

ASSESSMENT

INTERPRETATION

Functional Resistance (Fig. 4-30)

The athlete uses one finger on the plinth top for balance, then goes up and down on the toes of each foot 20 times (if possible). This may be repeated with the knee flexed.

Resistance with a flexed knee tests the soleus muscle, and resistance with the knee extended tests the gastrocnemii muscles. In weight-bearing, 15 to 20 repetitions is normal. Weakness and/or pain can be caused by an injury to the muscle or to its nerve supply (see Active Talocrural Plantar Flexion). A peroneal strain or subluxation problem can also cause pain and weakness when toe raises are performed. Rupture of the Achilles tendon will reveal gross weakness with or without pain with resisted manual plantar flexion. The athlete can walk despite a ruptured Achilles because plantaris, flexor hallucis longus, flexor digitorum longus, and the intrinsics of the foot can plantar flex. The athlete's gait will be altered, with a very flat foot throughout the stance phase. A plantaris rupture or medial gastrocnemius strain (tennis leg) will also cause pain and maybe weakness when heel raises are performed. Pain can also come from tibialis posterior or flexor hallucis longus lesions when heel raises are performed.

Common causes of weakness without pain include the following:

- L5 disc herniation or protrusion that causes an S1, S2 nerve root irritation
- damage to the tibial nerve
- direct contusion to the sciatic nerve

A superficial posterior compartment (gastrocnemius, soleus) trauma or overuse syndrome will also cause weakness here.

Active Toe Flexion (Fig. 4-31)

Ask the athlete to flex his or her toes fully while you hold the foot proximal to the metatarsophalangeal joints.

Pain, weakness, or limitation of range of motion can be caused by an injury to the prime movers or to their nerve supply. The prime movers of the great toe (I) are:

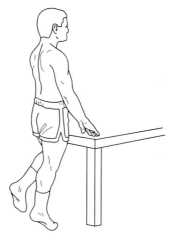

Fig. 4-30 Resisted talocrural plantar flexion.

ASSESSMENT   INTERPRETATION

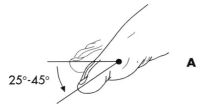

25°-45°

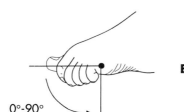

0°-90°

Fig. 4-31 Active great toe flexion. **A,** M.P. flexion. **B,** I.P. flexion.

The great toe (I) flexion range of motion is 45° at the MP joint and 90° at the IP joint. In toes II through V the flexion range of motion is 40° at the MP joint, 35° at the PIP joint, and 60° at the DIP joint.

- Flexor hallucis brevis—tibial N. (L4, L5, S1)
- Flexor hallucis longus—tibial N. (L5, S1, S2)

The prime movers of the toes II to V are:

- Flexor digitorum brevis—tibial N. (L4, L5, S1)
- Flexor digitorum longus—tibial N. (L5, S1)
- Quadratus plantae—tibial N. (S1, S2)
- Lumbrical I—tibial N. (L4, L5, S1) (MP flexion, IP extension)
- Lumbricals II, III, IV—tibial N. (S1, S2) (MP flexion, IP extension)
- Plantar interossei—tibial N. (S1, S2)

A flexor tendonitis may cause pain on active toe flexion. This is especially true of the flexor digitorum longus and the flexor hallucis longus in athletes like ballet dancers and gymnasts who spend long periods of time on their toes. These athletes will have pain behind the medial malleolus or at the base of the sesamoid bones.

If loss of range of motion or pain only occurs in the great toe, it should be tested separately.

Great Toe (Hallux) Flexion and Extension

Hallux limitus is described as a mild to moderate limitation of flexion and extension of the metatarsophalangeal joint of the great toe. Hallux rigidus is described as a severe limitation at the metatarsophalangeal joint of the great toe for flexion and/or extension. During walking gait approximately 80° to 90° of hallux metatarsophalangeal extension is needed in the push off of the stance phase prior to toe off—if this range is not available the metatarsophalangeal joint will be jammed and resupination will be affected. During walking, the hallux metatarsophalangeal joint must then flex to allow for normal push off and resupination.

ASSESSMENT

INTERPRETATION

Acute hallux limitus can be caused by direct trauma or inflammatory disease, which can cause hypomobility of the joint. Chronic hallux limitus, which can progress to rigidus, can be caused by the following:

- structural congenital or acquired abnormalities
- long first metatarsal bone
- hypermobility of the first ray with prolonged pronation problem
- metatarsus primus elevatus
- prolonged immobilization
- degenerative joint disease of the hallux metatarsophalangeal joint
- degenerative sesamoids on the plantar surface of the great toe

Passive Toe Flexion (I to V)

Passively flex the athlete's toes with one hand until an end feel is reached or until pain stops the movement. Stabilize the metatarsals with your other hand.

The passive range of motion may be limited and/or painful because of the following:

- toe extensor tendonitis, strain, or avulsion
- metatarsophalangeal, proximal interphalangeal, or distal interphalangeal joint synovitis sprain or tear
- metatarsal or phalangeal fracture
- retinaculum that has adhered to the extensor tendons

The metatarsophalangeal, proximal interphalangeal, and distal interphalangeal joints should be tested separately if they are injured. If the range of motion is restricted only in the great toe, it should be tested separately. A capsular end feel is normal.

Resisted Toe Flexion (I to V)

The athlete attempts to flex the toes while you resist under the toes with one hand and stabilize the metatarsophalangeal joints with the other hand. The MP and talocrural joints should remain in the resting position.

Weakness and/or pain can be caused by an injury to the muscle or to its nerve supply (see Active Toe Flexion). If weakness is found only in the great toe, the great toe should be tested separately. Powerful toe flexion is needed during the propulsion phase of walking and running. Toe flexion strength is particularly important for the proprioception and ground control that is necessary during sporting events. Good proprioception of the foot in turn will affect the entire lower limb.

Active Toe Extension (I to V) (Fig. 4-32)

Ask the athlete to extend the toes

Pain, weakness, or limitation of range of motion can be

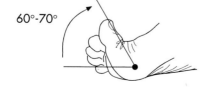

60°-70°

Fig. 4-32 Active toe extension. M.P. extension.

ASSESSMENT

INTERPRETATION

fully while you hold the metatarsal joints proximally.

The great toe (I) extension range of motion is 70° at the MP joint and negligible at the IP joint. Toes II through V extension range of motion is 40° at the MP joint and 30° at the DIP joint. Extension of the PIP joint is minimal.

caused by an injury to the prime movers or to their nerve supply. The prime movers are the:

- Extensor digitorum longus—peroneal N. (L4, L5, S1)
- Extensor digitorum brevis—deep peroneal N. (L4, L5, S1)
- Extensor hallucis longus—deep peroneal N. (L4, L5, S1)
- Extensor hallucis brevis—deep peroneal N. (L4, L5, S1)
- Lumbricals—tibial N. (L4, L5, S1, S2) (MP extension)
- Dorsal interossei—tibial N. (S1, S2)

Toe extensor tendonitis or strain will cause problems with gait—these conditions are fairly common in race walkers and swimmers (backstrokers) because of the repeated dorsiflexion required in their sport. Approximately 65° of metatarsophalangeal extension is needed for normal walking gait prior to propulsion.

Passive Toe Extension (I to V)

With one hand, passively extend the athlete's toes until an end feel is reached or until pain limits the range of motion, while the other hand stabilizes the metatarsals.

The total amount of metatarsophalangeal passive extension needed is 60° to 70°—this is important for normal supination of the foot.

The passive range of motion may be limited and/or painful because of the following:

- toe flexor tendonitis or strain
- plantar fasciitis
- flexor hallucis longus tendonitis or strain
- metatarsal or phalangeal fracture
- metatarsophalangeal, proximal interphalangeal, or distal interphalangeal sprain or tear

Hyperextension sprains of the first metatarsophalangeal joint (turf toe) are becoming common in the football player because of thin flexible shoes and synthetic turf. The metatarsophalangeal, proximal interphalangeal, and distal interphalangeal joints should be tested separately if they are injured. If the range of motion is restricted only in the great toe, it should be tested separately. A restriction in dorsiflexion of the toes or of the first metatarsal will lead to metatarsalgia or sesamoiditis. Hallux rigidus often leads to joint capsule problems and a limitation in the push-off phase of gait and during squatting.

Resisted Toe Extension (I to V)

Ask the athlete to extend the toes while you resist extension with one hand over the toes and stabilize the metatarsophalangeal joints with the other hand (the MP and talocrural joints should remain in the resting position).

Weakness and/or pain can be caused by an injury to the muscle or to its nerve supply (see Active Toe Extension). The extensor digitorum brevis is often injured during a plantar flexion and inversion ankle sprain.

SPECIAL TESTS

Drawer Sign (Fig. 4-33)

The athlete's knee is flexed to an

A positive forward movement of the talus in the mortise indi-

ASSESSMENT   INTERPRETATION

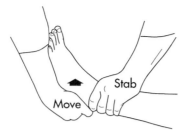

Fig. 4-33 Anterior drawer sign.

angle of 90° to alleviate the pull of the Achilles tendon by relaxing the gastrocnemius.

Method 1

The athlete's legs should dangle over the end of the plinth. Place one hand on the anterior aspects of the athlete's lower tibia while the palm of the other hand grips the calcaneus. The ankle joint is in the resting position (slight plantar flexion). Attempt to draw the calcaneus and talus anteriorly while stabilizing the tibia.

A positive test allows the talus to come forward.

Method 2

The athlete flexes the knee with the foot resting on the plinth.

Put one hand around the athlete's foot to hold it firmly on the plinth; the other hand pushes the tibia backward.

If the tibia moves backward and the talus comes forward, the test is positive.

NOTE: The athlete must be relaxed in both methods. The test may be negative if there is sufficient joint effusion (intracapsular or extracapsular) even though the ligament is torn.

Posterior Talofibular Ligament Test (Lapenskie)

While the athlete is sitting or lying, passively dorsiflex the ankle fully. While maintaining this position, attempt to externally rotate the rearfoot.

cates a tear in the anterior talofibular ligament and capsule. There may even be a "clunk" heard and felt as the talus slides forward. Pain can indicate an anterior talofibular ligament sprain.

If the rearfoot can rotate, there is a sprain, partial tear, or torn posterior talofibular ligament.

ASSESSMENT

INTERPRETATION

Talar Tilt

The talar tilt test should mainly be done at the time of injury to determine the degree of injury and the resulting laxity. It should not be done on an acute sprain that is healing. This test can also be done on an ankle that has fully healed to determine the amount of persisting instability.

If there is gapping during the test, the calcaneofibular ligament is torn and maybe the anterior talofibular ligament is damaged, resulting in lateral ankle instability. If the end feel is mushy the ligament may be completely torn. The posterior talofibular ligament can only be torn as a result of massive ankle trauma such as dislocation. A young child seldom sprains his or her ankle; children are more likely to fracture the fibula through the epiphyseal plate because the ligaments are stronger than the bone at this age.

Lateral Ligaments

Turn the athlete's foot into a position of plantar flexion and inversion. Invert the calcaneus and palpate to see if the talus gaps and rocks in the mortise.

Medial Ligaments

Stabilize the athlete's tibia and calcaneus with one hand while the other hand everts the foot. Palpate on the medial site for joint opening.

If the ankle joint gaps medially, there is a deltoid ligament tear. There is often a fracture or an avulsion fracture on the medial malleolus with this sprain.

Wedge Test (Anterior Inferior Tibiofibular Ligament)

The athlete's foot is in neutral. Press the talus up superiorly into the mortise with one hand while the other hand stabilizes the ankle joint. Pain indicates a positive test.

The wedge test forces the talus up into the mortise. If the anterior inferior tibiofibular ligaments are torn, the talus will wedge the mortise open and the torn or sprained ligaments will cause pain. Pain with this test will also be elicited with a dome of the talus fracture.

Inferior Tibiofibular Joint Stability Test (Lapenskie)

With the athlete supine lying, flex the knee, bringing the heel as close to the buttocks as possible. The ankle should be tightly dorsiflexed. Put one hand on the dorsum of the foot to fix the forefoot. Your other hand is placed behind the foot with the heel of your hand (base of the thumb) against the posterior aspect of the lateral malleolus (fibula). Attempt to move the fibula in an anterior direction.

If the fibular joint moves anteriorly, there is some inferior tibiofibular instability (sprain or partial tear). If the ankle joint dislocated with a tibiofibular diastasis and then spontaneously reduced, the mortise may open excessively and the athlete will have difficulty weight-bearing. An x-ray that measures the width of the diastasis must be done.

Anterolateral Subluxation of the Talus (Lapenskie)

Have the athlete stand and take

If the talus shifts in this anterolateral direction, there is pain

ASSESSMENT

INTERPRETATION

weight on to the anterolateral aspect of the plantar flexed and inverted foot and ankle.

Deformity of the talus moving anterior into the sinus tarsi area will be seen and felt at the base of the extensor digitorum brevis muscle.

and a feeling of "giving way." This injury can follow an inversion ankle sprain of the calcaneofibular ligament.

Subtalar Joint Irritation (Lapenskie)

Have the athlete lie prone with the ankle in full plantar flexion. Hold the foot in this position and gently tap the plantar aspect of the calcaneus upward. If pain is elicited and it radiates up the Achilles tendon, it is positive.

Subtalar irritation can occur after an inversion ankle sprain or due to compressive forces through the joint from overuse. Athletes on their toes, or landing on the toes, repeatedly can lead to subtalar irritation also (e.g. gymnastics, ballet).

Homan's Sign

The athlete sits with his or her legs over the edge of the plinth. Dorsiflex the foot and extend the knee. Pain will be experienced in the calf with deep palpation of the calf muscle.

If this test is positive and the athlete experiences pain on calf palpation, deep-vein thrombophlebitis (a serious medical problem) exists. This requires immediate referral to a physician.

Thompson Test (Achilles Tendon Rupture) (Fig. 4-34)

The athlete lies prone with legs extended and relaxed. Squeeze the calf muscle and the ankle should plantar flex. A positive test is indicated by the absence of plantar flexion.

When the calf is squeezed, the ankle joint will plantar flex if the Achilles tendon is intact. The absence of plantar flexion indicates that the tendon is ruptured. A visible and/or palpable depression may be felt in the tendon. The athlete may still be able to walk with an Achilles rupture but the foot will remain flat during toe off.

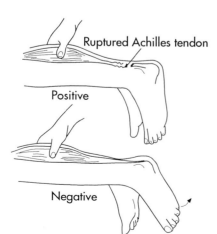

Fig. 4-34 Thompson test (Achilles rupture test).

ASSESSMENT

INTERPRETATION

Longitudinal Arch Mobility Tests (Fig. 4-35)

Toe Raise

The athlete is asked to go up on his or her toes while holding the plinth in the front for balance. Observe the calcaneus and foot from behind.

When the athlete goes up on his or her toes the calcaneus should go into inversion with the longitudinal arch supported. The navicular moves up and the cuboid moves down. If the calcaneus, navicular, or cuboid has lost the ability to perform these accessory movements or if the arch is not supported, normal foot mechanics are not occurring. The function of the peroneals is directly affected by the position of the cuboid.

If the calcaneus does not invert, it may be due to some boney abnormality within the subtalar mechanism. These abnormalities may be tarsal coalition or degenerative arthritis.

The calcaneus may not invert and balance may be very poor if the tibialis posterior, gastrocnemius, or peroneals are weak or injured.

Squat

The athlete is asked to squat with the feet flat on the floor. Observe the calcaneus and arch.

When the athlete lowers into the squat position the calcaneus should evert and the subtalar joint should pronate. During this pronation the navicular should move down and the cuboid should move upward. This compresses the talus in the mortise and any injuries to the talus, mortise, or inferior tibiofibular joint will also cause pain.

Legs-crossed Weight Transfer

The athlete stands with his or her legs and feet crossed. Ask the athlete to shift his or her weight over one foot and then the other.

This test (Lapenskie method) can also be done by observing the rearfoot and forefoot from the anterior and pos-

As the athlete shifts his or her weight over one foot, the arch should lower (pronate) and then rise (supinate) as the weight is transferred off that foot. This can be used to grade the arch mobility.

If the arch does not depress and re-elevate but stays rigid as in a rigid cavus foot, the shock-absorbing properties of that foot are reduced, and stress-related conditions can develop.

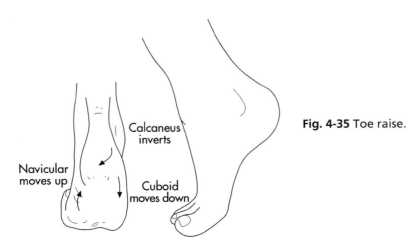

Navicular moves up

Calcaneus inverts

Cuboid moves down

Fig. 4-35 Toe raise.

ASSESSMENT

INTERPRETATION

terior view without the legs crossed, but with the athlete rotating the body to the right and then left (Lapenskie).

If there is pain during this test, the arch support ligaments and musculature should be examined for injury. The arch support ligaments are the following:

- plantar calcaneonavicular (spring) ligament
- medial talocalcaneal (deep to deltoid) ligament
- cuneometatarsal ligament
- cuneonavicular ligament

The flatter the arch, the less mobility it can achieve; this causes pronation conditions to develop (see Prolonged Pronation Problems; Table 4-3).

Lapenskie Method—During right rotation the right foot should supinate and the left pronate. Compare the amount of mobility in each direction.

Standing Superior Tibiofibular Mobility (Lapenskie)

Have the athlete stand in full weight-bearing. On the right leg, palpate the distance from the tibial tubercle to the head of the fibula. Ask the athlete to rotate at the trunk to the left, the distance between the tubercle and fibular head should increase. Ask the athlete to rotate to the right and the distance should decrease. Repeat with the other leg.

This test determines if there is normal superior tibiofibular joint movement necessary for full fibular motion. If there is hypo or hypermobility, the inferior tibiofibular joint will also go into dysfunction.

Hypomobility can lead to a supinator problem, while hypermobility can lead to pronator problems.

Mobility of the Tibia and Fibula Around the X-axis (Lapenskie)

Place the index finger and thumb in the sinus of the talocrural joint, just anterior to the tibia and fibula. Ask the athlete to rotate his or her body to the right and left. Determine if the motion is equal in both directions.

The amount of motion of the talus in the mortise should be equal in each direction and on each ankle. Ligamentous tears, scarring, or joint hypomobility should be recorded so that it can be addressed in rehabilitation.

Swelling Measurements

Using boney landmarks (medial or lateral malleolus) measure above and below the joint and around the foot to determine the amount of swelling and joint effusion that is present.

Comparing the degree of swelling helps determine the degree of injury. Increases in measurements at the joint line indicate the presence of swelling in the joint. Increases in the forefoot measurements suggest forefoot injury or tracking from the ankle or lower leg.

Longitudinal Arch Height Measurement

Feiss Line (Fig. 4-36)

Measure in weight-bearing the relation of the medial malleolus, the navic-

The closer the navicular measurement is to the ground, the greater the pronation during gait and the more the pronation

ASSESSMENT

INTERPRETATION

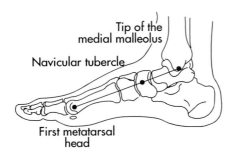

Fig. 4-36 Normal Feiss line.

ular, and the head of the first metatarsal (MP joint).

Put a mark on each of the anatomic landmarks to check whether they line up in a straight line.

Problems arise when the navicular drops.

problems that can develop. If the athlete is totally flat-footed (pes planus) it usually presents no problems, but problems develop as the support structures of the arch become lax or weak. This is a static measurement and the foot must be observed dynamically to see what happens to the navicular and the arch during weight-bearing.

Proprioception Testing

Ask the athlete to stand and balance on each leg for 30 seconds with the eyes open and then repeat for 30 seconds with the eyes closed.

Wavering or the necessity of putting the opposite foot down to regain balance gives a positive test. The test is easier with the eyes open; therefore an alteration in balance with the eyes open indicates a more substantial balance problem than with the eyes closed.

Kinesthetic awareness decreases in athletes with multiple ankle sprains (Garn and Newton). Any substantial injury to the foot and ankle can affect the kinesthetic awareness of the joint involved. This test helps to determine the degree of proprioceptive awareness in the foot and ankle, which has a direct effect on the entire lower quadrant. Good proprioception is needed to prevent injury and prevent reoccurrences of injury throughout the entire lower extremity.

Neurological Scan

Dermatomes (Fig. 4-37)

Run a sharp object, like a pin, over the dermatome areas of the ankle and foot to determine if there is any sensory loss. If a pin is used, at least 10 different points in each dermatome should be tested. The athlete must look away or close eyes during the sensory testing. Sensations must be compared bilaterally. If sensations are not the same on both sides, repeat the tests using objects at different temperatures (e.g., hot and cold test tubes) or objects with different textures (e.g., cotton balls and paper clips).

Sensory loss in a dermatome usually indicates a nerve-root irritation. The dermatomes for the entire limb should then be tested. Dermatomes vary in each individual; therefore several locations must be tested on each dermatome.

ASSESSMENT

Cutaneous Nerve Supply (Fig. 4-38)

You can use a pin to determine local cutaneous nerve problems. Several locations in each cutaneous area should be tested.

General Results

INTERPRETATION

The sensation of each peripheral nerve (lateral cutaneous, saphenous, deep and superficial peroneal, and sural) should be tested, as well as the dermatomes. Each of the peripheral nerves can be tested because any problem with these nerves will cause local cutaneous effects.

According to Cyriax the following is true:
- Paresthesia of the big toe is attributable to the L4, L5 nerve root or the saphenous nerve.
- Paresthesia of the big toe and second toe is attributable to the L5 nerve root, tight tibial fascial compartment, or pressure on the second digital nerve.
- Paresthesia of the big toe and the two adjacent toes is attributable to the L5 nerve root.
- Paresthesia of all of the toes is attributable to compression of the peroneal nerve at the fibula and combined pressure at L5 and S1.
- Paresthesia of the second, third, and fourth toes is attributable to the L5 nerve root.
- Paresthesia of the fourth and fifth toes is attributable to the S1 nerve root and Morton's metatarsalgia.
- Paresthesia of the heel, calf, and posterior thigh is attributable to the S2 nerve root.

Pressure paresthesia in both limbs may indicate the following:
- spondylolisthesis
- spinal claudication
- cervicothoracic disc lesions protruding centrally
- spinal neoplasms (benign or malignant)
- lumbar central disc protrusion

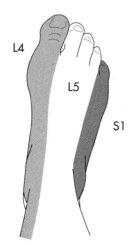

Fig. 4-37 Dermatomes.

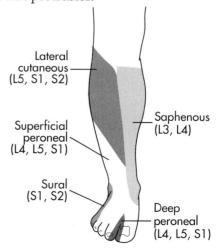

Fig. 4-38 Cutaneous nerves.

ASSESSMENT

INTERPRETATION

Achilles Tendon Reflex (S1)

The athlete sits with the legs dangling over the edge of the plinth.

Put the athlete's ankle in slight dorsiflexion, then tap the Achilles tendon with the flat side of a hammer while the hand palpates the plantar flexion action of the foot.

The tendon can be tapped 10 times to check tendon fatigability.

The Achilles tendon reflex is a deep tendon reflex supplied by nerves emanating from the S1 cord level. The nerve root could be compressed by L5, S1 disc herniation. If the S1 root is severed or compressed, the reflex is absent. Slight compression can cause a diminished reflex or a reflex that fatigues readily.

Circulatory Scan (Fig. 4-39)

Posterior Tibial Artery

Palpate the posterior tibial artery, which is the main source of blood supply to the foot, and the dorsal pedal artery for their pulses. These pulses should be palpated with the foot in a nonweight-bearing position and with the tendons relaxed.

The posterior tibial artery supplies the entire foot and any diminution of this pulse may indicate arterial occlusion. The artery lies between the flexor digitorum longus and flexor hallucis longus tendons, behind the medial malleolus.

Dorsal Pedis Artery

The dorsal pedis artery is absent 12% to 15% of the time, but because it is more subcutaneous it is easier to detect when present. This artery is the secondary blood supply to the foot. If the pulse is diminished, it may be because of a vascular disease or vascular occlusion. The artery lies between the extensor digitorum longus and the extensor hallucis longus tendons. Repeated monitoring of these pulses is needed if you suspect occlusion. Any occlusion or a diminished pulse is considered an emergency and the athlete should be sent to the nearest physician or hospital for further care.

These circulatory tests are important when you suspect an anterior compartment syndrome, circulatory occlusion due to a fracture or a tight cast, or compression or laceration injuries to the limb's arterial supply.

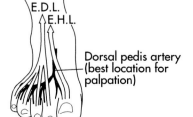

Fig. 4-39 Dorsal aspect of the foot.

ASSESSMENT

BIOMECHANICAL ANALYSIS

Nonweight-bearing (Table 4-2)

Talocrural Joint Range (Fig. 4-40)

The athlete is lying prone with the knee extended. Put the talocrural joint at an angle of 90° of dorsiflexion, keeping the calcaneus (or subtalar joint) in neutral or slight inversion.

If the calcaneus everts during dorsiflexion, pronation occurs and true dorsiflexion is not achieved. Apply an overpressure and passively dorsiflex the talocrural joint until an end feel is reached.

A goniometer may be used with one arm of the goniometer in line with the tibia, its center just below the lateral malleolus, and the other goniometer arm along the shaft of the fifth metatarsal. There must be 10° of dorsiflexion beyond 90° for normal talocrural function with the knee extended.

Repeat this procedure with the knee flexed. There must be 15° of dorsiflexion for the talocrural joint with knee flexion.

According to Elvern et al., measurements of talocrural passive range of motion are moderately reliable when taken by the same therapist over a relatively short period of time.

Clinical measurements of passive plantar flexion may be moderately reli-

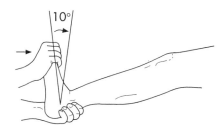

Fig. 4-40 Talocrural dorsiflexion.

INTERPRETATION

Examination of the foot and ankle at rest (nonweight-bearing) is done to find structural and functional ability before weight-bearing compensations occur.

During the midstance phase of gait the foot must reach an angle of 10° dorsiflexion in relation to the tibia, otherwise the subtalar or the midtarsal joint will compensate by overpronating. A tight triceps surae (functional talipes equinus) or an inherited talipes equinus can cause a limitation so that 10° of dorsiflexion is not possible. If this occurs in nonweight-bearing the foot should be re-examined in weight-bearing and during gait to see if prolonged pronation is occurring (Fig. 4-41).

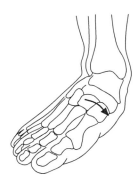

Fig. 4-41 Need 10° of dorsiflexion in the talocrural joint or the forefoot will collapse, causing overpronation.

ASSESSMENT   INTERPRETATION

able when done by different examiners, but measurements of passive dorsiflexion done by different examiners has lower reliability.

Subtalar Joint Range (Determination of Neutral Position)

The athlete lies prone with his or her foot 6 to 8 inches over the end of the plinth. The athlete's other knee is flexed, which puts the hip in an abducted, flexed, and externally rotated position.

Push up on the fourth and fifth metatarsal heads and gently dorsiflex the foot until resistance is met (soft end feel; Fig. 4-42).

Your other hand stabilizes the tibia.

Maintaining the dorsiflexion, move the foot into inversion and eversion through its entire range.

As the subtalar joint is moved into inversion and eversion, there is a position at which the joint tries to come to rest. This is the neutral position (Wernick and Langer's technique).

The talar head can be palpated with the other hand while the foot is moved into inversion and eversion.

During inversion the talar head will bulge laterally; during eversion it will bulge medially (Fig. 4-42).

When the foot is positioned so that the talar head does not bulge to either side, the foot is said to be in the neutral position.

To get an exact measurement of the

It is important to determine the neutral position of the subtalar joint because the position of the calcaneus in relation to the tibia can help determine what will happen in the subtalar joint and midtarsals during gait. The normal subtalar neutral position is at an angle of 0°. Active subtalar (or calcaneal) inversion should be a total of 20° and active subtalar (or calcaneal) eversion should be a total of 10°.

At a normal neutral position the functioning of the subtalar and midtarsal joints is most efficient and the amount of muscle or ligamentous stress is minimal.

If the calcaneus is fixed in an inverted position or if the range into eversion is very restricted while inversion is full, a *subtalar varus* problem exists. This condition will elicit a negative value on calculations of neutral position. On weight-bearing you can determine if this is a *compensated* or an *uncompensated subtalar varus*.

If the calcaneus is fixed in an everted position or if the range in inversion is restricted while eversion is full, a subtalar valgus problem exists. This condition will elicit a positive number on calculations. On weight-bearing you can determine if this is *compensated* or *uncompensated subtalar valgus*.

According to Percy and Mann, if the subtalar motion is very limited in both directions, a talocalcaneal coalition can be the cause. This usually occurs in the posterior or medial area and often causes a peroneal spastic flat foot (rigid pes planus with forefoot abduction and excessive calcaneal valgus with the athlete weight-bearing).

According to Lattanza et al., if excessive passive eversion exists, the subtalar joint may be abnormally compensating for some other structural problem, such as forefoot varus. Too little

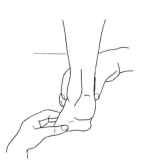

Fig. 4-42 Palpation of the talar head with inversion and eversion.

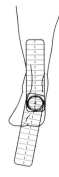

Fig. 4-43 Measurement of calcaneal position and subtalar range.

ASSESSMENT

neutral position (Root et al. technique) draw a line to bisect the posterior surface of the calcaneus (do not allow the fat pad alteration or boney exostosis to affect the marking; Fig. 4-43).

Draw another line to bisect the distal third of the leg from the center of the tibia through the musculotendinous junction of the triceps surae to the base of the ankle mortise (ignore the position of the Achilles tendon). Measure the angle of the subtalar joint with a goniometer. Place the center of the goniometer over the subtalar joint with one arm on the upper tibial line and the other arm lined up with the calcaneal line (Fig. 4-44). Move the subtalar joint into full calcaneal eversion by pushing up on the fourth and fifth metatarsal head with dorsiflexion, eversion, and abduction of the foot.

Record the subtalar eversion range in degrees. Move the subtalar joint into full calcaneal inversion by plantar flexing, inverting, and adducting the foot. Record the subtalar inversion range in degrees.

Use the following formula to compute the neutral position: Neutral position = maximum eversion minus one third of the total range of motion.

Midtarsal Relation of Forefoot to Hindfoot

With the athlete in the prone position, move the subtalar joint into the neutral position. Looking down from above (directly over the posterior calcaneus), observe the relationship of the forefoot to the hindfoot (Fig. 4-44).

INTERPRETATION

eversion indicates that the subtalar joint is unable to compensate for other structural problems.

The metatarsal heads of the forefoot should form a line that is directly perpendicular to the line through the calcaneus. If the forefoot is twisted in relation to the calcaneus so that the lateral metatarsal heads are lower than the medial metatarsal heads, the forefoot is in *forefoot varus*. Whether this is *compensated* or *uncompensated forefoot varus* will be determined in weight-bearing.

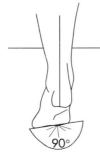

Fig. 4-44 Measurement of forefoot alignment, subtalar joint in neutral.

ASSESSMENT

INTERPRETATION

If the forefoot is twisted so that the medial metatarsal heads are lower than the lateral heads, the forefoot is in *forefoot valgus*.

If only the first metatarsal is lower or higher, a *hypermobile first ray* may be present. This will be tested next.

Mobility of First Ray

With the athlete in the prone position, move the first metatarsal head superiorly and inferiorly to see the amount of movement in the first ray.

The first ray is made up of the first metatarsal and the cuneiform. The articulations include the movement between the navicular and the first cuneiform, and the first cuneiform and the first metatarsal. If the first metatarsal has more than 2 cm of anterior or posterior movement, a hypermobile first ray exists. The first ray is usually dorsiflexed and hypermobile. This hypermobility is often the result of the inability of peroneus longus to stabilize the first ray. A hypermobile first ray is unable to carry its share of the weight and, as a result, more weight is shifted to the second or third metatarsal heads. Weight-bearing forces are thus thrown laterally; this can cause the following:
- stress fractures of the second metatarsal
- metatarsalgia
- collapsed transverse arch
- overpronation problems
- callus or keratosis under the head of the second metatarsal

The first ray may become hypermobile secondary to a hallux valgus. Hallux rigidus (rigid first metatarsal) causes a severe lack of extension in the metatarsophalangeal joint during the latter half of midstance—this causes twisting of the foot and related rotational problems up the limb. During gait, the hallux should extend at least 90°; 60° of extension is considered hypomobile. Hallux limitus is a mild or moderate limitation of flexion and extension of the metatarsophalangeal joint. For further discussion of hallux rigidus and limitus refer to the section on Active Toe Flexion.

Weight-bearing (see Table 4-2)

If an alignment problem was found in a nonweight-bearing position, re-examine the athlete's standing and walking gait to see if the body or foot compensates for this alignment deficiency. It is also important to determine the foot type because different overuse conditions develop with each foot type, depending on where the weight is borne, how the body compensates, and where the forces are transferred. Lattanza et al. determined that the subtalar joint eversion range was significantly greater during weight-bearing than with passive manual testing; therefore, the subtalar joint must also be tested during weight-bearing.

Tibial Varum (Mcpoil and Brocato Technique)

With the athlete standing, observe the posterior calcaneus at eye level, if

With a tibial varum deformity the distal tibia is closer to the midline than the proximal portion; this is frontal plane deformi-

ASSESSMENT

INTERPRETATION

possible. Place the subtalar joint in the neutral position by palpating the talus and asking the athlete to medially and laterally rotate the tibia. Palpate the talus with your thumb and index finger until the talus sits in the mortise and cannot be felt medially or laterally.

The posterior calcaneus and lower third of the tibia is already bisected from the nonweight-bearing subtalar measurements done earlier. One arm of the goniometer rests on the supporting surface in the frontal plane with the arm projecting past the lateral malleolus. The other arm of the goniometer lines up with the distal third of the tibia. The amount of deviation from 90° or from the vertical position is the amount of tibial varum that exists.

Talocrural Joint

If there is less than 10° to 15° of dorsiflexion, the foot and ankle should be re-examined while the athlete is standing. With the athlete standing and walking, determine how the body compensates for the limitation in dorsiflexion. You should determine whether the foot type is *uncompensated talipes equinus* or *compensated talipes equinus.*

Uncompensated Talipes Equinus

Compensated Talipes Equinus

ty. The normal position is approximately 0° to 10° from the perpendicular. A tibial varum deformity causes a bow-legged position or bowing in the lower third of the tibia, which should not be confused with genu varum. During walking and running gaits, this deformity leads to overpronation and its related conditions (see Prolonged Pronation Problems; Table 4-3).

The decreased dorsiflexion can cause uncompensated or compensated talipes equinus.

If the athlete cannot get his or her heel down to the ground and is virtually a toe-walker, severe uncompensated talipes equinus exists. This is very rare and usually surgically correctable. There are varying degrees of uncompensated talipes equinus but the heel will always rise prematurely in midstance.

If the necessary dorsiflexion did not exist when testing in a nonweight-bearing position, and if the foot pronates excessively in midstance, a compensated talipes equinus may exist. If the tibia cannot move anteriorly over the dome of the talus during midstance, the talus will move anteriorly to achieve the necessary range of motion, causing forefoot collapse. The metatarsal joints can even sublux to gain the range of motion, which leads to a rocker-bottom foot (vertical talus). Problems that can develop in association with a compensated talus equinus include:
- medial arch pain

ASSESSMENT

INTERPRETATION

- plantar fasciitis
- Achilles tendonitis
- for other problems, refer to Prolonged Pronation Problems; Table 4-3.

Compensated talipes equinus can develop in the athlete who does a great deal of running or jumping without maintaining flexibility in the triceps surae group. A restriction of dorsiflexion from a talar or tibial exostosis can also lead to this problem.

Subtalar Joint

With the athlete standing, evaluate the position of the calcaneus in relation to the lower tibia (a skin marker can be used to bisect the calcaneus) (Fig. 4-45). Ask the athlete to walk while you observe the calcaneus from the anterior and posterior view. Determine the athlete's foot type.

During normal standing and in early midstance of the walking gait, the calcaneus everts slightly. The subtalar joint pronates and the midtarsal joints unlock to allow the foot to adapt to the terrain.

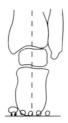

Fig. 4-45 Good forefoot and hindfoot alignment.

Compensated Subtalar Varus (Fig. 4-46)

The compensated subtalar varus foot type rests in an inverted position in nonweight-bearing. During standing or early midstance, the foot compensates for this calcaneal position by unlocking the talus, causing the subtalar joint to overpronate so that the forefoot can contact the ground. The midtarsal joints unlock to allow the foot to become flexible and mold to the terrain. Because of the overpronated position of the subtalar joint it can not resupinate to lock the midtarsal joint for a stable foot for the push off. Therefore the push off occurs through a pronated flexible foot.

If the athlete had subtalar varus in a nonweight-bearing position, it is necessary to determine if the foot overpronates during midstance in weight-bearing. If pronation occurs, the forefoot has compensated by collapsing so as to allow the metatarsals to reach the ground because the calcaneus cannot evert. This condition is called compensated subtalar varus. It causes overpronation during walking and running and leads to several overuse problems in the foot, ankle, knee, and even the low back (see Prolonged Pronation Problem; Table 4-3) because the foot does not get resupinated for push off. Compensated subtalar varus problems that can develop with overuse include the following:

- shearing forces under the forefoot
- hypermobility in first ray
- calluses under the second, second and third, or the second, third, and fourth metatarsal heads
- Achilles bowing (Hebling's sign) leading to Achilles tendonitis
- tibialis posterior tendonitis
- hallux valgus

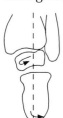

Fig. 4-46 Compensated subtalar varus (common).

ASSESSMENT

INTERPRETATION

Uncompensated Subtalar Varus (Fig. 4-47)

In this foot type the calcaneus is already inverted and the subtalar joint is supinated.

During standing or in the early midstance of walking gait, the calcaneus does not evert and the subtalar joint does not achieve the required pronation. The subtalar joint remains supinated and the forefoot remains rigid throughout the stance phase.

The weight-bearing forces continue through the lateral calcaneus and the lateral side of the foot.

Fixed supination problems can develop (see chart on fixed supination problems; Table 4-4).

If subtalar varus was determined in nonweight-bearing and the foot stays supinated throughout the stance phase, the condition is *uncompensated subtalar varus*. This is a semirigid foot that lacks shock-absorbing capabilities because the subtalar joint does not pronate and does not allow the arch to absorb shock or adapt to the terrain in midstance. Weight distribution is more lateral on this foot. The problems or overuse conditions that develop with this type foot include the following:

- calluses under the fifth metatarsal head (and sometimes the fourth)
- tailor's bunion
- medial pinch callus under the great toe because of abnormal roll-off during push off
- stress fractures of the fifth metatarsal
- lateral compartment syndrome

Other conditions are presented in Fixed Supination Problems, Table 4-4.

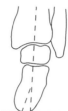

Fig. 4-47 Uncompensated subtalar varus.

Subtalar Valgus (Fig. 4-48)

The calcaneus is already everted so in standing or in midstance the subtalar joint is already in full pronation. The longitudinal arch may be totally collapsed, resulting in a "flat foot." The midtarsal joints may dorsiflex in midstance. This condition rarely has any symptoms.

If it is determined in nonweight-bearing that the subtalar joint is in valgus, and if the calcaneus remains everted and the longitudinal arch is totally flat while the athlete is standing and walking, the athlete has subtalar valgus foot. In this condition the foot is flat without talar compensations. This is an uncommon foot type and can occur with talocalcaneal coalition.

This foot type stays pronated during gait. Surprisingly, it has few symptoms or problems related to it other than irritation from the arch support and heel cup footwear.

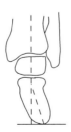

Fig. 4-48 Uncompensated or compensated subtalar valgus (rare).

Forefoot

The forefoot and subtalar joints are also observed during gait to determine if excessive pronation or supination exists and to determine the type of forefoot the athlete has.

ASSESSMENT

INTERPRETATION

Compensated Forefoot Varus (Fig. 4-49)

During the stance phase the calcaneus everts excessively to allow the forefoot to bear weight evenly. With this calcaneal eversion the subtalar joint overpronates and does not get resupinated for push off. Prolonged pronation problems can develop.

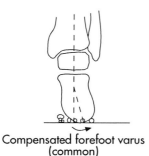

Compensated forefoot varus
(common)

Fig. 4-49 Compensated forefoot varus (common).

If forefoot varus was determined in nonweight-bearing and the foot pronates excessively in standing and walking, the athlete has a compensated forefoot varus. The presence of normal subtalar motion allows the inverted forefoot to be compensated for by pronation. To get the medial forefoot to the ground the calcaneus everts excessively and the subtalar joint overpronates during midstance. The subtalar joint cannot get resupinated. With the subtalar joint pronated, the cuboid and navicular remain unstable and the peroneus longus cannot stabilize the first ray or assist in plantar flexing it. Because of the unstable cuboid bone, this first ray starts to become hypermobile and dorsiflexes out of the way.

A common problem in this type of foot is a stress fracture of the fibular sesamoid bone. The second metatarsal takes more weight as the first ray swings out of the way, leading to calluses or keratosis under the second metatarsal head. This is a fairly common foot problem, which leads to extensive foot and postural problems because of the pronation. The tibia remains internally rotated as well, so knee and hip dysfunction can also develop.

The medial foot structures are elongated and the lateral foot structures are compressed. See the chart on Prolonged Pronation Problems, Table 4-3.

Uncompensated Forefoot Varus (Fig. 4-50)

During the stance phase, while the subtalar joint is in neutral, the forefoot is in varus. During propulsion, most of the weight-bearing forces go through the fourth and fifth metatarsals.

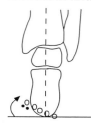

Fig. 4-50 Uncompensated forefoot varus.

If there is a forefoot varus determined in nonweight-bearing and the foot does not pronate when the athlete is standing or walking, an uncompensated forefoot varus exists. This is very rare, but when it does occur the inverted forefoot position is fixed and propulsion occurs through the fourth and fifth metatarsals. The uncompensated forefoot produces lateral instability that can result in the following (Fig. 4-50):
- ankle sprains
- peroneal tendonitis
- stress fractures of the metatarsals (especially the fifth metatarsal)

See Fixed Supination Problems (Table 4-4).

Forefoot Valgus

If forefoot valgus is diagnosed in nonweight-bearing and the foot has a high-arched cavus foot in weight-bearing, forefoot valgus exists.

Uncompensated Forefoot Valgus (Fig. 4-51)

During standing and in early midstance the subtalar joint everts normally but the forefoot cannot fully pronate because the first metatarsal hits the

There is eversion of the forefoot on the rearfoot with the subtalar joint in neutral. The subtalar joint cannot pronate the necessary amount because the great toe hits the ground before the subtalar joint can unlock.

ASSESSMENT   INTERPRETATION

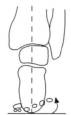

Fig. 4-51 Uncompensated forefoot valgus (very rare).

ground first, preventing the metatarsals from gradually bearing weight. During standing and gait the foot appears as a very high-arched "cavus foot." Fixed supination problems can develop. The great toe can suffer the brunt of the weight-bearing forces, causing sesamoiditis and calluses under the first metatarsal head.

Compensated Forefoot Valgus (Fig. 4-52)

During standing and in early mid-stance the subtalar joint inverts to allow all the metatarsals to bear weight. The subtalar joint remains supinated because of the inverted calcaneus. Often, the first ray compensates and becomes plantar flexed and/or everted. This foot type develops fixed supination problems.

In uncompensated forefoot valgus the foot is rigid (there is no subtalar compensation) and there is direct pressure under the first metatarsal, which can cause the following:
- inversion ankle sprains
- sesamoiditis (medial sesamoid bone)
- calluses (first metatarsal)
- supination related conditions

Such a foot is not a good shock absorber, therefore stress fractures and related stress conditions can develop.

This everted forefoot is more flexible than the uncompensated forefoot yet it is still high arched. The subtalar joint compensates by inverting the calcaneus during gait. The first ray is hypomobile and the metatarsals go into an equinus position. This foot again does not get pronated enough in midstance to absorb shock but remains supinated. There is considerable torque within the foot and localized forces on the sole of the foot. The overuse conditions seen with this type of foot include the following:
- calluses
- metatarsalgia
- plantar fasciitis
- lateral ankle sprains
- arch strain
- spring ligament sprain
- Achilles tendonitis

See Fixed Supination Problems, Table 4-4.

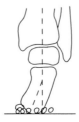

Fig. 4-52 Compensated forefoot valgus.

ASSESSMENT

INTERPRETATION

ACCESSORY MOVEMENT TESTS

Superior Tibiofibular Joint
Anterior-Posterior Glide (Fig. 4-53)

The athlete lies with the hip and knee flexed and the foot resting on the plinth.

Sit on the athlete's foot to stabilize it and grasp the proximal head and neck of the fibula with the thumb and index finger of one hand. Your other hand rests on the proximal upper surface of the tibia to stabilize it.

The fibula is moved gently anteriorly and posteriorly to see that movement is present and is equal bilaterally.

Anterior-posterior movements of the superior tibiofibular joint are needed because the head of the fibula must move forward on knee flexion and backwards on knee extension. The head of the fibula must move upward and posteriorly with talocrural dorsiflexion and downward and anteriorly with plantar flexion.

If plantar flexion or dorsiflexion is limited during the functional testing, the accessory movements of the superior and inferior tibiofibular joints should be tested.

Inferior Tibiofibular Joint

Anterior-Posterior Glide (Fig. 4-54)

The athlete is lying prone with the foot over the edge of the plinth and a rolled towel under the front of the ankle joint. Stabilize the plantar aspect of the foot with one hand while the other hand goes around the distal end of the fibula. Use the thenar eminence to the heel of the hand to push forward gently on the fibula for an anterior glide. Your index finger can pull the fibula backward for a posterior glide.

Anterior-posterior movements are important for normal talocrural and ankle function. The inferior tibiofibular restriction usually limits range of motion and causes pain after an ankle joint effusion or post cast. A limitation here causes decreased dorsiflexion because the ankle mortise is unable to open.

Superior-Inferior Glide

Palpate the head of the fibula for superior and inferior motion as you passively plantar flex, dorsiflex, invert, and evert the foot and ankle.

With subtalar inversion, the head of the fibula slides inferiorly and posteriorly; with subtalar eversion, the fibular head slides superiorly and anteriorly. If the fibula becomes fixed in a superior position, the ankle joint often compensates with overprona-

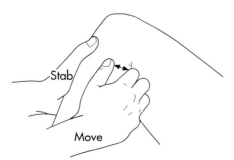

Fig. 4-53 Superior tibiofibular joint anterior-posterior glide.

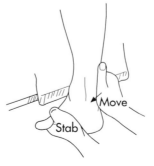

Fig. 4-54 Inferior tibiofibular joint anterior-posterior glide.

ASSESSMENT   INTERPRETATION

tion. If the fibula becomes fixed in an inferior position the foot may be unable to pronate and therefore stay supinated. These altered fibular movements will not only alter foot and ankle mechanics but can also influence the knee and lower quadrant mechanics.

Talocrural Joint

Posterior Glide of Tibia on Talus (Fig. 4-55, A)

The athlete is lying supine with the hip flexed to an angle of 45°, the knee at an angle of 90°, and the foot relaxed at about 20° of plantar flexion (the resting position of the joint). Stabilize the foot and subtalar joint with one hand around the talus distal to the malleoli. Your other hand is around the tibia just above the joint line. Your hand around the tibia is moved posteriorly to see if joint-play movement is present.

If the posterior glide movement of the tibia on the talus is not full, the athlete is often incapable of full plantar flexion range of motion.

Anterior Glide of Talus on Tibia (Fig. 4-55, B)

The athlete is lying supine with his or her foot over the end of the plinth. The ankle is plantar flexed about 20°. Cup one hand around the calcaneus while the opposite hand is on the distal anterior aspect of the tibia. Move the calcaneus anteriorly to push the talus anteriorly under the tibia.

This is very similar to the anterior drawer test—any limitation of this movement will often limit talocrural dorsiflexion range of motion.

Fig. 4-55 A, Talocrural joint posterior glide of tibia on talus. **B,** Talocrural joint anterior glide of talus on tibia.

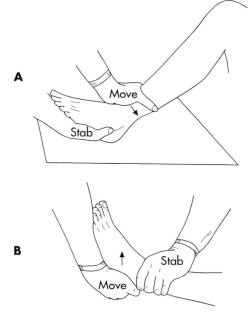

ASSESSMENT

INTERPRETATION

Subtalar Joint

Distraction (Fig. 4-56)

The athlete is lying supine with the knee flexed to an angle of 90° and the hip flexed slightly and abducted. Sit on the plinth with your back to the athlete. Wrap the athlete's leg around your body with your iliac crest pushing into the athlete's posterior thigh. Grasp the talus just below the malleoli with both hands. With the thumb under the medial malleolus and the other fingers under the lateral malleolus gently push the talus out of the mortise inferiorly to see how much joint play there is. Lean back with your body to help traction the joint.

You should see how hypomobile or hypermobile the subtalar joint is. Hypermobility can be the result of the following:
- chronic instability: ligamentous and capsular
- inherited joint laxity

Hypomobility can be the result of the following:
- talus coalition
- osteoarthritic subtalar joint
- rigid cavus foot type
- ankle post-cast restriction

Distraction with Passive Inversion and Eversion (Fig. 4-57)

In the position described above, tilt the calcaneus into inversion and eversion to see the available joint play.

An increased amount of calcaneal inversion can be the result of the following:
- chronic lateral ankle laxity
- compensated subtalar varus foot type

A decreased calcaneal inversion can be the result of the following:
- uncompensated subtalar varus foot type
- osteoarthritic or degenerative joint problems
- ankle post-cast restriction

An increased calcaneal eversion can be the result of the following:
- subtalar valgus foot type
- chronic overpronating foot

A decreased calcaneal eversion can be the result of the following:
- uncompensated subtalar varus ankle
- osteoarthritis or degenerative joint problems
- ankle post-cast restriction

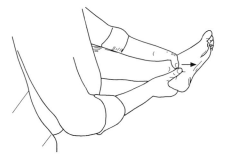

Fig. 4-56 Subtalar joint distraction.

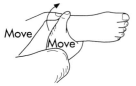

Fig. 4-57 Subtalar joint distraction with inversion and eversion.

ASSESSMENT

INTERPRETATION

Calcaneotalar Dorsal and Plantar Rock

Perform the same as above but stabilize the talus anteriorly with the web of one hand while the other hand is on the calcaneus, rocking it forward and upward.

Perform the same as above but your stabilizing hand and mobilizing hand switch functions. The hand on the foot slides to the navicular tubercle while the other hand moves posteriorly on the calcaneus. The calcaneus is rocked backward with slight foot plantar flexion with the forward hand while the posterior hand acts as a fulcrum.

Calcaneotalar dorsal and plantar rock is important for normal talar calcaneal movement during plantar flexion and dorsiflexion.

Midtarsal and Tarsometatarsal Joints

Dorsal-Plantar Midtarsal Glide (Fig. 4-58)

The athlete is lying supine with the knee flexed about 70° and the heel resting on the plinth. Stabilize the proximal row of tarsal bones (navicular and calcaneus) with the right hand while the other hand grasps the distal row of tarsal bones (cuboid and cuneiforms). Then oscillate in an anterior and posterior direction with the left hand.

These glide movements are done to test forefoot mobility. For normal supination the navicular must be able to move dorsally and the cuboid plantarly. For normal pronation the navicular must move plantarly and the cuboid dorsally.

Dorsal-Plantar Tarsometatarsal Glide

As above, but the right stabilizing hand fixes the distal row of tarsals (cuboid and cuneiforms) while the mobilizing hand is placed around the base of the metatarsals. A plantar and dorsal movement is made by the mobilizing hand.

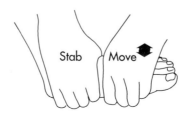

Fig. 4-58 Midtarsal joint anterior-posterior glide.

ASSESSMENT

INTERPRETATION

Tarsometatarsal Rotation (Fig. 4-59)

Perform in the same position as described on p. 317, but rotate the forefoot with the mobilizing hand.

Rotational components are needed in the forefoot so that during pronation the forefoot can adapt to the terrain.

Metatarsophalangeal, Proximal Interphalangeal, and Distal Interphalangeal Joints

All these joints are capable of dorsal-plantar glides (Fig. 4-60).
- Rotation
- Traction
- Side glide

Stabilize the proximal bone of the joint and move the distal bone in the above movements to determine if the movements are present, hypomobile, or hypermobile.

All these accessory movements are needed for toe flexion, extension, abduction, and adduction. If there was a problem with the functional tests at the toes, these accessory tests should be done. Forefoot swelling that has been present for a long time can also lead to hypomobility in these joints.

PALPATION

Palpate for point tenderness, temperature differences, swelling, muscle spasm, muscle tone, bone and muscle congruency, adhesions, crepitus, and calcium deposits.

Medial Structures

Boney
Head of the First Metatarsal

The following can occur at this site:
- bunions
- blisters
- boney exostosis (hallux valgus—bursa inflamed)
- scars, surgical repairs
- gout (urate crystals in the tissue about the joint)

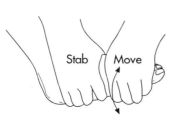

Fig. 4-59 Tarsometatarsal joint rotation.

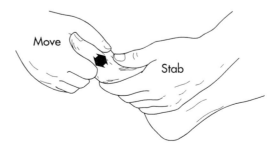

Fig. 4-60 Great toe metatarsophalangeal joint anterior-posterior glide.

ASSESSMENT	INTERPRETATION

First Cuneometatarsal

An exostosis can exist here in the presence of a high-arched mobile foot (cavus).

Navicular Tubercle

Tenderness from aseptic necrosis and tenderness from pressure with the shoe if there is os navicularis or prominent tubercle can occur here.

Medial Malleolus

The malleolus can be contused or fractured and the distal aspect may be point tender. An avulsion fracture of the distal medial tip can occur with an eversion injury.

Tibia

Point tenderness and swelling over the distal medial margin of the tibia occurs with tibial stress reaction (shin splints or stress fractures).

Soft Tissue (Fig. 4-61)
Cuneonavicular Ligaments

The cuneonavicular ligaments may be tender from overpronation because they help to support the longitudinal arch.

Cuneometatarsal Ligaments

Cuneometatarsal ligaments (dorsal or plantar) can be tender from overpronation or if they are sprained.

Spring Ligament

The spring ligament runs from the sustentaculum tali to the navicular to help support the talus. If the foot is losing its arch,

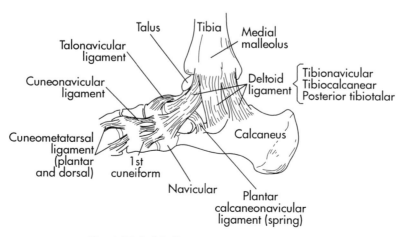

Fig. 4-61 Ankle ligaments. Medial view.

ASSESSMENT

INTERPRETATION

the spring ligament may become tender because it helps to support the longitudinal arch; prolonged jumping or running can also irritate this ligament.

Calcaneonavicular Joint

Point tenderness can occur over the calcaneonavicular joint, especially if a coalition is present here.

Tibialis Posterior Tendon and Muscle (Fig. 4-62)

The tibialis posterior tendon and muscle help to prevent the talus from rocking medially.

Tendonitis here will cause tenderness over the insertion of the tendon on the navicular or over the tendon behind the medial malleolus. Prolonged pronation will aggravate the tendon.

The tendon is protected in the groove by a synovial lining that can become inflamed.

Palpate as much of the muscle as possible for point tenderness and trigger points. According to Simons and Travell, there is a trigger point pain pattern for the tibialis posterior muscle that goes over the Achilles tendon and posterior calf into the sole of the foot.

Tibialis Anterior Tendon (Fig. 4-62)

Point tenderness at the point of insertion or along the tibialis anterior tendon can be caused by overpronation, especially from running or repeated jumping. The tibialis anterior is the primary muscle that supports the longitudinal arch.

Deltoid Ligament
- Posterior tibiotalar ligament
- Tibiocalcaneal ligament
- Tibionavicular ligament

The medial collateral ligament is just inferior to the medial malleolus—tenderness or pain elicited during palpation suggests an eversion ankle sprain. Palpate the posterior tibiotalar, tibiocalcaneal, and tibionavicular portions of the deltoid ligament for tenderness or swelling.

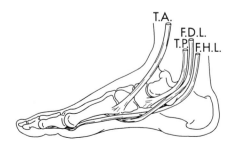

Fig. 4-62 Medial aspect of the foot. *F.H.L.*, Flexor hallucis longus tendon. *F.D.L.*, Flexor digitorum longus tendon. *T.P.*, Tibialis posterior tendon. *T.A.*, tibialis anterior tendon.

ASSESSMENT   INTERPRETATION

Flexor Hallucis Longus Tendon (Fig. 4-62)

The flexor hallucis longus tendon cannot usually be palpated. The athlete will indicate tenderness around the posterior aspect of the medial malleolus or just below the sustentaculum tali. This condition should not be confused with tibialis posterior tendonitis. This tendon can be irritated from excessive internal rotation during an inversion sprain. The tendon gets injured after the posterior tibiotalar ligament is torn. Pain is localized to the posteromedial aspect of the ankle at the posterior aspect of the talus.

Flexor Digitorum Longus Tendon (Fig. 4-62)

Tendonitis or tenosynovitis will cause point tenderness below the medial malleolus. This along with the flexor hallucis longus, can become inflamed from repeated takeoff and tiptoe (en pointe) movements. A flexor digitorum longus muscle strain can cause local pain and soreness along the posterior middle third of the tibia.

Tarsal Tunnel

The flexor retinaculum covers the tip of the medial malleolus and runs distally to join the deep fascia on the dorsum of the foot. It forms a tunnel that contains, from medial to lateral, the following structures:
- tibialis posterior tendon
- flexor digitorum longus tendon
- posterior tibial nerve and artery in a neurovascular bundle
- flexor hallucis longus tendon

The possible causes of tarsal tunnel syndrome are:
- prolonged pronation
- chronic tendonitis
- previous fracture with callus formation
- direct trauma
- rheumatoid arthritis

Entrapment of the lateral plantar nerve can result as the nerve passes through a fibrous opening between the abductor hallucis and the quadratus plantae muscles adjacent to the medial tubercle (calcaneal spur location). The spur can irritate the nerve. The athlete may then experience paresthesia, pain, or burning into the toes or sole of the foot when the tibial nerve is percussed.

Talocalcaneal Joint

Point tenderness in this area can be caused by a talocalcaneal coalition—there will be very limited subtalar movements and the athlete will have a very flat foot. Tenderness here can also occur when the joint is sprained or in dysfunction.

ASSESSMENT   INTERPRETATION

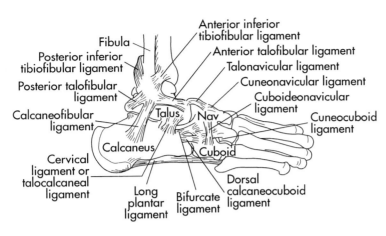

Fig. 4-63 Ankle ligaments. Lateral view.

Lateral Structures (Fig. 4-63)

Boney
Lateral Malleolus

Tenderness on the tip of the lateral malleolus can suggest periosteal contusion or fracture. The tip of lateral malleolus can be avulsed with an inversion ankle sprain.

Fifth Metatarsal Bone

The base of the fifth metatarsal can be fractured through trauma or overuse at the styloid process where the peroneus brevis inserts (complication of ankle sprain). The bursa over the process may also become inflamed and tender.

Soft Tissue
Fifth Metatarsophalangeal Joint

This may be point tender at the fifth metatarsophalangeal joint from a tailor's bunion or blister, which is caused by wearing shoes that are too narrow. This joint can also be tender if the joint has been sprained or dislocated.

Lateral Ligaments
- Anterior talofibular ligament
- Calcaneofibular ligament
- Posterior talofibular ligament

The lateral ligaments will be point tender if they are sprained or partially torn. The anterior talofibular ligament has the highest incidence of sprain because it is stressed the most with plantar flexion and inversion. The calcaneofibular ligament is the next ligament to take the stress with an inversion sprain. The posterior talofibular ligament is only injured in very severe ankle sprains or a dislocation.

Bifurcate Ligaments

The calcaneocuboid or calcaneonavicular part of the bifurcate ligament will be tender if sprained or partially torn from a plantar flexion injury mechanism.

ASSESSMENT	INTERPRETATION

Peroneal Tendons

A tear in the fascial band that holds the tendons in the groove (peroneal retinaculum) may allow the tendons to sublux or dislocate. This snapping and dislocating of the tendons can cause point tenderness here.

The tendons can develop tenosynovitis as they wrap under the malleolus—this can develop with overuse, especially in the cavus foot.

Peroneal Muscles

The peroneal muscles may be tender from overuse. According to Simons and Travell, there is a trigger point near the head of the fibula with referred pain into the lateral lower leg behind the lateral malleolus and into the lateral aspect of the foot. These muscles can also be tender if the muscle is strained. This can occur, especially to peroneus brevis, with a significant inversion ankle sprain.

Lateral Compartment

Tenderness of the lateral compartment can be because of an acute or chronic compartment syndrome. It contains peroneus longus and brevis muscles. A lateral compartment syndrome can cause pain and tightness in the lateral leg with eversion weakness and changes in anterolateral skin sensation. An acute compartment syndrome is a medical emergency and the athlete should be transported to a medical facility as soon as possible.

Superior Tibiofibular Joint

Any dysfunction in the superior or inferior tibiofibular joint can make it point tender. Forced inversion, eversion, plantar flexion, or dorsiflexion can sprain this joint. Direct trauma can result in dislocation, subluxation, or sprain.

Dislocation occurs with a lateral blow to the joint while weight-bearing on a flexed knee, according to Radovich and Malone.

Posterior Structures

Boney
Calcaneus

This structure will be acutely tender if there is a compression fracture or a growth-plate fracture (epiphysitis) in young children. It can be moderately tender with a contusion or periosteitis.

Soft Tissue (Fig. 4-64)
Achilles Tendon
- Achilles tendonitis

Tenderness will be present if there is Achilles tendonitis, an

ASSESSMENT

INTERPRETATION

- Calcaneal bursa
- Achilles tendon strain or partial tear
- Retrocalcaneal bursa

Achilles tendon strain or partial tear, calcaneal bursitis, or retro-calcaneal bursitis.

Achilles tendonitis can cause a warm, inflamed site of pain, with a nodule or snowball crepitus if severe.

The Achilles tendon can strain or partially tear. Palpate the length of the tendon for any gap in the tendon's continuity. The healthy tendon rarely tears but an older athlete with a history of chronic Achilles tendonitis or a tendon with previous cortisone injections can rupture when stressed.

Retrocalcaneal bursitis can occur from trauma and will be present deep to the Achilles tendon over the posterior calcaneus.

Calcaneal bursitis exists just under the skin and usually gets inflamed or enlarged because of oversized or tight shoes.

Gastrocnemius
- Medial head
- Lateral head

Ruptures or strains of the gastrocnemius usually occur to the medial muscle belly where the Achilles tendon joins the belly. There is point tenderness and swelling; sometimes a gap can be felt in the muscle tissue. According to Simons and Travell, the myofascial trigger point for the gastrocnemius muscle is located in the upper medial belly. Its referred pain pattern centers in the longitudinal arch but extends from the popliteal space to the posteromedial calf and the plantar surface of the foot.

Soleus

The soleus muscle is deep to the gastrocnemius muscle but it can be gently palpated below the gastrocnemius muscle belly on the calf's medial and lateral aspect. According to Simons and Travell, the trigger point is deep to the distal medial gastrocne-mius muscle belly. Its referred pain pattern centers on the plan-tar aspect of the calcaneus but extends down the lower postero-medial calf.

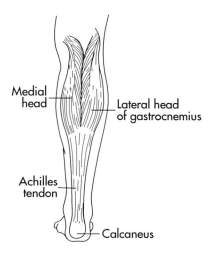

Medial head — Lateral head of gastrocnemius

Achilles tendon

Calcaneus

Fig. 4-64 Posterior structures.

ASSESSMENT

INTERPRETATION

Plantar Structures (Fig. 4-65)

Boney
Calcaneus

A calcaneal bursa may be locally tender on the plantar surface of the calcaneus. A calcaneal spur develops on the medial tubercle of the calcaneus and will cause pain during heel strike. A calcaneus periostitis (bone bruise) will cause point tenderness over the calcaneus.

Sesamoid Bones

The two sesamoid bones that lie within the flexor hallucis brevis tendon may become tender and inflamed (sesamoiditis). They also can be fractured, especially the medial sesamoid bone; there is local swelling and point tenderness. In the presence of a Morton's foot the sesamoid bones can become displaced and tender.

Metatarsal Head

If a metatarsal head is more prominent, it may bear more weight. This dropped metatarsal is usually the second metatarsal and calluses develop under the head because of the added stress.

Metatarsalgia can develop if the transverse arch collapses, causing painful metatarsal heads and pinched digital nerves.

A painful spot between the third and fourth metatarsal heads is a Morton neuroma.

Plantar warts can develop on the weight-bearing areas on the sole of the foot.

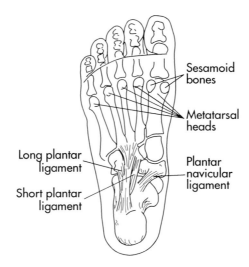

Fig. 4-65 Plantar ligaments.

ASSESSMENT

INTERPRETATION

Soft Tissue (Fig. 4-65)
Plantar Fascia

Fasciitis can develop close to the calcaneus or down the medial side of the fascia. Nodules in the fascia can be Dupuytren's contracture.

Long and Short Plantar Ligaments (Plantar Calcaneocuboid Ligaments)

These ligaments help support the longitudinal arch of the foot. If foot strain, sprain, or prolonged pronation occurs, these ligaments may be acutely point tender.

Spring Ligament (Plantar Calcaneonavicular)

This ligament also helps to support the arch and can become strained and painful from overuse.

Plantar Flexor Muscles

Any strain or contusion to the plantar flexor muscles will cause local point tenderness. Gait will be affected, especially during midstance and toe off.

Dorsal Structures

Boney
Sinus Tarsi

Ankle sprains usually cause tenderness just anterior to the lateral malleolus because the cavity may be edematous or the extensor digitorum brevis may be strained. Deep tenderness within the sinus tarsi is evidence of some problem in the subtalar complex and can be indicative of fracture.

Metatarsals, Phalanges, and Local Soft Tissue

Corns between the toes cause discomfort. Psoriasis of the skin may be obvious here and cause some discomfort. Pain between the third and fourth metatarsal that radiates sharp pain into the toes can be a Morton neuroma. The toes involved can also experience numbness.

Any fracture of the metatarsals or phalanges will cause local point tenderness.

Contusions of the dorsum of the foot will cause local swelling and point tenderness.

Soft Tissue (Fig. 4-66)
Anterior Inferior Tibiofibular Ligament

Point tenderness over the anterior inferior tibiofibular ligament can occur from a ligament sprain or tear.

Tibialis Anterior Tendon and Muscle

Tendonitis can develop as the tendon crosses the front of the ankle joint or as it passes under the arch; the tendon will be ten-

ASSESSMENT   INTERPRETATION

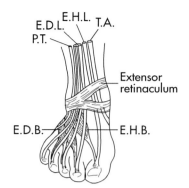

E.D.L. E.H.L. T.A.
P.T.

Extensor
retinaculum

E.D.B.   E.H.B.

Fig. 4-66 Dorsal structures. *E.H.B.*, Extensor hallucis brevis. *T.A.*, Tibialis anterior. *E.H.L.*, Extensor hallucis longus. P.T., Peroneus tertius. *E.D.B.*, Extensor digitorum brevis. *E.D.L.*, Extensor digitorum longus.

der and there may be palpable creaking or crepitus. Local point tenderness over the muscle can occur from a muscle strain or overuse. According to Simons and Travell, the trigger point for tibialis anterior is in the proximal muscle belly. The referred pain pattern is centered at the great toe and can radiate over the anteromedial lower leg.

Anterior Compartment Syndrome

If the entire anterior compartment is tight, swollen, tender, and warm, this is a sign of an acute anterior compartment syndrome. It can occur after trauma, surgery, tight cast, or overexercising the muscles of this compartment (tibialis anterior, extensor hallucis longis and extensor digitorum longus). The first dorsal web can show diminished cutaneous sensation and, if severe, foot dorsiflexion and toe extension may be diminished or absent. If this occurs it is a medical emergency and the athlete must be transported to the nearest medical facility as soon as possible.

This compartment problem can be chronic and usually arises only after exertion. In the chronic case, there will be no circulatory, neural, or motor involvement, yet the compartment may continually develop tenderness after exertion (i.e., joggers, soccer players, football players).

Extensor Digitorum Longus

Tendonitis or tenosynovitis can develop from overuse, especially in the race walker and the swimmer who uses the back stroke a great deal.

Extensor Digitorum Brevis

Tendonitis can develop from overuse of the extensors. This muscle can be strained with a plantar flexion inversion ankle sprain.

Extensor Hallucis Longus and Brevis

Tendonitis or strain can injure these muscles, especially the longus, because it crosses both the toe and ankle joints.

ASSESSMENT

INTERPRETATION

Extensor Digiti Minimi and Peroneus Tertius

These can be strained with an inversion mechanism especially if the foot rolls, pinning the fifth metatarsal and the phalanges.

REFERENCES

Acker JH and Drez D: Nonoperative treatment of stress fractures of the proximal shaft of the fifth metatarsal (Jones' fracture), Foot and Ankle 7(3):152, 1986.

Anderson JE: Grant's Atlas of anatomy, Baltimore, 1983, Williams & Wilkins.

Ankle sprains—a round table discussion, The Physician and Sportsmedicine 14(2):101, 1986.

APTA Orthopaedic Section Review for advanced orthopedic competencies: the foot, Dan Riddle, Chicago, Aug 11, 1989.

Bassett F et al: Talar impingement by the anteroinferior tibiofibular ligament, J Bone Joint Surg 72(A):55, 1990.

Bauer M, Johnell O, Redlund-Johnell I: Supination-eversion fractures of the ankle joint—changes in incidence over 30 years, Foot and Ankle 8(1):26, 1987.

Bazzoli A and Pollina F: Heel pain in recreational runners, The Physician and Sportsmedicine 17(2):55, 1989.

Berman David: Etiology and management of hallux valgus in athletes, The Physician and Sportsmedicine 10(8):103, 1982.

Beskin J et al: Surgical repair of Achilles tendon ruptures, Am J Sports Med 15(1):1, 1987.

Booher JM and Thibodeau GA; Athletic injury assessment, Toronto, 1985, The CV Mosby Co.

Brodsky A and Khalil M: Talar compression syndrome, Am Sports Med 14(6):472, 1986.

Bruckner J: Variations in the human subtalar joint, J Ortho Sports Phy Therapy 8(10):489, 1987.

Calliet R: Foot and ankle pain, Philadelphia, 1968, FA Davis Co.

Caspi I et al: Partial apophysectomy in Sever's Disease, J Orthop Sports Phy Therapy 10(9):370, 1989.

Clanton TB, Butter J, Eggert A: Injuries to the metatarsophalangeal joints in athletes, Foot and Ankle 7(3):162, 1986.

Cyriax J: Textbook of orthopedic medicine—diagnosis of soft tissue lesions, vol 1, London, 1978, Bailliere Tindall.

Daniels L and Worthingham C: Muscle testing techniques of manual examination, Toronto, 1980, WB Saunders.

DeLee JC et al: Acute posterolateral rotary instability of the knee, Am J Sports Med 11(4):199, 1983.

Donatelli R: Normal biomechanics of the foot and ankle, abnormal biomechanics of the foot and ankle, Orthop Sports Phy Ther 7(3):91, 1985.

Donatelli R: Abnormal biomechanics of the foot and ankle, J Orthop Sports Phy Therapy, 9(1):11, 1987.

Donatelli R and Wooden M: Orthopedic physical therapy, New York, 1989, Churchill Livingstone.

Doxey G: Calcaneal pain: a review of various disorders, J Orthop Sports Phy Therapy 9(1):25, 1987.

Elkus R: Tarsal coalition in the young athlete, Am J Sports Med 14(6):477, 1986.

Elvern R et al: Geometric reliability in a clinical setting—subtalar and ankle joint measurements, Phy Therapy 68(5):672, 1988.

Elvern R et al: Methods for taking subtalar joint measurements—a clinical report, Phys Therapy 68(5):678, 1988.

Fricker PA and Williams JP: Surgical management of os trigonum and talar spur in sportsmen, Brit J Sports Med 13:55, 1979.

Fowler PJ: Foot problems in athletes, CATA J 6:3, 1979.

Garn SN and Newton RA: Kinesthetic awareness in subjects with multiple ankle sprains, Phys Therap 68(11):1667, 1988.

Garth W and Miller S: Evaluation of claw toe deformity, weakness of the foot intrinsics, and posteromedial shin pain, Am J Sports Med 17(6):821, 1989.

Gould JA and Davieg GJ: Orthopaedic and sports physical therapy, Toronto, 1985, Mosby.

Gross T and Bunch R: A mechanical model of metatarsal stress fracture during distance running, Am J Sports Med 17(5):669, 1989.

Hagmeyer R and Van der Wurff P: Transchondral fractures of the talus on an inversion injury of the ankle: a frequently overlooked diagnosis, J Orthop Sports Phy Ther 1:362, 1987.

Hontas M, Haddad R, Schlesinger L: Conditions of the talus in runners, Am J of Sports Med 14(6):486, 1986.

Harbourn TE and Ross HE: Avulsion fracture of the anterior calcaneal process, Physician and Sportsmedicine 15(4):73, 1987.

Hardaker W, Margello S, Goldner L: Foot and ankle injuries in theatrical dancers, Foot Ankle 6(2):59, 1985.

Harper M: Deltoid ligament: an anatomical evaluation of function, Foot and Ankle 8(1):19, 1987.

Heim M et al: Case study: persistent ankle pain—the os trigonum duly conquered, J Orthop Sports Phy Therapy 8(8):402, 1987.

Hlavac H: The foot book, California, 1977, World Publications.

Hontas M, Haddad R, Schlesinger L: Conditions of the talus in the runner, Am J Sports Med 14(6):486, 1986.

Hoppenfeld S: Physical examination of the spine and extremities, New York, 1976, Appleton-Century Crofts.

Jacobs D et al: Comparison of conservative and operative treatment of Achilles tendon rupture, Am J Sports Med 6(3):107, 1978.

Kapandji IA: The physiology of the joints, vol II, Lower limb, New York, 1983, Churchill Livingstone.

Kendall FP and McCreary EK: Muscles testing and function, Baltimore, 1983, Williams & Wilkins.

Kessler RM and Hertling D: Management of common musculoskeletal disorders, Philadelphia, 1983, Harper and Row.

Kisner C and Colby L: Therapeutic exercise—foundations and techniques, Philadelphia, 1987, FA Davis Co.

Kosmahl E and Kosmahl H: Painful plantar heel, plantar fasciitis, and calcaneal spur: etiology and treatment, J Orthop Sports Phys Ther 9(1):17, July 1987.

Kulund D: The injured athlete, Toronto, 1982, JB Lippincott.

Lapenskie Garry: Subtalar joint rehabilitation workshop, 1991, University of Western Ontario, London, Ontario, Canada.

Lattanza L, Gary G, Kantner R: Closed versus open kinematic chain measurements of the subtalar joint eversion: implications for clinical practice, J Orthop Sports Phys Ther 3:310, 1988.

Leach RE and Corbett M: Anterior tibial compartment syndrome in soccer players, Am J Sports Med 4:258, 1979.

Leach RE, James S, Wasilewski S: Achilles tendonitis Am J Sports Med 9(2):93, 1981.

Lillich JS and Baxter DE: Common forefoot problems in runners, Foot and Ankle 7(3):145, 1986.

Lillich JS and Baxter DE: Bunionectomies and related surgery in the elite female middle-distance and marathon runners, Am J Sports Med 14(6):491, 1986.

Mack R: American Academy of Orthopaedic Surgeons Symposium on the foot and leg in running sports, Toronto, 1982, Mosby.

Magee DJ: Orthopaedics conditions, assessments, and treatment, vol II, Alberta, 1979, University of Alberta Publishing.

Magee DJ: Orthopaedic physical assessment, Toronto, 1987, WB Saunders.

Maitland GD: Peripheral manipulation, Toronto, 1977, Butterworth & Co. Malone T and Hardaker W: Rehabilitation of foot and ankle injuries in ballet dancers, J Sports Phys Therap 11(8):355, 1990.

Mandelbaum B et al: the anterior capsule impingement syndrome in the ankle of the athlete: methods of evaluation and treatment (abstracts of the annual meeting of the American Orthopaedic Society for Sports Medicine), Am J Sports Med 15(6):619, 1987.

Mann RA and Hagy J: Biomechanics of walking, running, and sprinting, Am J Sports Med 8(5):345, 1980.

Mann RA et al: Running symposium, Foot and Ankle 1:190, 1981.

Mann RA: Biomechanical approach to the treatment of foot problems, Foot and Ankle 2(4):205, 1982.

Mannheimer JS and Lampe GN: Clinical transcutaneous electrical nerve stimulation, Philadelphia, 1986, FA Davis Co.

Matheson G et al: Stress fractures in athletes—a study of 320 cases, Am J Sports Med 15(1):46, 1987.

McConkey JP and Favero KJ: Subluxation of the peroneal tendons within the peroneal tendon sheath, Am J Sports Med 15(5):511, 1987.

McConkey JP: Ankle sprains, consequences, and mimics in foot and ankle in sport and exercise, New York, 1987, Karger.

Montgomery L et al: Orthopedic history and examination in the etiology of overuse injuries, Med Sci Sports Exercise 21(3):237, 1989.

Miller WA: Rupture of the musculotendinous junction of the medial head of the gastrocnemius muscle, Am J Sports Med 5(5):191, 1977.

Myerson MS and Shereff MJ: The pathological anatomy of claw and hammer toes, J Bone Joint Surg 71A(1):45, 1989.

Nicholas J and Hershman EB: The lower extremity and spine in sports medicine, St Louis, 1986, Mosby.

Nigg BM and Morlock M: The influence of lateral heel flare of running shoes on pronation and impact forces, Med Sci Sports Exerc 19(3):294, 1987.

Nitz A, Dobner J, Kersey D: Nerve injury and grades II and III sprains, Am J Sports Med 13(3):177, 1985.

Norkin C and Levangie D: Joint structure and function, Philadelphia, 1987, FA Davis Co.

O'Donaghue D: Treatment of injuries to athletes, Toronto, 1984, WB Saunders.

Olney BW et al: Excision of symptomatic coalition of the middle facet of the talocalcaneal joint, J Bone J Surg 69A(4):539, 1987.

O'Neill D and Micheli L: Tarsal coalition: a followup of adolescent athletes, Am J Sports Med 17(7):544, 1989.

Parisien J: Arthroscopic treatment of osteochondral lesions of the talus, Am J Sports Med 14(3):211, 1986.

Percy EC and Mann DL: Tarsal coalition: a review of the literature and presentation of 13 cases, Foot and Ankle 9(1):40, 1988.

Radovich M and Malone T: The superior tibiofibular joint: a forgotten joint, J Sports Phys Therapy 3(3):129, 1982.

Reid DC: Functional anatomy and joint mobilization, Alberta, 1970, University of Alberta.

Reid DC: Sports injury assessment and rehabilitation, New York, Churchill Livingstone, 1992.

Renstrom P et al: Strain in the lateral ligaments of the ankle, Foot and Ankle 9(2):59, 1988.

Root M et al: Biomechanical examination of the foot, vol 1, Los Angeles, 1971, Clinical Biomechanics Corp.

Root ML, Orien WP, Weed JH: Normal and abnormal biomechanics of the foot. Clinical biomechanics, vol 2, ed 1, Los Angeles, 1977, Clinical Biomechanics Co.

Sarrafian S: Functional characteristics of the foot and plantar aponeurosis under tibiotalar loading, Foot and Ankle 8(1):4, 1987.

Savastano A: Articular fractures of the dome of the talus, Phys Sports Med 10(10):113, 1982.

Schepsis A and Leach R: Surgical management of Achilles tendonitis, Am J Sports Med 15(4):308, 1987.

Scranton PE: The management of superficial disorders of the forefoot, Foot and Ankle 2(4):238, 1982.

Scranton PE: Treatment of symptomatic talocalcaneal coalition, J Bone Joint Surg 69A(4):533, 1987.

Seder JI: Heel injuries incurred in running and jumping, Phys Sports Med 10:70, 1976.

Siegler S, Block J, Schneck C: The mechanical characteristics of the collateral ligaments of the human ankle joint, Foot and Ankle 8(5):234, 1988.

Simons D and Travell JG: Myofascial origins of low back pain. 3, Pelvic and lower extremity muscles, Post grad Med 73:99, 1983.

Sinton W: The ankle: soft tissue injuries, J Sports Med 1(3):47, 1973.

Styf J and Korner L: Chronic anterior-compartment syndrome of the leg, J Bone J Surg 68A(9):1338, 1986.

Subotnick SI: Podiatric sports medicine, New York, 1975 Futura Publishing.

Subotnick SI: Sports medicine of the lower extremity, New York, 1989, Churchill Livingstone.

Taylor P: Osteochondritis dissecans as a cause of posterior heel pain, Phys Sports Med 10(9):53, 1982.

Torg JS et al: Stress fractures of the tarsal navicular, J Bone Joint Surg 64A(5):700, 1982.

Travell J and Simons D: Myofascial pain and dysfunction—the trigger point manual, Baltimore, 1983, Williams & Wilkins.

Wernick J and Langer S: A practical manual for a basic approach to biomechanics, New York, Langer Acrylic Lab, Vol 1, 1972.

Wiley JP et al: A primary case perspective of chronic compartment syndrome of the leg, Phys Sports Med 15(3):111, 1987.

Williams PL and Warwick R: *Gray's anatomy*, New York, 1980, Churchill Livingstone.

Yocum L: Clinics in sports medicine, vol 7:1, Philadelphia, 1988, WB Saunders.

Index